# Concise
# Dermatology,
# Venereology and
# Leprology

W0235473

# Concise
# Dermatology,
# Venereology and
# Leprology

## Srikantha Daga Rathi
MBBS, DDVL, DNB, MNAMS (DVD)

Assistant Professor
Department of Dermatology, Venereology and Leprology
SVS Medical College
Mahabubnagar, AP, India

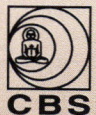

**CBS**

## CBS Publishers & Distributors Pvt Ltd

New Delhi • Bengaluru • Chennai • Kochi • Kolkata • Mumbai
Hyderabad • Nagpur • Patna • Pune • Vijayawada

**Disclaimer**

Science and technology are constantly changing fields. New research and experience broaden the scope of information and knowledge. The author has tried his best in giving information available to him while preparing the material for this book. Although, all efforts have been made to ensure optimum accuracy of the material, yet it is quite possible some errors might have been left uncorrected. The publisher, printer and the author will not be held responsible for any inadvertent errors or inaccuracies.

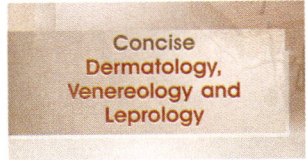

**Concise Dermatology, Venereology and Leprology**

**ISBN:** 978-93-85915-65-9

Copyright © Author and Publisher

**First Edition:** 2017

All rights reserved. No part of this book may be reproduced or transmitted in any form or by any means, electronic or mechanical, including photocopying, recording, or any information storage and retrieval system without permission, in writing, from the author and the publisher.

Published by Satish Kumar Jain and produced by Varun Jain for

**CBS Publishers & Distributors Pvt Ltd**

4819/XI Prahlad Street, 24 Ansari Road, Daryaganj, New Delhi 110 002, India.
Ph: 23289259, 23266861, 23266867    Website: www.cbspd.com
Fax: 011-23243014    e-mail: delhi@cbspd.com; cbspubs@airtelmail.in.
*Corporate Office:* 204 FIE, Industrial Area, Patparganj, Delhi 110 092
Ph: 4934 4934    Fax: 4934 4935    e-mail: publishing@cbspd.com; publicity@cbspd.com

*Branches*

- **Bengaluru:** Seema House 2975, 17th Cross, K.R. Road,
  Banasankari 2nd Stage, Bengaluru 560 070, Karnataka
  Ph: +91-80-26771678/79    Fax: +91-80-26771680    e-mail: bangalore@cbspd.com
- **Chennai:** No. 7, Subbaraya Street, Shenoy Nagar, Chennai 600 030, Tamil Nadu
  Ph: +91-44-26680620/26681266    Fax: +91-44-42032115    e-mail: chennai@cbspd.com
- **Kochi:** Ashana House, No. 39/1904, AM Thomas Road, Valanjambalam, Ernakulam 682 018,
  Kochi, Kerala
  Ph: +91-484-4059061-65, 67    Fax: +91-484-4059065    e-mail: kochi@cbspd.com
- **Kolkata:** 6/B, Ground Floor, Rameswar Shaw Road, Kolkata-700 014, West Bengal, India
  Ph: +91-33-22891126, 22891127, 22891128    e-mail: kolkata@cbspd.com
- **Mumbai:** 83-C, Dr E Moses Road, Worli, Mumbai-400018, Maharashtra
  Ph: +91-22-24902340/41    Fax: +91-22-24902342    e-mail: mumbai@cbspd.com

*Representatives*

- **Hyderabad**    0-9885175004        • **Nagpur**    0-9021734563
- **Patna**    0-9334159340        • **Pune**    0-9623451994
- **Vijayawada**    0-9000660880

*Printed at:* Goyal Offset Printes, GT Karnal Road, Industrial Area, Delhi, India

# Foreword

A brief and introductory book, very well written and covers comprehensively the subject of dermatology. I am quite sure that this book will be very useful to undergraduate students and the candidates appearing in different postgraduate entrance examinations as it has relevant and apt questions and multiple choice questions (MCQs). It will also be useful to postgraduate students in dermatology to start with and to revise the subject before the examination.

A well executed maiden venture. I am happy to write the Foreword to this book.

All the best !

**Dr V Gowri** MD (Dermatology)
ex-Professor and Head
Department of Dermatology
Osmania Medical College
Hyderabad, India

# *Preface*

While there are many excellent books available on dermatology, it is inevitably assumed that the reader already has a working knowledge of the subject, and it becomes difficult to read and retain the matter, especially by the residents and the aspiring postgraduates. I have tried to write this book in simple words as one would speak if asked to deliver a lecture covering succinctly the basic concepts of dermatology. This book would be of great help to the medical students to understand and memorise the very basic concepts of dermatology and venereology.

There is hardly any concise shortbook for dermatology which can be read in a few days and at the same time make essentials of dermatology clear. I believe that this handbook would appropriately fill up the dearth and would especially be indispensable for those preparing for postgraduate medical entrance examination and for the dermatology residents.

In view of human or technical errors, suggestions for enhancement of the book are most welcome.

**Srikantha Daga Rathi**
DDVL, DNB (DVD)
sacshri@gmail.com

# Acknowledgments

Mr Abhishek Rathi BE (Computers)

Dr Arun S Rathi MS (Surg)

Dr Sachin V Daga
Surgical Gastroenterologist and Liver Transplant Surgeon

Dr Bipin V Daga MD, DNB, FRCR (London)

Dr Aditi B Daga BDS

# Contents

# 1 Introduction to Dermatology

Dermatology may be defined as the study of the skin and its diseases.

## Cell Cycle (Fig.1.1)

- It is time interval between two successive mitoses.
- The multiplying cells pass through four phases:
  - ➢ M: Mitosis
  - ➢ $G_1$: Interphase/postmitotic growth phase
  - ➢ S: Active DNA synthesis
  - ➢ $G_2$: Short resting/premitotic phase
- The correct sequence of cell cycle is: $G_0$-$G_1$-S-$G_2$-M
- Mitotic divisions occur in the keratinocytes every 18–19 days.
- G0 = Cells which have stopped multiplying. Temporarily leave the cycle and remain quiescent and potentially fertile.

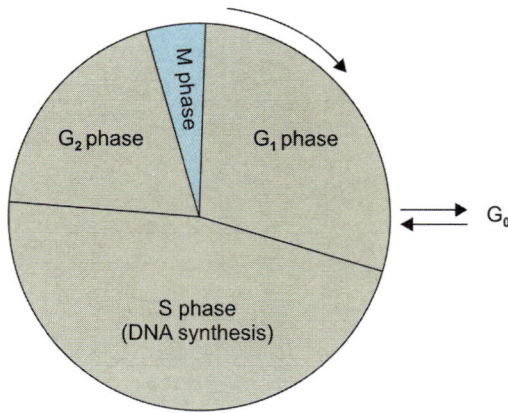

**Fig. 1.1:** Cell cycle

## Structure of Skin (Fig. 1.2)

- The skin has three layers—the epidermis, dermis, and fat layer (also called the subcutaneous layer).

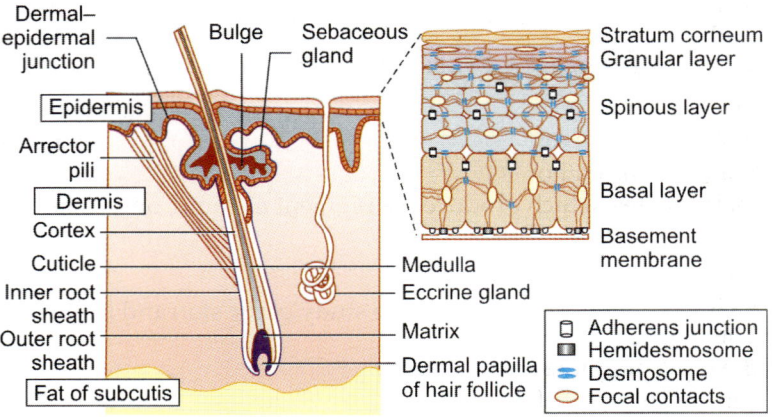

**Fig. 1.2:** The skin and its appendages

## EPIDERMIS

- The epidermis is the relatively thin, tough, outer layer of the skin.
- The thickness of the epidermis varies in different types of skin. It is the thinnest on the eyelids at .05 mm and the thickest on the palms and soles at 1.5 mm.
- Most of the cells in the epidermis are keratinocytes. They originate from cells in the deepest layer of the epidermis called the basal layer. New keratinocytes slowly migrate up toward the surface of the epidermis. Once the keratinocytes reach the skin surface, they are gradually shed and are replaced by younger cells pushed up from below.
- The epidermis contains 5 layers. From bottom to top the layers are named:
  - ➢ Stratum basale
  - ➢ Stratum spinosum
  - ➢ Stratum granulosum
  - ➢ Stratum lucidum
  - ➢ Stratum corneum
- The outermost portion of the epidermis, known the stratum corneum, is relatively waterproof, and when undamaged, prevents most bacteria, viruses, and other foreign substances from entering the body.

- Stratum lucidum is a translucent zone between stratum corneum and stratum granulosum, present only in palmar and plantar skin.
- Stratum granulosum contains granular cells which are 3–4 layered.
- Stratum spinosum contains polygonal cells with intercellular bridges.
- Stratum basale contains columnar cells arranged in a single layer.
- The epidermis (along with other layers of the skin) also protects the internal organs, muscles, nerves, and blood vessels against trauma.
- Scattered throughout the basal layer of the epidermis are cells called melanocytes, which produce the pigment melanin, one of the main contributors to skin color. Melanin's primary function, however, is to filter out ultraviolet radiation from sunlight, which can damage DNA, resulting in numerous harmful effects, including skin cancer.
- The epidermis also contains Langerhans' cells, which are part of the skin's immune system. Although these cells help detect foreign substances and defend the body against infection, they also play a role in the development of skin allergies.
- The normal turnover time of epidermis is 28 days (4 wks).
- The turnover time is psoriasis = 4 days
- Stratum corneum is permeable in preterm infants and becomes similar to the adult and full term infant after 2–3 weeks, postnatal maturation.

## Langerhans' Cells (Antigen Presenting Cells)

- Langerhans' cells are dendritic cells similar to melanocytes but are Dopa negative and ATPase positive.
- Derived from bone marrow.
- Distributed in basal, spinous, and granular cell layers.
- Electron microscopy: They have rod/racquet shaped granules (*Birbeck granules*)
- Play a vital role in antigen presentation and phagocytosis.

## Merkel Cells

- These cells are found in the basal layer and originate from either neural crest or epidermal keratinocytes.
- They are numerous on fingertips and in the oral cavity and play a role in sensation.

## Keratinocytes

- Secrete a variety of cytokines (e.g. interleukins, gamma-interferon, tumor necrosis factor alpha) in response to tissue injury or in certain skin diseases.

- These play a role in specific immune function, cutaneous inflammation and tissue repair.

## Melanocytes

- Melanocytes are dendritic cells.
- Are derived from neural crest.
- Involved with melanin synthesis (eumelanin or pheomelanin)
- Distributed among basal cells in a nonrandom fashion.
- Melanocytes have
  - Pale staining cytoplasm
  - Ovoid nucleus
  - Pigment containing melanosomes
- Melanocytes are in contact with keratinocytes through their processes.
- One melanocyte is in contact with about 36 basal and suprabasal keratinocytes (epidermal melanin unit)
- These protect against UV irradiation.
- Racial differences are due to variation in melanin production not melanocyte numbers.

## DERMIS

- The dermis, the skin's next layer, is a thick layer of fibrous and elastic tissue (made mostly of collagen, elastin, and fibrillin) that gives the skin, its flexibility and strength.
- The dermis contains nerve endings, sweat glands and oil glands, hair follicles, and blood vessels.
- Dermis can be divided into upper papillary dermis and deeper reticular dermis.
- Collagen constitutes about 70% of the dry weight of the dermis. Elastic fibers constitute about 3% of the dry weight of the dermis.
- Ground substance is an amorphous material that consists mainly of water, electrolytes, plasma proteins and mucopolysaccharides.
- Other cells in dermis include mast cells and fibroblasts.

## EPIDERMAL APPENDAGES

- The sweat glands produce sweat in response to heat and stress. Sweat is composed of water, salt, and other chemicals. As sweat evaporates off the skin, it helps cool the body. Specialized sweat glands in the armpits and the genital region (apocrine sweat glands) secrete a thick, oily sweat that produces a characteristic body odor when the sweat is digested by the skin bacteria in those areas.

- The sebaceous glands secrete sebum into hair follicles. Sebum is an oil, that keeps the skin moist and soft and acts as a barrier against foreign substances.
- The hair follicles produce the various types of hair found throughout the body. Hair not only contributes to a person's appearance but has a number of important physical roles including regulating body temperature, providing protection from injury, and enhancing sensation. A portion of the follicle also contains stem cells capable of regrowing damaged epidermis.
- Nail unit consists of nail matrix underneath the proximal nail fold which gives rise to the nail plate which is a keratinized structure. The nail plate rests on a nailbed and is bounded by lateral nail folds on two sides. The distal portion of nail is free.

## BLOOD VESSELS AND LYMPHATICS

- The blood vessels form two plexuses—superficial plexus in the upper part of reticular dermis just beneath the papillary dermis (subpapillary plexus) and deep plexus in the lower part of reticular dermis.
- The blood vessels of the dermis provide nutrients to the skin and help regulate body temperature. Heat makes the blood vessels enlarge (dilate), allowing large amounts of blood to circulate near the skin surface, where the heat can be released. Cold makes the blood vessels narrow (constrict), retaining the body's heat.
- Lymphatics are parallel to the plexuses.

## NERVES

- The somatic sensory system mediates pain, light touch, itch, vibration, proprioception, pressure and temperature.
- Fingertips and toes contain many nerves and are extremely sensitive to touch.
- The autonomic motor nerves control cutaneous vascular tone, pilomotor responses and sudomotor activity.
- Specialized receptors of dermis include pacinian corpuscles, Meissner's corpuscles and mucocutaneous end organs.

## MUSCLES

- Errector pilorum
- Dartos of the scrotum
- In areolae around the nipples.

## SUBCUTANEOUS FAT

- Consists of adipocytes.
- Functions:
  - ➢ Shock absorber
  - ➢ Facilitates mobility of skin over structures that underlie it.
  - ➢ Cosmetic role
  - ➢ Stores triglycerides which serve as fuel for energy
  - ➢ Insulator for heat

## BLASCHKO'S LINES

- The lines of Blaschko were delineated over 100 years ago; First described by Blaschko in 1901.
  - ➢ The pattern is attributed to the lines of migration and proliferation of epidermal cells during embryogenesis (i.e. the bands of abnormal skin represent clones of cells carrying a mutation in a gene expressed in the skin).
- The lines do not correspond to any known nervous, vascular or lymphatic structures, but **represent the developmental growth pattern of the skin**.
- Generally longitudinally oriented on the limbs and circumferential on the trunk, but not perfectly linear.
- Implies a mosaic disorder (e.g. incontinentia pigmenti, inflammatory linear verrucous epidermal nevus).

### QUESTIONS FROM PREVIOUS EXAMINATIONS

1. Blood supply of the skin
2. Functions of skin
3. Complement system of skin
4. HP of psoriasis, TV, EMF
5. Pallisading granulomas
6. Mast cells
7. Apocrine glands
8. Civatte bodies
9. Process of keratinization
10. Function of eccrine glands
11. Langerhans' cells
12. Cutaneous innervations
13. Odland bodies

– Biopsy procedures
– Basophilic degeneration
– Epidermopoiesis
– HPE of Bowen's disease
– Dermoepidermal junction
– Permeability of skin
– Lamina lucida
– Wood's lamp
– Immunofluorescence testing
– Patch test
– S-100 protein
– Normal cutaneous flora
– X-linked recessive inheritance

14. The skin as a barrier            – Price curve
15. Basal lamina                     – Pigmentary incontinence
16. Dermoscopy                       – IL-2
17. Touton giant cells               – Kamino bodies
18. Attachment plaque                – Fibers of the dermis
19. Epidermal growth factor          – Chalone
20. Birbeck's granules               – Raper Mason Scheme
21. Fibronectin                      – Meckel's end organs
22. Cytodiagnosis                    – Acantholysis
23. Scanning electron microscope     – Sensory end organs
24. Desmosomes                       – HLA antigen
25. Cardinal signs of inflammation   – Special stains

## MULTIPLE CHOICE QUESTIONS

1. **Melanocytes are present in:**                    *(PGI 09)*
   (a) Stratum corneum      (b) Stratum basale
   (c) Stratum granulosum   (d) Dermis

2. **Langerhans' cells in skin are:**                 *(AI 06)*
   (a) Antigen presenting cells   (b) Pigment producing cells
   (c) Keratin synthesizing cells (d) Sensory nerves

3. **The correct sequence of cell cycle:**            *(DNB 07)*
   (a) $G_0$-$G_1$-S-$G_2$-M      (b) $G_0$-$G_1$- $G_2$-S-M
   (c) $G_0$-M-$G_2$-S-$G_1$      (d) $G_0$-$G_1$-S-M-$G_2$

4. **Delayed hypersensitivity in skin tests, is assessed by:**
                                                       *(AIIMS 02)*
   (a) Erythema       (b) Bulla
   (c) Necrosis       (d) Induration

5. **Normal turnover rate of epidermis:**             *(AIIMS 01)*
   (a) 2 wks          (b) 4 wks
   (c) 6 wks          (d) 8 wks

6. **Which layer of epidermis is underdeveloped in VLBW infants in the initial 7 days?**                          *(AIIMS Nov 02)*
   (a) Stratum germinativum   (b) Stratum granulosum
   (c) Stratum lucidum        (d) Stratum corneum

7. **Langerhans' cells play a crucial role in:**      *(JK 2009)*
   (a) Healing of wound       (b) Distribution of melanin pigment
   (c) Contact sensitization  (d) Body temperature regulation

8. **Wood's lamp is used to diagnose:**    *(MH 05)*
   (a) Psoriasis    (b) *Tinea versicolor*
   (c) pityriasis rosae    (d) Erysipelas
9. **Yellow fluorescence on Wood's lamp:**    *(MH 07)*
   (a) Tuberous sclerosis    (b) Pseudomonas infection
   (c) *Tinea capitis*    (d) Erythrasma
10. **Diascopy is very helpful in diagnosis of:**    *(MH 09)*
   (a) Cutaneous vasculitis    (b) Nevus anemicus
   (c) Lupus vulgaris    (d) All of the above
11. **Wavelength of UV rays used in Wood's lamp:**    *(Bihar 07)*
   (a) E. 360 nM    (b) F. 460 nM
   (c) G. 660 nM    (d) H. 760 nM
12. **All the following about skin are true *except:***    *(PGI 06)*
   (a) Skin is stratified squamous epithelium
   (b) Melanocytes and Merkel cells are immigrant cells
   (c) Keratin filaments are hallmark of epidermal cells
   (d) Keratinization causes hydration of cells
   (e) Spines of spinous cells are formed from housekeeping organelle
13. **Wood's lamp is used in diagnosis of:**    *(PGI 2006)*
   (a) *P. versicolor*    (b) Vitiligo
   (c) Porphyria    (d) Psoriasis
   (e) Lichen planus
14. **Blashco's lines are present along:**    *(AIIMS 2011)*
   (a) Nerves    (b) Lymphatics
   (c) Vessels    (d) Lines of development

## Answers

1. **Ans. (b)** Stratum basale *(Ref. IDVL Textbook of Dermatology, 2nd edn/ 12)*
2. **Ans. (a)** Antigen presenting cells *(Ref. IDVL Textbook of Dermatology, 2nd edn/ 12)*
3. **Ans. (a)** ($G_0$-$G_1$-S-$G_2$-M) *(Ref. IDVL Textbook of Dermatology, 2nd edn/11)*
4. **Ans. (d)** Induration *(Ref. IDVL Textbook of Dermatology, 2nd edn/ 43)*
5. **Ans. (b)** 4 weeks *(Ref. Roxburgh's Common Skin Diseases, 17th edn/ 136)*
6. **Ans. (d)** Stratum corneum *(Ref. Physical Diagnosis in Neonatology, 109)*

7. **Ans. (c)** Contact sensitization *(Ref. Robbin's Pathology, 7th edn/1172; Fitzpatrick Dermatology, 6th edn/130)*

8. **Ans. (b)** *Tinea versicolor*

9. **Ans. (c)** *Tinea capitis*

10. **Ans. (d)** All of the above *(Ref. Rook's Textbook of Dermatology, 7th edition/5.10)*

11. **Ans. (a)** E. 360 nM *(Ref. Rook's Textbook of Dermatology, 7th edn/5.10)*

12. **Ans. (d)** Keratinization causes hydration of cells, and **(e)** spines of spinous cells are formed from housekeeping organelle *(Ref. Fitzpatrick's Dermatology, 6th edn/58–62).*

13. **Ans. (a, b, c)** *(Ref. Rook's Textbook, 7th end/5.11–5.14).*

14. **Ans. (d)** Lines of development *(Ref. Rook's Textbook of Dermatology, 8th edn/page 15.6).*

# 2 Type of Lesions

## TYPE OF CUTANEOUS LESIONS

1. Primary lesions
2. Secondary lesions
3. Special lesions

## Primary Lesions

*Macule*　　A circumscribed alteration in the color of the skin.

*Papule*　　A circumscribed palpable elevation, less than 0.5 cm in diameter.

*Plaque*　　An elevated area of skin, usually defined as 2 cm or more in diameter. It may be formed by the extension or coalescence of either papules or nodules as in psoriasis and granuloma annulare, respectively. Small plaque is sometimes used for such lesions 0.5–2 cm in diameter.

*Nodule*　　A solid mass in the skin, which can be observed as an elevation or can be palpated. It is more than 0.5 cm in diameter. It may involve epidermis and dermis, dermis and subcutis, or subcutis alone. It may consist of fluid, other extracellular material (e.g. amyloid), inflammatory or neoplastic cells.

*Vesicles and bullae*　　Visible accumulations of fluid within or beneath the epidermis. Vesicles are small (less than 0.5 cm in diameter) and often grouped. Bullae may be of any size over 0.5 cm.

*Pustule*　　A visible accumulation of free pus. It may occur within a pilosebaceous follicle or a sweat duct, or less often, on glabrous skin. Most commonly due to infections, but some eruptions typically cause sterile pustules.

*Wheal*　　A transient area of dermal or dermal and hypodermal edema, pale or erythematous, compressible and usually evanescent. It is the characteristic lesion of urticaria.

*Cyst*　　A sac that contains liquid or semisolid material.

## Secondary Lesions

- These lesions are due to subsequent changes which take place on the primary lesions.
  - ➤ **Erosion:** Superficial ulceration involving epidermis only which heals without scarring.
  - ➤ **Ulcer (of skin ):** A loss of dermis and epidermis, often with loss of the underlying tissues.
  - ➤ **Crust:** Dried up exudate like serum, pus or blood.
  - ➤ **Scale:** A flat plate or flake of stratum corneum.

| Type of scale | Features | Example |
|---|---|---|
| Collarette scale | is a fine, peripherally attached and centrally detached scale at the edge of an inflammatory lesion. | **Pityriasis rosea** |
| Annular scaling | is also seen in porokeratosis. | |
| Furfuraceous or pityriasiform | scales are fine and loose. | |
| Ichthyotic scales (fish-like) | are large and polygonal. | |
| Silvery scales | are characteristic of processes involving parakeratosis, especially psoriasis. | |
| Greasy adherent scales | are seen in seborrheic dermatitis. | |

- **Excoriation:** Superficial erosion or ulcer caused by scratching.
- **Fissure:** Linear crack in the skin which may be superficial or deep to the dermis.
- **Lichenification:** Thickening of skin with increased skin markings and pigmentation.
- **Scar:** Replacement by fibrous tissue of another tissue that has been destroyed by injury or disease. An atrophic scar is thin and wrinkled. A hypertrophic scar is elevated, with excessive growth of fibrous tissue. A cribriform scar is perforated with multiple small pits.
- **Sclerosis:** Diffuse or circumscribed induration of the subcutaneous tissues. It may also involve the dermis, when the overlying epidermis may be atrophic. It is characteristically seen in scleroderma.

## Special Lesions

- **Comedones:** It is a plug of keratin and sebum formed in the follicular canal of pilosebaceous unit. It may be open or closed.

- **Burrow:** Seen in Scabies. S-shaped brownish black lesions which have a papule at their distal end homing the mite.
- **Telangiectasia:** Visible, dilated and tortuous blood vessels. *Petechia (pl. petechiae):* A punctate hemorrhagic spot, approximately 1–2 mm in diameter.
- **Poikiloderma:** The association of cutaneous pigmentation, atrophy and telangiectasia.
- **Sinus:** A cavity or track with a blind ending.
- **Target lesions:** These are less than 3 cm in diameter and have three or more zones, usually a central area of dusky erythema or purpura, a middle paler zone of edema, and an outer ring of erythema with a well-defined edge.

## BASIC DERMATOPATHOLOGICAL TERMS

### Acantholysis

- **Acantholysis** is the term used to describe loss of cohesion between keratinocytes, due to breakdown of intercellular bridges. It results in the formation of intraepidermal clefts, vesicles and bullae.

  *Primary:* Pemphigus and its variants, Darier's disease, transient and persistent acantholytic dermatosis and warty dyskeratoma. The site of acantholysis in these disorders is important.

  > In pemphigus foliaceus and pemphigus erythematosus, acantholysis is usually confined to the upper portion of the epidermis, whereas in pemphigus vulgaris the split is formed at a lower level in the epidermis. In **benign familial pemphigus** (Hailey-Hailey disease), although acantholysis is often focal or incomplete, where it does occur it tends to affect the full thickness of the epidermis.

  *Secondary:* Bullous impetigo, viral disorders, solar keratoses and some forms of squamous cell carcinoma.
- A typical acantholytic lower spinous cell is rounded with a round vesicular nucleus, a perinuclear halo and peripheral condensation of cytoplasm and lacks desmosomal connections with adjacent keratinocytes.
- An acantholytic granular cell is oval or elongated and lacks desmosomal bridges.
- **Acanthosis**
  > This term is used to describe an increase in number of cells in the malpighian or prickle cell layer of the epidermis.

> Acanthosis is commonly accompanied by other histological changes such as *hypergranulosis, hyperkeratosis and papillomatosis*. When reactive epidermal proliferation is marked, the process may simulate an epithelial carcinoma, and in this situation is referred to as pseudoepitheliomatous hyperplasia.

- **Anaplasia**
  > This is a term used to describe variations in nuclear size, dense and clumped heterochromatin, and nuclear contour angulation typical of malignant cells, as in metastatic melanoma.

- **Apoptosis**
  > This is a morphologically distinct type of cell degeneration and death, usually applied to keratinocytes that become homogeneous and eosinophilic and are extruded into the underlying upper dermis. These eosinophilic bodies (known as **civatte or colloid bodies**), and the process of apoptosis, occur characteristically in lichenoid tissue reactions.

- **Colloid body**
  > This term, usually regarded as synonymous with civatte body, describes the homogeneous eosinophilic rounded body resulting from degeneration and death of keratinocytes, particularly in the lower layers of the epidermis. This structure is found in various lichenoid tissue reactions and is involved in the process of apoptosis.

- **Degenerations**
  *Dermal*

| Type of dermal degeneration | Refers to | Seen in |
| --- | --- | --- |
| *Colloid degeneration* | The deposition of extracellular homogeneous gelatinous material of variable composition. | Colloid **milium**, Also in certain epithelial tumours. |
| *Elastotic degeneration* | The d**egenerative** changes that develop with increasing age, particularly in the upper part of the dermis in sun-exposed skin. | **Degenerative changes,** especially involving sun-exposed skin. |
| *Fibrinoid degeneration* | The deposition in tissue of eosinophilic, granular or fibrillary material resembling fibrin. | – |

*Contd.*

*Contd.*

| Type of dermal degeneration | Refers to | Seen in |
|---|---|---|
| **Hyaline degeneration** | The presence of homogeneous eosinophilic degenerative material in dermal connective tissue, or in relation to blood vessels. The material has a glassy and refractile appearance. | **Porphyria**, lipoid **proteinosis** and sometimes in **lichenoid** tissue reactions. |
| **Myxoid degeneration** | The deposition or replacement of dermal connective tissue by amorphous, stringy, basophilic material. | Localized **myxedema**, papular **mucinosis**, **scleroderma** and **dermatomyositis**. |

### Epidermal

➢ *Ballooning degeneration:* This form of degeneration of keratinocytes is associated with marked swelling and pallor of individual cells, with loss of intercellular bridges. A blister forms as a result of the consequent acantholysis. Ballooning degeneration along with reticular degeneration is characteristic of virus disorders affecting epithelia, such as **herpesvirus** infections.

➢ *Hydropic degeneration:* This is also known as liquefaction degeneration, and refers to a vacuolar change that affects the basal cell layer of the epidermis. Associated with **pigmentary incontinence**, and when marked may lead to subepidermal blister formation. It occurs typically in the whole range of **lichenoid** tissue reactions, including lupus erythematosus, lichen planus, dermatomyositis, poikiloderma atrophicans vasculare and lichen sclerosus.

➢ *Reticular degeneration:* This indicates the development of large, multiple, intraepidermal vesicles, where there remains a ragged network of epidermal cell remnants.

• **Dyskeratosis:** This term relates to some abnormality in the process of epidermal cell keratinization. The changes usually consist of nuclear pyknosis and bright pink condensation of the cytoplasm of keratinocytes. The process occurs in two main contexts. Firstly, in malignant and premalignant epithelial lesions, such as **squamous cell carcinoma, Bowen's disease and solar keratosis**. Secondly, in various forms of acantholytic disorder such as **Darier's** disease.

• **Exocytosis:** This term describes the migration of inflammatory cells from the blood vessels of the dermis into the overlying epidermis. The process may be associated with spongiosis, as in eczema, or occur in the absence of spongiosis, such as may be seen in mycosis fungoides. In the later setting, the word epidermotropism is usually preferred.

- **Granuloma:** A granuloma describes circumscribed foci of inflammation containing monocytes, macrophages, lymphocytes and epithelioid cells. Multinucleated giant cells of foreign body, Langhans or Touton type may also be observed.
- **Grenz zone:** A narrow zone of normal dermis between the epidermis and pathological changes in the underlying dermis.
- **Hypergranulosis:** This refers to an increase in thickness of the granular layer of the epidermis, and is commonly accompanied by hyperkeratosis and acanthosis.
- **Hyperkeratosis:** Hyperkeratosis refers to increased thickness of the stratum corneum, and may be associated with acanthosis of the malpighian layer.
  - ➢ *Epidermolytic hyperkeratosis:* There is an increase in the thickness of the granular layer, where keratinocytes appear to contain an increased number of keratohyaline granules. Perinuclear vacuolization occurs in this area, and the cell boundaries may be indistinct.
  - ➢ The vacuolization may be marked, in some cases appearing lead to intraepidermal vesicle formation. Seen in bullous ichthyosiform erythroderma and many other inherited and acquired conditions, including a form of palmoplantar keratoderma, so-called epidermolytic acanthoma, and some forms of linear epidermal nevus.
  - ➢ *Follicular hyperkeratosis:* This describes varying degrees of hyperkeratosis and plugging of the ostia of hair follicles, and this change may be associated with the rupture of the follicular wall. It occurs in many conditions including pityriasis rubra pilaris, lupus erythematosus, lichen planopilaris and lichen sclerosus.
- **Kamino bodies (eosinophilic globules):** This term describes the eosinophilic globules seen in the epidermis or in the region of the dermal–epidermal junction in spindle and epithelioid cell (**spitz**) nevi.
- **Karyorrhexis:** This refers to the fragmentation of cell nuclei, and the process may be seen in various forms of neutrophilic dermatoses and cutaneous pyoderma.
- **Necrosis:** This term describes the death of cells or tissues.
- **Papilloma:** This term indicates a tumor or tumor-like proliferation exhibiting both papillomatosis and hyperkeratosis. Acanthosis is also present. Examples of skin papillomas include viral warts, seborrheic keratoses and some epidermal nevi.

- **Papillomatosis:** This change is characterized by elongation upwards of the dermal papillae, giving an accentuated and sometimes irregular, undulating configuration to the dermal–epidermal junction.

- **Parakeratosis:** Parakeratosis can be defined as the retention of keratinocyte nuclei within the horny cell layer. It represents a disturbance of keratinization, and is normally associated with an absence or reduction in thickness of the granular cell layer. It is commonly seen in psoriasis and subacute eczematous reactions, and in conditions such as pityriasis lichenoides.

- **Pigmentary incontinence:** This refers to the loss of melanin from cells of the basal layer of the epidermis, and the accumulation of melanin, both free and within dendritic macrophages, in the underlying dermis. It is associated with damage to keratinocytes of the lower epidermis, and is commonly seen in lichenoid tissue reactions.

- **Microabscesses**

| | |
|---|---|
| **Kogoj's spongiform pustule** | This describes the multilocular micropustules that form in the superficial portions of the epidermis in pustular psoriasis. They form in a similar manner to Munro microabscesses but the process is more extensive. |
| **Munro microabscesses** | These lesions are small collections of neutrophil polymorphs usually found within the stratum corneum. They are normally seen in lesions of chronic established psoriasis. |
| **Papillary tip microabscesses** | These are small focal collections of neutrophil. polymorphs or occasionally eosinophils, in the tips of dermal papillae. Although they are characteristic of dermatitis herpetiformis, they may occur in other bullous eruptions such as epidermolysis bullosa acquisita and the bullous form of lupus erythematosus. |
| **Pautrier microabscesses** | These small, intraepidermal collections of lymphoid cells in the absence of marked spongiosis are characteristic of mycosis fungoides. |
| **Subcorneal pustules** | Large, subcorneal collections of neutrophil polymorphs usually represent either impetigo or subcorneal pustular dermatosis. |

- **Saw-toothing:** This refers to an alteration in the pattern of the dermal–epidermal junction where dermal papillae are expanded and the tips of the rete pegs are pointed. The resulting pattern bears a superficial resemblance to the teeth of a saw and the change is seen in lichen planus and other lichenoid reactions.
- **Spongiosis:** Spongiosis is also known as intercellular edema, and describes the widening of intercellular spaces between keratinocytes due to fluid accumulation. Spongiosis is the characteristic histopathological change seen in acute and subacute eczematous reactions.
- **Theque:** This term is derived from French and Greek words for a box (thèque, θηκη) and is conventionally used in dermatopathology to describe small aggregates or nests of cells, particularly the collections of nevus cells at, and in the region of, the dermal–epidermal junction.
- **Villi**
  - ➤ This term refers to elongated dermal papillae covered usually with a single layer of epidermal cells, and which form the base of a blister cavity that has resulted from the process of suprabasal acantholysis.
  - ➤ Villi are seen in the various forms of pemphigus and Darier's disease, warty dyskeratoma, and transient and persistent acantholytic dermatosis.

## QUESTIONS FROM PREVIOUS EXAMINATIONS

1. Describe the role of skin in thermoregulation
2. Dermoepidermal junction and its pathophysiology
3. Odland bodies
4. Melanocytes
5. Dermatoglyphics
6. Immunological function of keratinocytes
7. Vater–Pacini corpuscle
8. Describe the dynamics of epidermal cell cycle and discuss the control of epidermopoiesis
9. Skin as defence organ
10. Apocrine gland
11. Type I skin vs type II
12. Ultrastructure and function of Langerhans' cells
13. Cutaneous microbial flora

14. Cytokines in dermatology
15. Cell adhesive molecule in dermatology
16. Keratin: Origin, site, function of keratinocyte and discuss keratinization
17. What is Melanin? Discuss origin, site, function of melanocyte and discuss melanization
18. Discuss microanatomy and physiology of mast cells
19. Percutaneous absorption, routes of percutaneous absorption, factors influencing. What are penetration enhancers? Properties of penetration enhancers
20. Lipid interaction, protein modification, partitioning promoter's concept
21. Structure of the lower part of the hair shaft
22. Biosynthesis of keratin
23. Phototoxic vs photoallergic response
24. Anatomy of nail
25. Dermal connective tissue
26. Melanogenesis and racial differences in the skin
27. Structure of peripheral nerve
28. Merkel cells
29. Dendritic cells of the epidermis
30. Antigen presenting cells of the epidermis
31. Structure of apocrine gland and hidradenitis suppurative
32. Acantholysis
33. DEJ + mention the lines of cleavage and pathogenetic factors in blistering disorders
34. Barrier functions of the skin
35. Write note with diagram of normal skin
36. Dermatological purpura
37. Epidermal growth factors
38. Epidermal cell kinetics
39. Pharmacological control of sebum
40. Discuss role of immunofluorescence in diagnosis of dermatological disorders
41. Subcutaneous tissue
42. Sunlight and skin
43. Epidermal melanin unit
44. Basal cell degeneration

45. Cycles of sebaceous activity and changes brought thereby
46. Structure of dermis and its organization and function
47. Various phases of hair cycle
48. Epidermotropism
49. Basement membrane zone
50. T helper cells
51. Development of the skin
52. Structure and physiology of nail
53. Skin as sensory organ
54. Different types of dyskeratosis, various dyskeratotic cells in histopathology with examples
55. Structure innervations and function of apocrine glands
56. Nail matrix
57. Different microabscess in skin
58. Describe hair follicle and hair cycle
59. Eccrine sweat glands and role in thermoregulation
60. Mediators of pruritus in skin
61. Bartholin gland
62. Classify proteoglycans and mention about the functions
63. Changes in collagen with aging
64. Giant cells in dermatology
65. Glomus bodies
66. Embryology of nail
67. HLA in dermatology
68. Mechanism of sweating and sweat test and its application
69. Degerming capacity of the skin and normal flora.
70. Complement and skin

## MULTIPLE CHOICE QUESTIONS

1. **Type of scale observed in pityriasis rosea is:**    *(MH'2014)*
   (a) Mica-like
   (b) Powdery
   (c) Silvery
   (d) Collarette-like

2. **Kamino bodies are seen in:**    *(AI/NEET 2013)*
   (a) Melanoma
   (b) Lichen planus
   (c) Spitz nevus
   (d) Miliaria rubra

3. **Acanthosis nigricans histologically show:**    *(MH'2010)*
   (a) Papillomatosis
   (b) Marked acanthosis
   (c) Hypermelanosis
   (d) All of the above

4. A 2-month-old female child is brought with chief complains of linear verrucous rash on the lower abdomen (trunk). On microscopic examination, the lesions showed vaccuolar degeneration of the keratinocytes in stratum spinosum and in stratum granulosum. What is the diagnosis?

*(AIIMS Nov 2008; May 2011)*

(a) Linear Darier's disease
(b) Incontinentia pigmenti
(c) Verrucous epidermal nevus
(d) Delayed hypersensitivity reaction

## Answers

1. **Ans. (d)** Collarette-like
2. **Ans. (c)** Spitz nevus
3. **Ans. (d)** All of the above *(Ref. Robbin's and Cotran Pathologic Basis of Disease, 7th edn, Table 7–12; p. 335)*
4. **Ans. (c)** Verrucous epidermal nevus. Linear verrucous lesions, with characteristic histopathological feature of granular degeneration of epidermis favor the diagnosis of **verrucous epidermal nevus**.

# 3 Diagnostic Techniques in Skin Diseases

## SKIN BIOPSY

### Indications

1. To confirm a clinical diagnosis or in the establishment of a diagnosis where clinical diagnosis is not apparent.
2. Excisional biopsy for the treatment of benign and malignant lesions.
3. Used for immunofluorescence studies, immunohistochemistry, and enzyme immunohistochemistry.

### Procedure

Written consent is taken from the patient. In this procedure, a small area of skin is anesthetized with 1% lidocaine with or without epinephrine. The lesion biopsied should be an early and untreated lesion.

### Techniques

*Elliptical surgical biopsy:* The skin lesion in question can be excised with a scalpel.

*Punch biopsy:* A punch (usually 5 mm) is pressed against the surface of the skin and rotated with downward pressure until it penetrates to the subcutaneous tissue. The circular biopsy is then lifted with forceps, and the bottom is cut with iris scissors. Biopsy sites may or may not need suture closure, depending on size and location.

*Shave biopsy*

*Excisional biopsy*

## POTASSIUM HYDROXIDE (KOH) PREPARATION

KOH dissolves keratin of keratinocytes, hair and nails but not fungus and allows easier visualization of fungal elements.

### Indications

A potassium hydroxide (KOH) preparation is performed on scaling skin lesions where a fungal etiology is a possibility.

## Procedure

- The edge of such a lesion is scraped gently with a scalpel blade, and the removed scale is collected on a glass microscope slide and treated with 1 to 2 drops of a solution of 10 to 20% KOH.
- Specimen is covered with a cover slip.
- Wait for 2–5 minutes. For hair wait for half an hour and nail 24 hrs.
- Brief heating of the slide accelerates dissolution of keratin.
- When the preparation is viewed under the microscope under low power magnification, the refractile hyphae will be seen more easily when the light intensity is reduced and the condenser is lowered.
- This technique can be utilized to identify hyphae in dermatophyte infections, pseudohyphae and budding yeast in Candida infections, and fragmented hyphae and spores in tinea versicolor (spaghetti and meatballs appearance/banana and grapes appearance).

|  | Clinical features | Etiologic agent | Treatment |
|---|---|---|---|
| **Impetigo** | Honey-colored crusted papules, plaques, or bullae | Group A *Streptococcus* and *Staphylococcus aureus* | Systemic or topical antistaphylococcal antibiotics |
| **Dermato-phytosis** | Inflammatory or noninflammatory annular scaly plaques; may have hair loss; groin involvement spares scrotum; hyphae on KOH preparation | *Trichophyton, Epidermophyton*, or *Microsporum* sp. | Topical azoles, systemic griseofulvin, terbinafine, or azoles |
| **Candidiasis** | Inflammatory papules and plaques with satellite pustules, frequently in intertriginous areas; may involve scrotum; pseudohyphae on KOH preparation | *Candida albicans* and other *Candida* species | Topical nystatin or azoles; systemic azoles for resistant disease |
| **Tinea versicolor** | Hyperpigmented or hypopigmented scaly patches on the trunk; characteristic mixture of hyphae and spores on KOH preparation (*spaghetti and meatballs*) | *Malassezia furfur* | Topical selenium sulfide lotion or azoles |

## TZANCK SMEAR

A Tzanck smear is a cytologic technique most often used in the diagnosis of herpesvirus infections (simplex or varicella-zoster) and also done in vesicular and bullous lesions. The material is placed on a glass slide, air-dried, and stained with Giemsa or Wright's stain. Multinucleated epithelial giant cells suggest the presence of herpes, but culture or immunofluorescence testing must be performed to identify the specific virus.

### Procedure

a. An early vesicle, not a pustule or crusted lesion, is unroofed, and the base of the lesion is scraped gently with a scalpel blade.
b. The material is placed on a glass slide, air-dried, and stained with Giemsa or Wright's stain.
c. Smear is examined under oil immersion field.

### Results

a. Multinucleated epithelial giant cells suggest the presence of herpes, but culture or immunofluorescence testing must be performed to identify the specific virus.
b. Pemphigus demonstrates acantholytic cells. These are rounded cells with large nuclei, peripheral condensed cytoplasm and perinuclear halo. Pemphigus vulgaris and Hailey-Hailey disease show plenty of rounded acantholytic cells with large nuclei, whereas in pemphigus foliaceous and pemphigus erythematosus the acantholytic cells are fewer, oval with smaller nuclei.
c. Molluscum contagiosum lesions show intracytoplasmic inclusion bodies known as **Henderson-Patterson bodies**.

## DIASCOPY (VITROPRESSION)

Diascopy is designed to assess whether a skin lesion will blanch with pressure as, for example, in determining whether a red lesion is hemorrhagic or simply blood-filled. For instance, urticaria will blanch with pressure, whereas a purpuric lesion caused by necrotizing vasculitis will not. Diascopy is performed by pressing a microscope slide or magnifying lens against a lesion and noting the amount of blanching that occurs. Granulomas often have an "apple jelly" appearance on diascopy.

*Useful in*

• **Lupus vulgaris:** Granulomatous nodules have translucent brownish color ("apple jelly nodules").
• To differentiate **nevus anemicus** from nevus depigmentosus.

- Application of medium pressure to a **spider nevus** can compress radiating arterioles and allow visualization of pulsatile flow in the feeding vessel.
- In vasculitis lesions—lesions are not blanchable (**purpura**).

## WOOD'S LAMP

It is a low intensity ultraviolet light (360 nm) emitted by a high pressure mercury-lamp fitted with a special filter made up of nickel oxide and silica.

| Disease (360 nm UV light used) | Color on Wood's lamp |
|---|---|
| 1. Erythrasma (*Corynebacterium minutissimum*) | Coral red color |
| 2. Tinea versicolor | Golden yellow |
| 3. Tinea capitis (*Microsporum canis or M. audouini*) | Yellow fluorescence |
| 4. *Trichophyton schoenleini* | Pale green |
| 5. *Pseudomonas aeruginosa* | Pale blue/aquagreen |
| 6. Tuberous sclerosis appears white | Ash-leaf-shaped spot |
| 7. Porphyria cutanea tarda | Pink to pink-orange |
| 8. Leprosy | Blue white |
| 9. Hypopigmentation | Pale white |
| 10. Hyperpigmentation | Purple brown |
| 11. Depigmentation—vitiligo | Totally white |
| 12. Albinism | Bright white |
| 13. Pigmented lesions of the epidermis such as freckles | are accentuated under a Wood's light |
| 14. Lesions dermal pigment such as postinflammatory hyperpigmentation | Fades under a Wood's light |

## PATCH TEST

- Patch testing is the only scientific method to detect the cause of contact dermatitis.
- Introduced by Jadassohn.
- Patches are commonly applied on upper back for 48 hrs.
- First reading is taken after 48 hrs and 2nd reading on day 4 to day 7 because over 50% error is likely if only one reading is taken at day 2.

### Indications for Patch Testing

- Eczematous disorders where contact allergy is suspected or is to be excluded.
- Eczematous disorders failing to respond to treatment as expected
- Chronic hand and foot eczema

- Persistent or intermittent eczema of the face, eyelids, ears and perineum
- Varicose eczema

## Evaluation of Patch Test Reading

| Grading | Evaluation | Clinical findings |
|---------|-----------|-------------------|
| ± or ? | Doubt reaction | Faint erythema |
| + | Weak (nonvesicular) +ve reaction | Erythema, infiltration, and discrete papules |
| ++ | Strong (vesicular) +ve reaction | Erythema, infiltration, papules, and vesicles |
| +++ | Extreme (bullous) +ve reaction | Intense erythema, infiltration, and coalescing vesicles |

## Intradermal Test for Delayed Hypersensitivity

- Usually employed for infectious diseases.
- Antigen is prepared from the respective infective agents and injected intradermally.
- Significantly indurated nodule after 48 hrs is considered to indicate delayed hypersensitivity to the antigen.
- Test continues to remain positive even after the infection has subsided, though active infections usually produce more severe reactions.
- In overwhelming infections the test can completely become negative because of the suppression of delayed hypersensitivity.

## Some Stains Used in Dermatology

| Special stains | Tissue constituent |
|----------------|--------------------|
| Periodic acid–Schiff (PAS) | Glycogen mucopolysaccharides |
| van Gieson | Collagen muscle nerve |
| Congo red | Amyloid |
| Acid orcein—Giemsa | Elastic fiber collagen melanin hemosiderin Amyloid mast cell granules |
| Masson's trichrome | Collagen muscle + fibrin |
| Aldehyde fuchsin | Elastic fiber |
| Gomori | Reticulin |
| Alcian blue (pH 4.5, 0.5) and toluidine blue | Acid mucopolysaccharides |
| Perls' prussian blue | Iron (hemosiderin) |
| Masson and Fontana | Melanin |
| von Kossa | Calcium salts |
| Grocott | Fungus wall |
| Methenamine silver | Bacteria Gram-positive and Gram-negative |
| Ziehl-Neelsen/Wade-Fite | Acid-fast bacilli |

## QUESTIONS FROM PREVIOUS EXAMINATIONS

1. Patch test
2. Wood's lamp
3. Diascopy

## MULTIPLE CHOICE QUESTIONS

1. A 10-yer-old boy presented with painful boggy swelling of scalp, multiple sinuses with purulent discharge, easily pluckable hair, and lymph nodes enlarged in occipital region. Which one of the following would be most helpful for diagnostic evaluation?
   *(AIIMS Nov 09; May 2013)*
   (a) Biopsy           (b) Bacterial culture
   (c) KOH mount        (d) Patch test

2. 'Coral red' fluorescence on Wood's lamp is seen in:
   *(MH 2008; DNB 12)*
   (a) Erythrasma        (b) Erysipelas
   (c) *Pityriasis versicolor*   (d) *Tinea corporis*

3. "Apple jelly" appearance on diascopy:        *(AI 2014)*
   (a) Purpura           (b) Lupus vulgaris
   (c) Nevus anemicus    (d) Leprosy

### Answers

1. **Ans. (c)** KOH mount *(Ref. Harrison's Medicine, 17th edn, Table 54–5; Chapter 53, 54, 199).*
2. **Ans. (a)** Erythrasma *(Ref. Harrison's Medicine, 17th edn/p. 312).*
3. **Ans. (b)** Lupus vulgaris.

# 4 Nutritional and Metabolic Skin Disorders

## PELLAGRA

### Etiology

- Dietary deficiency of nicotinic acid or its precursor tryptophan.
- Seen in people with staple diet—maize and jowar.
- Maize is poor source of both nicotinic acid and tryptophan and a part of nicotinic acid is in a bound form that is not assimilated in GIT.
- Jowar contains adequate amounts of niacin and tryptophan but it also has high content of leucine. The resultant imbalance between leucine and other related amino acids particularly isoleucine interferes with conversion of tryptophan to nicotinic acid.
- Malabsorption
- Drugs like INH, 5FU, and 6-mercaptopurine.
- Carcinoid syndrome

### Clinical Features

- Middle aged persons

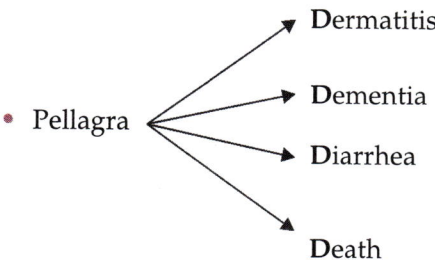

| Cutaneous | Mucous | GIT | CNS |
|---|---|---|---|
| • Sharply demarcated lesions on the upper central portions of chest and neck, form so called Casal's collar/necklace <br> • Common in sunexposed areas (Fig. 4.1) | • Cheilosis <br> • Scarlet tongue <br> • Angular stomatitis | • Esophagus, stomach, and colon affected <br> • Diarrhea, anorexia, dyspepsia, nausea, vomiting and abdominal pain | • Impairment of memory, insomnia, apathy, depression, psychosis, and coma <br> • Encephalopathy syndrome may be seen |

## Treatment

- Niacinamide 300–500 mg/day orally in divided doses.

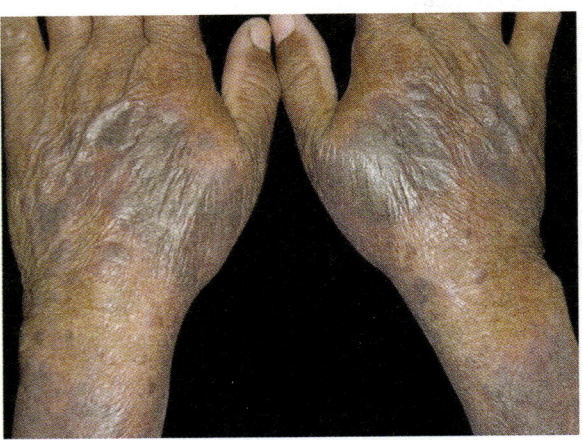

**Fig. 4.1:** Sharply demarcated erythematous scaly plaques on dorsum of hand

## ACRODERMATITIS ENTEROPATHICA

- AR inheritance
- Specific malabsorption defect of **zinc**.
- Presenting sign in cystic fibrosis or AIDS.
- Manifests between 3 wks and 18 months (usually weaning is started or earlier if baby is not breastfed)
  - Psorasiform lesions
  - Symmetrically distributed in periorificial regions, acral areas, and bony prominences (Fig. 4.2).

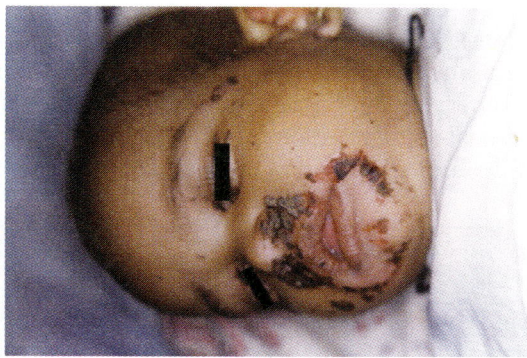

**Fig. 4.2:** Periorificial lesions in a child with acrodermatitis enteropathica

➢ Non-scarring alopecia of scalp is characteristic
➢ Chronic diarrhea
➢ Irritable and emotionally labile child
➢ Wound healing is poor and decreased resistance to infections
➢ Growth retardation is seen
➢ Child stops smiling early in the disease and this is always the first sign to return when the condition is brought under control.

Acrodermatitis enteropathica is a rare genetic disorder characterized by diarrhea, an inflammatory rash around the mouth and/or anus, and hair loss due to mutations in a gene (SLC39A4) that codes the zinc transporter protein—ZIP4. This results decreased zinc uptake and abnormal zinc metabolism.

➢ Oral zinc dose of 2–3 mg/kg/day cures all clinical manifestations, apart from hair and  nail growth, within a few days.
➢ Prolonged high-dose therapy up to adult age is necessary, then a continuous zinc supplementation is indicated, often with oral doses of 1–2 mg zinc/kg/day.

## KWASHIORKOR

• It occurs with protein deficiency but relatively adequate calorie intake.

• Essential features — Growth retardation
                     — Edema
                     — Mental apathy

Enamel-paint sign is seen in patients with kwashiorkor, a nutritional deficiency endemic in tropical and subtropical regions. Sharply demarcated hyperpigmented desquamating patches and plaques resembling enamel paint occur on the skin, predominantly in areas of pressure and irritation.

| Skin and mucous membrane lesions | Hair | Non-cutaneous features |
|---|---|---|
| • Enamel-paint spots (sharply demarcated hyperpigmented flat topped plaques with waxy feel seen over elbows, knees, ankle and intertriginous sites)<br>• Flaky paint or crazy paving (extensive skin peeling)<br>• Cheilitis, glossitis and cancrum oris | • **Flag sign** (hair grown during malnutrition is pale so that alternating bands of dark and pale hairs are seen in single strand). **This sign** is only rarely seen in older children who escape hair loss | • Anorexia<br>• Diarrhea<br>• Mental apathy<br>• Lassitude<br>• Drowsiness<br>• Irritability<br>• Growth failure<br>• Muscle wasting<br>• Pericardial, pleural, peritoneal effusion<br>• Hepatomegaly<br>• Gynecomastia<br>• Night blindness |

## MARASMUS (GREEK *MARASMOS,* WHICH MEANS WASTING)

- It is a result of severe protein and calorie deprivation for a prolonged period.
- Worldwide, marasmus is more frequent than kwashiorkor and is especially seen in developing countries where food is absent or scarce.
- *Clinical features:* Patients have a wrinkled, loose, dry skin. There is a substantial loss of subcutaneous fat tissue. 'Monkey facies' due to loss of the buccal adipose tissue.
- Follicular hyperkeratosis may be prominent in adults
- Poor hair and nail growth
- Child is irritable
- There is no peripheral edema.

## VITAMIN A DEFICIENCY

### Causes

- Inadequate intake
- Inadequate absorption
- Children with measles

## Clinical Features

- **Skin**
  - ➤ *Asteatosis*—earliest manifestation
  - ➤ *Phrynoderma (Toad skin disease):* Brown to dark brown, dry, rough, hyperkeratotic follicular papules with central keratotic horny spines are usual presentation.
  - ➤ Distributed bilaterally and symmetrically on anterolateral aspects of thighs and posterolateral aspects of arm.
  - ➤ Recent studies show that phyrnoderma is probably not directly due to EFA deficiency.
- **Eye**
  - ➤ Most common cause of blindness in India in children.
  - ➤ Night blindness and xerophthalmia
- **Nose and mouth**
  - ➤ Squamous metaplasia of nasal mucosa
  - ➤ Impaired spermatogenesis
  - ➤ Miscarriages
  - ➤ Malformations of fetus

## Treatment

- 30,000 IU/day orally for neonates (1–2 wks)
- 50,000 IU/day orally for children and adults.

## MENKES' KINKY HAIR SYNDROME

- X-linked metabolic disturbance of copper metabolism caused by mutations in the copper-transporting ATP7A gene. Affected infants have hypocupremia (low copper levels) and low circulating ceruloplasmin.
- *Clinically characterized by*
  - ➤ Progressive cerebral degeneration (mental retardation)
  - ➤ Growth retardation
  - ➤ Sparse brittle hair
  - ➤ Arterial lesions
  - ➤ Scurvy-like bone changes
  - ➤ Anemia and neutropenia
  - ➤ Failure to thrive
  - ➤ Pilitorti, trichorrhexis and monilethrix may occur
  - ➤ Children with this disease often die within 5 years because of dissecting aneurysms or cardiac rupture.

## SCURVY

### Etiology

- Limited access to fruits and vegetables
- Food faddism, alcoholism, and ignorance
- Teenagers living on processed food
- Chronic gastrointestinal disturbances
- Undiagnosed psychiatric illness

### Clinical Features

- Follicular keratosis with coiled hairs on the upper arms, back, buttocks and lower extremities.
- Later, perifollicular hemorrhage with blood pigment discoloration especially on the legs, swollen bleeding gums, stomatitis and epistaxis occur.
- Large skin hemorrhages may be seen
- Anemia is usually present, and the patient appears resentful and mentally disturbed.

### Treatment

Oral vitamin C 100 mg three times daily.

## ARIBOFLAVINOSIS

- Due to vitamin $B_2$ deficiency.
- Ariboflavinosis may occur in alcoholic liver cirrhosis
- Clinically, there is photophobia due to conjunctivitis, sometimes with corneal vascularization, angular stomatitis (perlèche) and sore lips, tongue and mouth. The tongue is purplish red and smooth.
- A scaly seborrheic dermatitis-like eruption may be seen around the nose, eyes, ears and genital area (oro-oculogenital syndrome).

### Treatment

Treatment consists of 5–15 mg riboflavine two to three times daily for 2 weeks and correction of dietary errors.

## PRIMARY LOCALIZED CUTANEOUS AMYLOIDOSIS

There is deposition of amyloid in previously apparently normal skin, with no evidence of deposits occurring in internal organs.

### Types

- Papular or lichen amyloidosis
  - ➢ Macular amyloidosis
  - ➢ Maculopapular amyloidosis

- Nodular or tumefactive
- Familial (dyschromic)

## Clinical Features

- The papular form (lichen amyloidosis) presents as a pruritic eruption of multiple, discrete, hyperkeratotic papules, scaly and often hyperpigmented, distributed principally on the shins.
- The calves, ankles, dorsa of the feet and thighs, and the extensor aspects of the arm may be involved.
- Papules may coalesce to form thickened plaques, closely simulating hypertrophic lichen planus or lichen simplex chronicus.
- The predominant sign in macular amyloidosis is clusters of small, pigmented macules, about 2 or 3 mm in diameter, which may coalesce to produce macular hyperpigmented areas.
- A reticulate or 'rippled' pattern of pigmentation is a characteristic diagnostic feature in many cases.
- The nodular or tumefactive form manifests as single or more commonly multiple nodules or plaques seen on the face, trunk, limbs, genitalia or palate. They vary in size from a few millimeters to several centimeters. The overlying skin is often atrophic, and there may be petechial hemorrhages within the nodules.

## Pathology

- In papular and macular forms of PLCA, the amyloid deposits are confined to the papillary dermis, and do not involve blood vessels or adnexal structures. The overlying epidermis shows considerable irregular acanthosis and hyperkeratosis.
- By contrast, in the nodular or tumefactive forms of PLCA the dermis, subcutis and blood vessel walls are diffusely infiltrated with amyloid. There is usually a perivascular infiltrate of plasma cells.

## Treatment

Topical steroids, hydrocolloid dressings, topical dimethyl sulfoxide, dermabrasion and $CO_2$ and pulsed dye lasers. Recurrence is likely.

## QUESTIONS FROM PREVIOUS EXAMINATIONS

1. Pellagra
2. Acrodermatitis enteropathica
3. Cutaneous amyloidosis
4. Kwashiorkor
5. Marasmus

## MULTIPLE CHOICE QUESTIONS

1. **"Casal's paint necklace" is seen in:**                    *(Delhi 08)*
   - (a) Lichen planus
   - (b) Pellagra
   - (c) Pernicious anemia
   - (d) SLE

2. **Acrodermatitis enteropathica occurs due to deficiency of:**
                                                                *(Delhi 08)*
   - (a) Zn
   - (b) Se
   - (c) Cu
   - (d) Cr

3. **Flaky-paint appearance of skin is seen in:**              *(AI 05)*
   - (a) Dermatitis
   - (b) Pellagra
   - (c) Kwashiorkor
   - (d) Marasmus

4. **Phrynoderma is a cutaneous manifestation of severe deficiency of:**
                                                                *(Delhi 03)*
   - (a) Vitamin A
   - (b) Vitamin B
   - (c) Vitamin C
   - (d) Vitamin D

5. **About 'Menkes' kinky hair' syndrome, which of the following is not true?**
                                                                *(AP' 2011)*
   - (a) Congenital deficiency of copper binding ATPase
   - (b) Increased levels of circulating ceruloplasmin
   - (c) Mutations in the copper-transporting ATP7A gene
   - (d) Dissecting aneurysms or cardiac rupture can cause death

6. **A middle-aged chronic alcoholic man complains of burning sensation in the mouth. On examination, he has thickened, dry, smooth tongue with absence of the filliform papillae. MCV is 100. Which of the following should be first-line of approach in the management of this patient?** *(AI 2008)*
   - (a) Estimation of vitamin $B_{12}$ levels
   - (b) Brush biopsy
   - (c) Start antifungal therapy
   - (d) Send patient to surgeon for incisional biopsy

7. **The most common cause of leg ulcers:**                    *(AP 05)*
   - (a) Leprosy
   - (b) Diabetes
   - (c) Arterial disease
   - (d) Chronic venous insufficiency

8. **The most common site of decubitus ulcer is area over:** *(WB 2002)*
   - (a) Sacrum
   - (b) Ischial tuberosities
   - (c) Greater trochanter
   - (d) Heel

9. **Wrong match:**                                    *(AI 2000)*
   (a) Mees lines: Arsenic poisoning
   (b) Pterygium: Lichen planus
   (c) Onycholysis: Psoriasis
   (d) Koilonychia: Megaloblastic anemia

10. **Which of the following is incorrect match?**
    (a) Copper: Menkes' kinky hair syndrome
    (b) Zinc: Acrodermatitis enteropathica
    (c) Chromium: Keshan-Bach's disease
    (d) Manganese: Ataxia

11. **Which of the following is false about acrodermatitis entero-pathica?**                          *(AIIMS 08; 2011)*
    (a) Low serum zinc levels
    (b) Symptoms relieved after zinc supplementation
    (c) Autosomal recessive inheritance
    (d) Triad of diarrhea, dementia, and dermatitis

## Answers

1. **Ans. (b)** Pellagra *(Ref. IADVL, 2nd edn/ 981)*
2. **Ans. (a)** Zinc *(Ref. IADVL, 2nd edn/987–989)*
3. **Ans. (c)** Kwashiorkor *(Ref. IADVL, 2nd edn/994–995)*
4. **Ans. (a)** Vitamin A *(Ref. IADVL, 2nd edn/975)*
5. **Ans. (b)** Increased levels of circulating ceruloplasmin *(Ref. Harrison, 18th edn/Ch 74; OP Ghai Paediatrics, 6th edn/132)*
6. **Ans. (a)** Estimation of vitamin $B_{12}$ levels.
7. **Ans. (d)** Chronic venous insufficiency *(Ref. Rook's Dermatology, 7th edn/11.12)*
8. **Ans. (b)** Ischial tuberosities > **(a)** Sacrum *(Ref. Bailey and Love, 25th edn/29; Rook's Dermatology, 7th edn/11.14)*
9. **Ans. (d)** Koilonychia: Megaloblastic anemia *(Ref, Roxburgh, 17th edn/41, 129)*
10. **Ans. (c)** Chromium: Keshan-Bach's disease.
11. **Ans. (d)** Triad of diarrhea, dementia, and dermatitis *(Ref. Harrison, 17th edn/pg. 449; 2061).*

# 5 Eczematous Disorders of Skin

## ECZEMA

- **Definition:** It is reaction pattern of inflammatory response of skin characterized clinically in acute stage by erythema, vesiculation, oozing and crusting and in chronic stages—scaling and lichenification.
- **Classification**

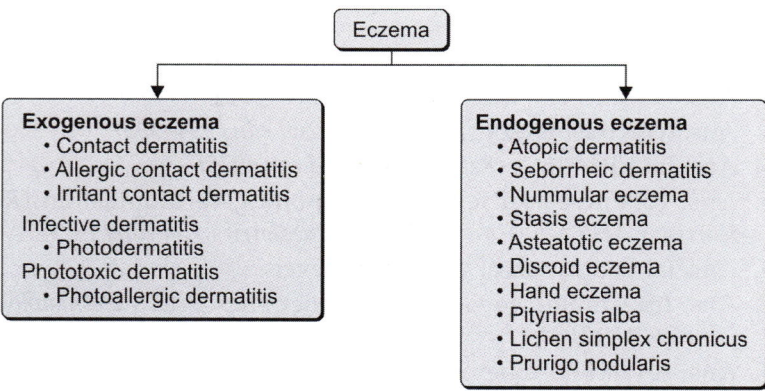

```
                          ┌──────────┐
                          │  Eczema  │
                          └──────────┘
```

**Exogenous eczema**
- Contact dermatitis
- Allergic contact dermatitis
- Irritant contact dermatitis

Infective dermatitis
- Photodermatitis

Phototoxic dermatitis
- Photoallergic dermatitis

**Endogenous eczema**
- Atopic dermatitis
- Seborrheic dermatitis
- Nummular eczema
- Stasis eczema
- Asteatotic eczema
- Discoid eczema
- Hand eczema
- Pityriasis alba
- Lichen simplex chronicus
- Prurigo nodularis

- **Histopathological features of eczema**
  - ➤ **Epidermis**

| | |
|---|---|
| 1. Acute eczema | In the epidermis, it is characterized by spongiosis, i.e. intercellular edema. Intraepidermal vesicles form by the disruption of intercellular attachments. |
| 2. Subacute phase | Parakeratotic stratum corneum forms and acanthotic process starts. The rete ridges broaden and get elongated. |
| 3. Chronic phase | Rete ridges broaden and elongate further. Hyperkeratosis replaces parakeratosis. |

> **Dermis:** Vasodilatation in the papillary dermis and accompanied by lymphohistiocytic infiltrate. Polymorphs and eosinophils are seen in acute eczema and in chronic stage infiltration is dense and mixed.

## Pityriasis Alba

- **Definition:** This is a pattern of dermatitis in which hypopigmentation is the most conspicuous feature. Some erythema and scaling usually precede the development of hypopigmentation but these are often relatively mild.

  **Aetiology:** Pityriasis alba is sometimes a manifestation of atopic dermatitis but it is certainly not confined to atopic individuals.

- **Pathology**
  > The histological changes are unimpressive acanthosis and mild spongiosis, with moderate hyperkeratosis and patchy parakeratosis. There may be follicular plugging, spongiosis and sebaceous gland atrophy.
  > On electron microscopy there are reduced numbers of active melanocytes and a decrease in number and size of melanosomes in affected skin.

- **Clinical features**
  > Pityriasis alba occurs predominantly in children between the ages of 3 and 16 years.
  > Sexes are equally susceptible.
  > The individual lesion is a rounded, oval or irregular plaque, which is red, pink or skin-colored and has fine lamellar or branny scaling.
  > Initially, the erythema may be conspicuous and there may even be minimal serous crusting. Later, the erythema subsides completely, and at the stage at which the lesions are commonly seen by a physician they show only persistent fine scaling and hypopigmentation.
  > There are usually several patches ranging from 0.5 to 2 cm in diameter, but they may be larger, especially on the trunk.
  > In children, the lesions are often confined to the face, and are most common around the mouth, chin and cheeks.
  > The course is extremely variable. Most cases persist for some months, and some may still show hypopigmentation for a year or more after all scaling subsides. Recurrent crops of new lesions may develop at intervals.

- **Differential diagnosis of pityriasis alba (P. alba)**
  - Vitiligo
  - Pityriasis versicolor
  - Leprosy
- **Treatment**
  - Mild topical corticosteroids are helpful if inflammation persists.
  - Topical tacrolimus and pimecrolimus are effective and well tolerated.

## Atopic Dermatitis

- **Definition:** It is an eczema characterized by intense itching and relapsing course in infants and children with a personal or family history of atopic disorders.
  - Coexists with asthma or rhinitis in 80% cases.
  - 70% of patients have family history of atopy.
- **Etiopathogenesis**
  - Genetically transmitted
  - Immunological dysfunction
  - 80% have raised total IgE.
- **Clinical features**
  - Itching is the basic symptom.

| | |
|---|---|
| 1. *Infantile phase* | – Up to 2 yrs.<br>– Appears usually at or after 3 months of age. Initial lesions are ill-defined erythematous patches on the cheeks.<br>– Later spread to scalp, upper trunk and extensor aspect of lower limbs. |
| 2. *Childhood phase* | – Flexural involvement is characteristic (antecubital and popliteal fossa)<br>– Presence of extensor involvement denotes poor prognosis. |
| 3. *Adolescent phase* | – Lichenification is main feature: Involvement of face, neck, flexures and upper trunk is characteristic.<br>– Excoriation due to scratching is important manifestation. |

- **Associated features**
  - Xerosis
  - Ichthyosis

➢ P. alba
➢ Dennie-Morgan fold
  – **Dennie-Morgan fold** is a single or double fold in the lower eyelid, due to eyelid edema.
  – Seen as associated feature in atopic dermatitis.
  – Infraorbicular folds are common in black children regardless of the atopic dermatitis.
➢ Periorbital darkening
➢ Cataract
➢ Keratoconus
➢ Lip lick cheilitis
➢ Hand and foot eczema
➢ Dirty neck sign refers to reticulate pigmentation of the neck seen in patients with chronic atopic dermatitis.

**Perioral pallor, pallor at nose and ears (head light sign) and dermographism** are characteristic of **atopic dermatitis**.

- **Investigations**
  ➢ The diagnosis of AD is essentially clinical.
  ➢ A biopsy is rarely necessary to diagnose eczema.
  ➢ Total serum IgE levels, RAST and prick tests do not establish anything besides as atopic diathesis.
- **Differential diagnosis**
  ➢ Seborrheic dermatitis
  ➢ Eczematized scabies
  ➢ Infective dermatitis
  ➢ Psoriatic lesions
  ➢ Wiskott-Aldrich syndrome
  ➢ Hartnup's disease
  ➢ Leiner's disease
- **Management**

1. First-line therapy
   – Emollients: Topical steroids
   – Topical anti-infectives
   – Antihistaminics
2. Second-line therapy
   – Systemic steroids
   – Immunomodulators (azathioprine, cyclosporine, interferons, tacrolimus)
   – Phototherapy

- **Diagnostic criteria for AD proposed by UK group**
  - ➤ **Major criteria:** Must have an itchy skin condition.
  - ➤ **Minor criteria**
    - History of flexural dermatitis or dermatitis of cheeks in children <10 yrs age.
    - Personal history of asthma or hay fever or atopy in a first degree relative, in children <4 yrs of age.
    - History of generalized dryness in last yr
    - Onset in the first 2 yrs of life if the child is older than 4 yrs
    - Visible flexural eczema or eczema of cheeks/forehead and outer limbs in children younger than 4 yrs.
  - ➤ Patients must have major criteria + 3 or more of minor criteria for diagnosis of AD.
- **Kaposi's variceliform eruption**
  - ➤ Eczema herpeticum
  - ➤ Generalized HSV eruptions
  - ➤ Seen mainly in infants of atopic dermatitis
  - ➤ Seen as vesiculopustular eruptions in which lesions show umbilication and often becomes hemorrhagic
  - ➤ The patient is toxic
  - ➤ There may be peripheral or central nervous system involvement.
  - ➤ It is also found in:
    - Burns, seborrheic dermatitis
    - Pemphigus, neurodermatitis
    - Ichthyosis vulgaris
    - Mycosis fungoides
    - Keratosis folicularis (Darrier's diasese)
    - Sézary syndrome.

## Treatment of Atopic Dermatitis

- Immunomodulators (calcineurin inhibitors) > 2-year-old
  - ➤ Pimecrolimus (Elidel®)
  - ➤ Tacrolimus (protopic)
- Antihistamines
  - ➤ Hydroxyzine (atarax)
  - ➤ Desloratadine (clarinex) one study 6–24 months
  - ➤ Cetinzine (zyrtec) approved > 6 months
  - ➤ Singulair 10 mg qhs (not FDA approved)
- Topical steroids—limit potency
- Control environment

## Seborrheic Dermatitis

- **Definition:** This is a chronic dermatitis that is difficult to define exactly, but it has a distinctive morphology (red, sharply marginated lesions covered with greasy-looking scales) and a distinctive distribution in areas with a rich supply of sebaceous glands, namely the scalp, face and upper trunk. In some cases the flexures are also involved, but this is not an essential diagnostic criterion.
  - ➤ It has bimodal occurrence—infancy and adolescence
  - ➤ In infants, it manifests as scaly plaque with dirty greasy scales over the vertex known as **cradle cap**.
  - ➤ In adults, lesions commonly originate in hairy skin, and involve the scalp, face, presternal and interscapular regions, and the flexures. The lesions tend to be dull or yellowish red in color and covered with greasy scales.
  - ➤ On the trunk, several forms of seborrheic dermatitis occur. Most common is the petaloid form.
- **Treatment**
  - ➤ Acute forms of seborrheic dermatitis on the face and trunk respond to mild steroid ointments.
  - ➤ Topical metronidazole, ciclopiroxolamine and tacalcitol have also been reported to be helpful.
  - ➤ For unresponsive cases, a course of UV B therapy may be helpful, or even a short-course of oral ketoconazole (200 mg/day for 14 days).
  - ➤ Oral itraconazole (100 mg/day for up to 21 days) is also effective, as is oral terbinafine.
  - ➤ Other topical preparations that have been shown to be effective include benzoyl peroxide and 5% lithium succinate ointment.
  - ➤ Generalized seborrheic dermatitis usually responds to the medications listed above, but in recalcitrant cases systemic steroids may be required. Prednisolone 30 mg/day usually produces a rapid response. Isotretinoin may also be helpful.

## Nummular Eczema

- Nummular eczematous is characterized by rounded coin-shaped eczematous lesions, papulovesicular and oozing or scaly erythematous, usually affecting extensors of the limbs.
- More common in adults >50 yrs of age.
- Mild to moderate itching
- Symmetrically distributed on dorsal aspects of the hands and feet, extensors of the arms and legs and occasionally on thighs and trunk.

- **Treatment**
  - Mid-potency topical steroid in a cream or lotion form.
  - Antihistaminics

## Asteatotic Eczema (Winter Eczema/Eczema Craquelé)

- Eczema developing in the very dry skin, usually elderly
- **Etiology:** Naturally 'dry' skin and a lifelong tendency to chapping; a further reduction in lipid with age, illness, malnutrition or hormonal decline; increased transpiration relative to the environmental water content; loss of integrity of the water reservoir of the horny layer; chapping and degreasing by industrial or domestic cleansers or solvents; low environmental humidity and dry, cold winds increasing convection loss; and repeated minor trauma, diuretics and myxedema can also cause.
- **Clinical features**
  - The condition occurs particularly on the legs, arms and hands. It tends to be more marked in the winter and in elderly people.
  - The asteatotic skin is dry and slightly scaly.
  - The surface of the backs of the hands is marked in a criss-cross fashion, as though the continuity and flexibility of the keratin had been disturbed.
  - The finger pulps are dry and cracked, producing distorted prints and retaining a prolonged depression after pressure ('parchment pulps').
  - On the legs, the pattern of superficial markings is more marked and deeper ('crazy-paving' pattern or eczema craquelé).
- **Treatment**
  - Emollient creams such as those based on lanolin or paraffins are generally helpful.
  - Weak topical corticosteroids are often prescribed.

## Pompholyx

- A form of eczema of the palms and soles, in which edema fluid accumulates to form visible vesicles or bullae.
- Because of the thick epidermis in these sites, the blisters tend to become larger than in other body areas before they burst.
- When pompholyx occurs on the palms, it may be called cheiropompholyx, and when on the soles, podopompholyx.
- **Clinical features**
  - An attack of pompholyx is characterized by the sudden onset of crops of clear vesicles, which appear deeply seated and 'sago-like'. Itching may be severe, preceding the eruption of vesicles (Fig. 5.1).

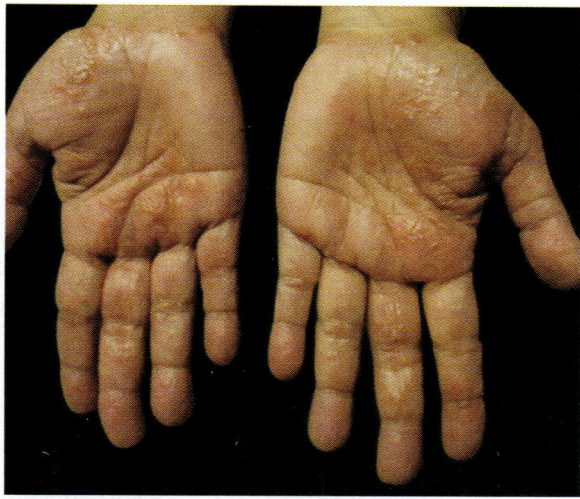

**Fig. 5.1:** Deep seated vesicles over palms giving "Sago grain appearance"

➤ The attack subsides spontaneously, and resolution with desquamation occurs in 2–3 weeks in most cases recurrence is common.

➤ In mild cases, only the sides of the fingers may be affected, but in a typical case the vesicles develop symmetrically on the palms and/or soles.

• **Treatment**

➤ In the acute phase, rest and bland applications are indicated.

➤ The hands or feet should be soaked three or four times a day in either Burow's solution (aluminum acetate 1%) or potassium permanganate solution (diluted 1 : 8000).

➤ Systemic antibiotics will be required if secondary bacterial infection develops. This is most likely to be staphylococcal, and flucloxacillin is usually effective.

➤ As the eruption subsides the soaks should be discontinued, and zinc cream or oily calamine lotion can be substituted.

➤ Topical steroids are useful in the subacute and chronic phases.

➤ In a few severe cases, a course of oral steroids may be justified.

## Stasis Dermatitis (Venous Eczema/Gravitational Eczema/ Varicose Eczema)

Eczema secondary to venous hypertension.

- **Clinical features**
  - ➤ Venous eczema is an erythematous, scaly and often exudative eruption usually seen around the ankle and lower leg (Figs 5.2 and 5.3).
  - ➤ It often occurs as a late result of deep vein thrombosis.
  - ➤ The eczema may develop suddenly or insidiously.
  - ➤ The patients are usually middle-aged or elderly and most often female.
  - ➤ The eczema is often accompanied by other manifestations of venous hypertension, including dilatation or varicosity of the

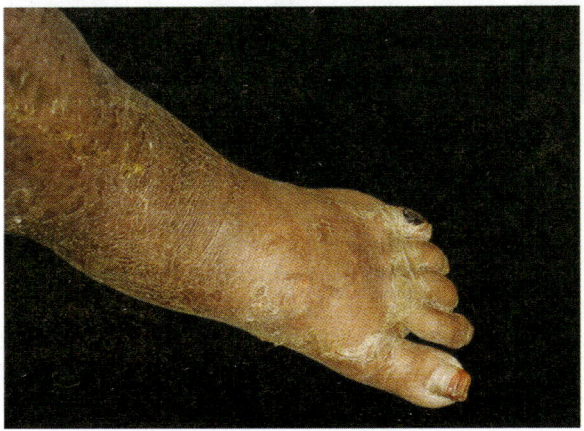

**Fig. 5.2:** Erythema and scaling over foot

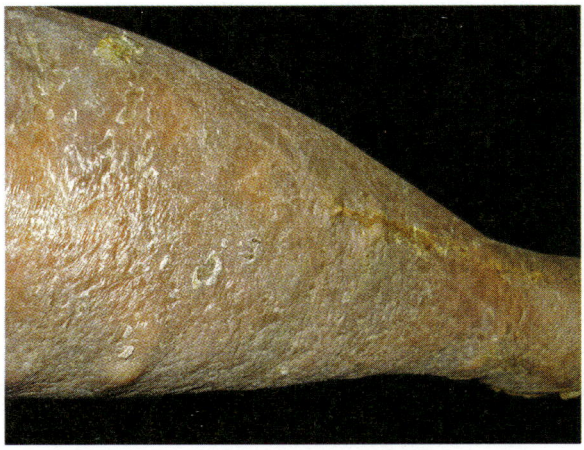

**Fig. 5.3:** Erythema, scaling and oozing over anterior aspect to leg

superficial veins, edema, purpura, hemosiderosis, ulceration, or small patches of white, atrophic, telangiectatic scarring ('atrophie blanche').

➢ Leashes of dilated venules around the dorsum of the foot or the ankle are particularly common.

➢ There may be a subepidermal vascular proliferation producing purple papules around the ankle, which may resemble Kaposi's sarcoma.

- **Treatment**
  ➢ The underlying venous hypertension should be controlled.
  ➢ Obese patients should be urged to lose weight.
  ➢ Well-fitted support stockings or firm bandages can be helpful if worn regularly.
  ➢ The legs should be elevated as effectively as possible.
  ➢ Mild topical steroids may be used to relieve irritation, but the use of potent steroids should be limited to short periods of a few days as they may cause cutaneous atrophy and increase the risk of ulceration.
  ➢ Topical tacrolimus has been reported to be effective.

## Lichen Simplex Chronicus

- Lichen simplex is an eczematous dermatosis characterized by a small number of heavily lichenified plaques or, very often, a single lesion.
- **Clinical features**
  ➢ Itching is predominant symptom
  ➢ 30–50 yrs of age
  ➢ Common in females
  ➢ Almost any area may be affected, but the commonest sites are those that are conveniently reached.
  ➢ The usual sites are the nape of the neck, the lower legs and ankles, the sides of the neck, the scalp, the upper thighs, the vulva, pubis or scrotum, and the extensor forearms.
- **Treatment**
  ➢ Break the itch-scratch cycle
  ➢ Sedative antihistaminics
  ➢ Potent topical steroids
  ➢ 5% doxepin cream
  ➢ Topical antibiotics if secondary infection.

## Prurigo Nodularis

- Characterized clinically by chronic, intensely itchy nodules and histologically by marked hyperkeratosis and acanthosis, with downward projections of the epidermis.
- **Etiology**
  - ➤ Emotional stress
  - ➤ Atopy
  - ➤ Insect bite (20%)
- **Clinical features**
  - ➤ Intense pruritus
  - ➤ 20–60 yrs of age
  - ➤ Both sexes equally affected
  - ➤ The individual lesions range from small papules to hard globular nodules, 1–3 cm in diameter, with a raised, warty surface.
  - ➤ Pigmentary changes are common
  - ➤ Lesions are common on extensor surfaces of distal parts of limbs.
- **Treatment**
  - ➤ Sedative antihistaminics
  - ➤ Topical and intralesional steroids
  - ➤ Topical capsaicin
  - ➤ Cryotherapy
  - ➤ Thalidomide, cyclosporine and azathioprine
  - ➤ PUVA and UV B

## Contact Dermatitis

- Contact dermatitis is an inflammatory process in skin caused by an exogenous agent or agents that directly or indirectly injure the skin.
- Injury by a direct toxic action on the skin—irritant contact dermatitis (ICD). An example of ICD would be dermatitis induced by a concentrated acid or base.
- Agents that cause allergic contact dermatitis (ACD) induce an antigen-specific immune response—a **T cell-mediated (type IV) hypersensitivity**.
- The clinical lesions of contact dermatitis may be acute (wet and edematous) or chronic (dry, thickened, and scaly), depending on the persistence of the insult (Table 5.1).

The most common presentation of contact dermatitis is hand eczema, and it is frequently related to occupational exposures.

**Table. 5.1:** Erythroderma (primary cutaneous disorders)

| | Initial lesions | Location of initial lesions | Other findings | Diagnostic aids | Treatment |
|---|---|---|---|---|---|
| **Psoriasis** | Pink-red, silvery scale, and sharply demarcated | Elbows, knees, scalp, and presacral area | Nail dystrophy, arthritis, and pustules | Skin biopsy | Topical glucocorticoids, vitamin D; UV B (narrowband); oral retinoid and/or PUVA; MTX, cyclosporine, anti-TNF agents |
| **Atopic dermatitis** | Acute: Erythema, fine scale, crust, indistinct borders Chronic: Lichenification (increased skin markings) | Antecubital and popliteal fossae, neck, and hands | Pruritus family history of atopy, including asthma, allergic rhinitis or conjunctivitis, and atopic dermatitis. Exclude secondary infection with *S. aureus*. Exclude superimposed irritant or allergic contact dermatitis | Skin biopsy | |
| **Contact dermatitis** | Local: Erythema, crusting, vesicles, and bullae | Depends on offending agent | Irritant—onset often within hours allergic—delayed-type hypersensitivity; lag time of 48 hrs. | Patch testing | |
| | Systemic: Erythema, fine scale, and crust | Generalized | Patient has history of allergic contact dermatitis to topical agent and then receives systemic medication that is structurally related, e.g. ethylenediamine (topical), aminophylline | Same as local | |

*Contd.*

**Table. 5.1:** Erythroderma (primary cutaneous disorders) *Contd.*

| | Initial lesions | Location of initial lesions | Other findings | Diagnostic aids | Treatment |
|---|---|---|---|---|---|
| **Seborrheic dermatitis** | Pink-red greasy scale | Scalp, nasolabial folds, eyebrows, and intertriginous zones | Flares with stress, HIV infection associated with Parkinson's disease | Skin biopsy | Topical glucocorticoids and imidazoles |
| **Stasis eczema (with autosensitization)** | Erythema, crusting, and excoriations | Lower extremities | Pruritus, lower extremity, edema, history of venous ulcers, thrombophlebitis, and/or cellulitis exclude superimposed contact dermatitis, e.g. topical neomycin | Skin biopsy | Topical glucocorticoids; open wet dressings; leg elevation; and pressure stockings |
| **Pityriasis rubra** | Orange-red and perifollicular | Generalized, but characteristic "skip" areas of normal skin | Wax-like keratoderma excludes cutaneous T cell lymphoma | Skin biopsy | Isotretinoin or acitretin and methotrexate |

- ICD is generally strictly demarcated and often localized to areas of thin skin (eyelids, intertriginous areas) or to areas where the irritant was occluded. Lesions may range from minimal skin erythema to areas of marked edema, vesicles, and ulcers.
- Chronic low-grade irritant dermatitis is the most common type of ICD, and the most common area of involvement is the hands.
- The most common irritants encountered are chronic wet work, soaps, and detergents.
- Ear lobe sign is observed in patients who develop contact dermatitis to a substance applied with the hand to the face and neck.
- Treatment should be directed to avoidance of irritants and use of protective gloves or clothing.
- ACD is a manifestation of delayed-type hypersensitivity mediated by memory T-lymphocytes in the skin. ACD  may be caused by a variety of allergens present in plants, cosmetics, shampoos, hair dyes, medicaments, shoes, soaps, detergents, etc.
- **Treatment**
  - ➤ If ACD is suspected and an offending agent is identified and removed, the eruption will resolve. Usually, treatment with high-potency fluorinated topical glucocorticoids is enough to relieve symptoms while the ACD runs its course. For those patients who require systemic therapy, daily oral prednisone beginning at 1 mg/kg, but usually not exceeding 60 mg/day, is sufficient. It should be tapered over 2 to 3 weeks, and each daily dose given in the morning with food.
  - ➤ Identification of a contact allergen can be a difficult and time-consuming task. Patients with dermatitis unresponsive to conventional therapy or with an unusual and patterned distribution should be suspected of having ACD. They should be questioned carefully regarding occupational exposures, topical medicaments, and oral medications. Common sensitizers include preservatives in topical preparations, nickel sulfate, potassium dichromate, thimerosal, neomycin sulfate, fragrances, formaldehyde, and rubber-curing agents.
  - ➤ **Patch testing** is helpful in identifying these agents, but should not be attempted on patients with widespread active dermatitis or on those taking systemic glucocorticoids.

## Photodermatitis

- **Phototoxic dermatitis:** Resembles an exaggerated sunburn reaction commonly due to phototoxic drugs like psoralens.
- **Photoallergic dermatitis:** Resembles allergic contact dermatitis but it occurs in photoexposed areas only.

## Parthenium Dermatitis

- In India, parthenium hysterophorus is the most notorious compositae weed known to produce contact hypersensitivity.
- The weed grows widely on waste lands, along canals, railway tracks and roads.
- Grows more profusely during the rainy season but the growth is almost perennial.
- The various dermatitis patterns described are:
  - Airborne contact dermatitis
  - Atopic dermatitis
  - Photodermatitis
  - Seborrheic dermatitis
  - Exfoliative dermatitis
- Eyelid involvement is common
- **Clinical features**
  - Lichenified lesions affecting the face, neck, upper trunk, and flexural aspects of the limbs.
  - Parthenium hysterophorus has been found to contain parthenin as well as hymenin, ambrosin, and coronopilin.

## QUESTIONS FROM PREVIOUS EXAMINATIONS

1. Patch test
2. Dermatopathic lymphadenitis
3. Nickel-induced eczema
4. Dermatosis cenicienta
5. Erythroderma
6. Seborrheic diasthesis
7. HPE of eczema
8. Pityrosporum ovale
9. Pompholyx
10. Dermatopathic lymphadenopathy
11. White dermographism
12. Acid immunology
13. Hardening
14. Atopic dermatitis
15. Non-eczematous industrial dermatosis
16. Chromium

17. Occupational dermatosis
18. Venous eczema
19. Asteatotic eczema
20. Eczemas in children (classification and management).

## MULTIPLE CHOICE QUESTIONS

1. **Spongiosis is seen in:**                              *(Delhi 07)*
   (a) Acute eczema            (b) Lichen planus
   (c) Psoriasis               (d) Pemphigus
2. **Babloo, a 5-year-old boy presents with small hypopigmented scaly macule on cheek. Some of his classmates also have similar lesions. Most probable diagnosis is:**    *(AIIMS 2000)*
   (a) Pityriasis rosea        (b) Pityriasis versicolor
   (c) Indeterminate leprosy   (d) Pityriasis alba
3. **A 5-year-old boy presents with multiple asymptomatic oval and circular hypopigmented macules with fine scaling on his face. What is the diagnosis?**
   (a) Pityriasis versicolor   (b) Indeterminate leprosy
   (c) Pityriasis alba         (d) Acrofacial RT
4. **True about pityriasis alba:**                          *(PGI 2001)*
   (a) No active Rx needed
   (b) Common in elderly
   (c) Variant of vitiligo
   (d) Common over face
   (e) Presents as scaly hypopigmented macules
5. **A 3-year-old child has eczematous dermatitis on extensor surfaces. His mother has history of bronchial asthma:**    *(AIIMS Nov 06)*
   (a) Atopic dermatitis
   (b) Contact dermatitis
   (c) Seborrheic dermatitis
   (d) Infantile eczematous dermatitis
6. **Characteristic feature of atopic dermatitis:**        *(MP 05)*
   (a) Pruritus                (b) Dennie's lines
   (c) Lichenification         (d) Rash
7. **Minor clinical feature in the diagnosis of atopic dermatitis:**
                                                            *(PGI 04)*
   (a) Dry skin                (b) Pruritus
   (c) Dennie-Morgan folds     (d) P. alba
   (e) White dermographism

8. **Kaposi varicelliform lesion is seen in:** *(PGI 05)*
   - (a) Atopic dermatitis
   - (b) Darrier's disease
   - (c) Lichen planus
   - (d) Varicella zoster

9. **An infant presented with erythematous lesions on cheek, and extensor aspect of limbs. Mother has history of asthma. Likely diagnosis:** *(AI 2007)*
   - (a) Airborne contact dermatitis
   - (b) Atopic dermatitis
   - (c) Seborrheic dermatitis
   - (d) Infectious eczematoid dermatitis

10. **Atopic dermatitis is diagnosed by:** *(AIIMS May 06)*
    - (a) Patch test
    - (b) Wood lamp examination
    - (c) Clinical examination
    - (d) Serum IgE levels

11. **Commonest cause of airborne contact dermatitis in India:** *(AI 99)*
    - (a) Parthenium
    - (b) Garden grass
    - (c) Oleander
    - (d) Yellow oleanders

12. **Diagnostic method of choice for contact dermatitis:** *(AI 92)*
    - (a) Clinical examination
    - (b) Skin biopsy
    - (c) Tzank smear
    - (d) Patch test

13. **Patch test is read after:** *(AI 99)*
    - (a) 2 hrs
    - (b) 2 days
    - (c) 2 wks
    - (d) 2 months

14. **A 10-year-old child has hypopigmented multiple scaly patches over face. The most possible diagnosis is:** *(AIIMS 2001)*
    - (a) *Tinea versicolor*
    - (b) Pityriasis alba
    - (c) Indeterminate leprosy
    - (d) Lupus vulgaris

15. **"Coin-shaped" eczema is:** *(Jharkhand 05)*
    - (a) Nummular eczema
    - (b) Atopic eczema
    - (c) Infantile eczema
    - (d) Endogenous eczema

16. **Dennie-Morgan fold is seen in:** *(Bihar 06)*
    - (a) Mastocytosis
    - (b) Seborrheic dermatitis
    - (c) Sarcoidosis
    - (d) Atopic dermatitis

17. **Berloque dermatitis occurs due to contact with:** *(AMU 07)*
    - (a) Metals
    - (b) Cosmetics
    - (c) Food
    - (d) Plants

18. **Commonest metal causing skin hypersensitivity:** *(AI 93)*
    - (a) Nickel
    - (b) Copper
    - (c) Iron
    - (d) Brass

19. Patch test is done to document:    *(AIIMS May 09)*
    (a) Type 1 hypersensitivity
    (b) Delayed type hypersensitivity
    (c) Autoimmune disease
    (d) Immunocomplex deposition

20. Plant-induced contact dermatitis occurs most commonly due to exposure to:    *(AIIMS May 08)*
    (a) Cotton fibers       (b) Parthenium
    (c) Poison ivy          (d) Ragweed

21. A 16-year-old boy presented with asymptomatic, multiple, erythematous, annular lesions with a collarette of scales at the periphery of the lesions which are present on trunk. Most probable diagnosis is:    *(AI 2005)*
    (a) Pityriasis rosea         (b) Pityriasis versicolor
    (c) Pityriasis rubra pilaris (d) Pityriasis alba

22. Regarding pityriasis rosea true is:    *(AI 07)*
    (a) Self-limiting condition   (b) Chronic relapsing condition
    (c) Dermatophytic infection   (d) Common in neonates

23. An 8-year-old boy from Bihar presents with a six months history of an ill-defined, oval hypopigmented slightly atrophic macule on his face. What is the most likely diagnosis:    *(AI 07)*
    (a) Pityriasis alba      (b) Indeterminate leprosy
    (c) Morphea             (d) Ca$^{++}$ deficiency

24. "White dermographism" is seen in:    *(JIPMER 07)*
    (a) Atopic dermatitis       (b) Airborne contact dermatitis
    (c) Chemical dermatitis     (d) Seborrheic dermatitis

25. Most common form of seborrheic dermatitis affecting trunk:
    *(Kerala 06)*
    (a) Petaloid            (b) Pityriasiform
    (c) Flexural           (d) Eczematous plaques
    (e) Follicular

26. A 5-year-old boy has multiple asymptomatic oval and circular faintly hypopigmented macules with fine scaling on his face. The most probable clinical diagnosis is:    *(AI 03)*
    (a) Pityriasis versicolor   (b) Indeterminate leprosy
    (c) Pityriasis alba        (d) Acrofacial vitiligo

27. The test likely to help in diagnosis of a patient who presents with an itchy annular plaque on the face is:    *(AI 03)*
    (a) Gram stain          (b) KOH mount
    (c) Tissue smear        (d) Wood's lamp examination

28. Multiple round to oval erythematous patches with fine central scale distributed along the skin tension lines on the trunk is highly suggestive of:                                   *(Orissa 2009)*
    (a) *Tinea versicolor*              (b) Pityriasis rosea
    (c) Lichen planus                  (d) Seborrheic dermatitis

29. A 55-year-old male with uncontrolled diabetes mellitus and hypertension and developed severe airborne contact dermatitis. The most appropriate drug for his treatment would be:
                                                    *(AIIM 2004)*
    (a) Systematic corticosteroids  (b) Thalidomide
    (c) Azathioprine               (d) Cyclosporine

30. Airborne contact dermatitis can be diagnosed by:
                                              *(AIIMS May 06)*
    (a) Skin biopsy                (b) Patch test
    (c) Prick test                 (d) Estimation of serum IgE levels

## Answers

1. **Ans. (a)** Acute eczema *(Ref. IADVL, 2nd edn/412)*
2. **Ans. (d)** Pityriasis alba *(Ref. IADVL, 2nd edn/428; Rook, 7th edn/39.58–39.59)*
3. **(c)** P. alba *(Ref. IADVL, 2nd edn/428; Rook, 7th edn/39.58–39.59)*
4. **Ans. (a, d, e)** *(Ref. Rook, 7th edn/17.37)*
5. **Ans. (a)** Atopic dermatitis *(Ref. IADVL, 2nd edn/416–427; Rook, 7th edn/18.1–18.30)*
6. **Ans. (a)** Pruritus *(Ref. IADVL, 2nd edn/ 416–427; Rook, 7th edn/18.1–18.30)*
7. **Ans. (a)** Dry skin *(Ref. IADVL, 2nd edn/423)*
8. **Ans. (a)** Atopic dermatitis *(Ref. IADVL, 2nd edn/423; Dermatology by Jean and Hoseph, 1st edn, 1237)*
9. **Ans. (b)** Atopic dermatitis *(Ref. Rook Dermatology, 7th edn/18.2; Table 18.1)*
10. **Ans. (c)** Clinical examination *(Ref. IADVL, 2nd edn/421)*
11. **Ans. (a)** Parthenium *(Ref. IADVL, 2nd edn/470)*
12. **Ans. (d)** Patch test *(Ref. IADVL, 2nd edn/485; Rook, 7th edn/Table 20.11)*
13. **Ans. (b)** 2 days *(Ref. IADVL, 2nd edn/485)*
14. **Ans. (b)** Pityriasis alba *(Ref. IADVL, 2nd edn/428; Rook, 7th edn/39.58 – 39.59)*
15. **Ans. (a)** Nummular eczema *(Ref. IADVL, 2nd edn/433)*
16. **Ans. (d)** Atopic dermatitis *(Ref. IADVL, 2nd edn/433)*

17. **Ans. (b)** Cosmetics *(Ref. IADVL, 2nd edn/640)*
18. **Ans. (a)** Nickel *(Ref. IADVL, 2nd edn/464)*
19. **Ans. (b)** Delayed type hypersensitivity
20. **Ans. (b)** Parthenium and **(c)** Poison ivy
21. **Ans. (a)** Pityriasis rosea *(Ref. Roxburgh's Dermatology, 17th edn/37; Behl, 8th edn/171: Pasricha, 4th edn/123–124, 189)*
22. **Ans. (a)** Self-limiting condition *(Ref. Behl, 8th/171: Pasricha, 4th edn/123–124, 189; Roxburgh, 17th/17, 37–39, 149)*
23. **Ans. (b)** Indeterminate leprosy *(Ref. Roxburgh's Common Skin Disease, 17th edn/37–38)*
24. **Ans. (a)** Atopic dermatitis *(Ref. Rook's Dermatology, 7th edn/18.12)*
25. **Ans. (a)** Petaloid *(Ref. Rook's Dermatology, 7th edn/17.12)*
26. **Ans. (c)** Pityriasis alba *(Ref. Behl, 7th edn/Pg–154)*
27. **Ans. (c)** KOH mount
28. **Ans. (b)** Pityriasis rosea *(Ref. Harrison's Medicine, 17th edn/ Table 53–5)*
29. **Ans. (c)** Azathioprine *(Ref. Harrison's Internal Medicine, Chapter 53)*
30. **Ans. (b)** Patch test.

# 6 Cutaneous Drug Eruptions, Urticaria and Angioedema

- An adverse drug reaction (ADR) may be defined as an undesirable clinical manifestation resulting from administration of a particular drug; this includes reactions due to overdose, predictable side effects and unanticipated adverse manifestations.
- Common in women than men
- Common in elderly age group and immunosuppressed.
- *Characteristics of drug eruptions*
  1. H/o drug intake prior to eruption
  2. Sudden in onset
  3. Often pruritic
  4. Usually bilaterally symmetrical (except FDE)
  5. Regression of eruption on withdrawal of drug
  6. Similar type of rash recurs on re-exposure to the same or drug from the class.

## CLASSIFICATION OF ADVERSE DRUG REACTIONS

### Nonimmunological

### *Predictable*

- Overdosage
- Side effects
- Cumulation
- Delayed toxicity
- Facultative effects
- Drug interactions
- Metabolic alterations
- Teratogenicity

- Nonimmunological activation of effector pathways
- Exacerbation of disease
- Drug-induced chromosomal damage

## *Unpredictable*
- Intolerance
- Idiosyncrasy

## Immunological (Unpredictable)
- IgE-dependent drug reactions (type I)
- Cytotoxic drug-induced reactions (type II)
- Immune complex-dependent drug reactions (type III)
- Cell-mediated reactions (type IV)

## Miscellaneous
- Jarisch-Herxheimer reactions
- Infectious mononucleosis–ampicillin reaction

## Types of Drug Eruptions (Table 6.1)
- Exanthematous (erythematous) reactions, or morbilliform (resembling measles) or maculopapular rash
- Erythroderma and exfoliative dermatitis
- Fixed drug eruption
- Urticaria and angioedema
- Serum sickness
- Pustular eruptions
- Acneiform
- Psoriasis and psoriasiform eruptions
- Purpura
- Erythema multiforme
- Stevens-Johnson syndrome
- Toxic epidermal necrolysis
- Pemphigus-like eruptions
- Phototoxic and photoallergic eruptions
- Pityriasis rosea-like eruptions
- Lichenoid drug eruptions

**Table 6.1:** Clinical features of selected severe cutaneous reactions often induced by drugs

| Diagnosis | Typical skin lesions | Mucosal lesions | Frequent signs and symptoms | Alternative causes not related to drugs |
|---|---|---|---|---|
| Stevens-Johnson syndrome | Small blisters on dusky purpuric macules or atypical targets; are areas of confluence; detachment 10% of body surface area | Erosions usually at two sites | Most cases involve fever | 10–20% cause not determined |
| Toxic epidermal necrolysis | individual lesions like those seen in Stevens-Johnson syndrome; confluent erythema; outer layer of epidermis separates readily from basal layer with lateral pressure; large sheet of necrotic epidermis; total detachment of >30% of body surface area | Erosions usually at two sites | Nearly all cases involve fever, "acute skin failure," leukopenia | 10–20% cause not determined |
| Hypersensitivity syndrome | Severe exanthematous rash (may become purpuric), exfoliative dermatitis | Infrequent | 30–50% of cases involve fever, lymphadenopathy hepatitis, nephritis, carditis eosinophilia, atypical lymphocytes | Cutaneous lymphoma |
| Acute generalized exanthematous | Initially nonfollicular small pustules overlying edematous erythema, sometimes leading to superficial ulcers | About 20% erosions—mouth and tongue | Fever, burning, pruritus, facial swelling, leukocytosis, and hypocalcemia | Infection |
| Serum sickness or reactions resembling | Morbilliform lesions, sometimes with urticaria | Absent | Fever, arthralgias and sickness | Infection |
| Anticoagulant-induced necrosis | Erythema then purpura and necrosis, especially of fatty areas | Infrequent | Pain in affected areas | Disseminated intravascular coagulopathy, septicemia |
| Angioedema | Urticaria or swelling of central part of face | Often involved | Respiratory distress, and cardiovascular collapse | Insect stings, and foods |

## Erythema Multiforme (EM)

- A vesiculobullous disease, generally with self-limiting course.
- Subdivided into *erythema multiforme major and minor*.
- The lesions are pink-red macules and edematous papules, the centers of which may become vesicular. The clue to the diagnosis of EM, as opposed to a morbilliform exanthem, is the development of a "dusky" violet color or petechiae in the center of the lesions.
- **Target or iris lesions** are also characteristic of EM and arise as a result of active centers and borders in combination with centrifugal spread. However, iris lesions need not be present for the diagnosis of EM.
- Preferred sites—distal extremities and mucous membrane.
- Lesions are bilaterally symmetrical
- Hemorrhagic crusts of lips characteristic (differential diagnosis— herpes simplex, pemphigus vulgaris, paraneoplastic pemphigus) Lesions resolve in 3–6 weeks
- **Etiology**
  - ➢ Drugs (sulphonamides, phenytoin, barbiturates, penicillin, carbamazepine).
  - ➢ Infection with herpes simplex **most common cause** in young.
  - ➢ Other causes—*Mycoplasma pneumoniae*, dimorphic fungus, viruses (echovirus, coxsackie, EBV, influenza), vaccination with BCG, polio, vaccinia, radiation and environmental toxins.

## Stevens-Johnson Syndrome (SJS)

- Induction of SJS is most often due to drugs, especially sulfonamides, phenytoin, barbiturates, penicillins, and carbamazepine.
- Widespread dusky macules and significant mucosal involvement are characteristic of SJS, and the cutaneous lesions may or may not develop epidermal detachment. If the latter occurs, by definition, it is limited to <10% of the body surface area (BSA).
- Constitutional symptoms and internal organ involvement is seen.
- Greater involvement leads to the diagnosis of SJS/TEN overlap (10–30% BSA) or TEN (>30% BSA).

## Toxic Epidermal Necrolysis (TEN)

- **Toxic epidermal necrolysis (TEN)** is characterized by bullae that arise on widespread areas of erythema and then slough. This results in large areas of denuded skin.
- The associated morbidity, such as sepsis, and mortality are relatively high and are a function of the extent of epidermal necrosis.

In addition, these patients may also have involvement of the mucous membranes and intestinal tract.

- Drugs are the primary cause of TEN, and the most common offenders are phenytoin, barbiturates, carbamazepine, sulfonamides, penicillins, and NSAIDs.
- Severe acute graft-versus-host disease (grade 4) can also resemble TEN.
- Nikolsky's sign is positive

### Exfoliative Dermatitis (Erythroderma)

- It is a generalized inflammatory disorder of skin manifesting with erythema and scaling.
- **Etiology**
  - ➤ *Preexisting skin diseases*
    - Atopic dermatitis
    - Contact dermatitis
    - Dermatophytosis
    - Eczema
    - Hailey-Hailey disease
    - Ichthyosis
    - Leiner's disease
    - Norwegian scabies
    - Pemphigus foliaceous
    - Pityriasis rubra pilaris
    - Psoriasis
    - Reiter's disease
    - Seborrheic dermatitis
    - Stasis dermatitis

  - ➤ *Systemic diseases*
    - Ca of lung and rectum
    - Acute and chronic leukemia
    - Angioimmunoblastic lymphadenopathy
    - Hodgkin's disease
    - SLE
    - Multiple myeloma
    - Mycosis fungoides
    - Reticulum cell sarcoma
    - Sézary syndrome
    - TSS

  - ➤ *Drugs*
    - Allopurinol
    - Arsenic
    - Antimalarials
    - Gold
    - Penicillin
    - Mercury
    - Antimalarials
    - Vitamin A
    - Tetracycline
    - INH
    - Quinine
    - Streptomycin
    - Phenothiazines
    - Dapsone
    - Iodine

➢ **Idiopathic**

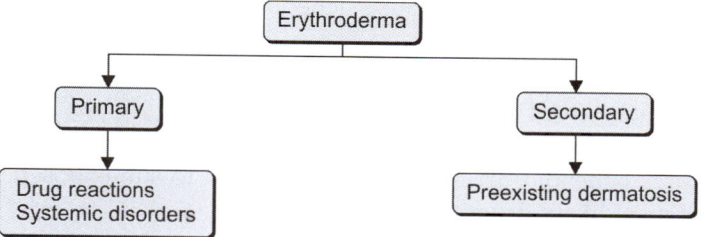

**Clinical features**
- Males > females
- Initially localized erythema but later involves >90% of body surface area.
- Scaling is seen.
- Hair loss in 25–30% cases.
- Nail changes more common showing dystrophy, ridging, and thickening.
- Palms and soles are involved.
- **Systemic manifestations**
  ➢ Malaise and bodyache
  ➢ Dermatophytic lymphadenopathy
  ➢ Hepatosplenomegaly
  ➢ Raised body temperature (40–80% cases)
  ➢ Hypoalbuminemia and edema
  ➢ Tachycardia and high cardiac output, cardiac failure
- Raised ESR, elevated IgE, and electrolyte abnormalities.

**Treatment**
- **Topical**
  ➢ Emollients
- **Systemic**
  ➢ Antibiotics for secondary infection.
  ➢ Systemic steroids (avoided if erythroderma is due to psoriasis)
  ➢ Cyclosporine
  ➢ Antimetabolites
- **General**
  ➢ Hospitalization
  ➢ Maintenance of temperature
  ➢ Fluid intake and output monitoring
  ➢ Nutritional support

### Lichenoid drug eruptions

- Many drugs can rarely cause lichenoid eruptions but the most common are:
  - Gold
  - Antimalarials
  - Captopril
- Actinic lichenoid drug eruption is confined to sun-exposed sites. The most likely drugs to cause this are:
  - Quinine
  - Thiazide diuretics
- Lichenoid drug eruptions clear up slowly when the responsible medication is withdrawn.

### Fixed drug eruptions

- Lesions develop soon after ingestion of the offending agent.
- Occur from 30 mins to 8 hours after the ingestion of drug (in previously sensitized individuals)
- Genital skin is the most commonly involved site.
- Nevertheless any site may be involved, conjunctiva, oropharynx, perioral or periorbital regions.
- Lesions begin as macules, become edematous forming plaques and may further evolve into vesicles and bullae and then into erosions
- Most commonly lesions are solitary but they may be multiple.
- Lesion heal with hyperpigmentation.
- 'After healing lesions show dark brown with violet hue postinflammatory hyperpigmentation'.
- Usually asymptomatic.
- May be pruritic, painful or burning.
- Painful when eroded.
- Lesions recur at same site every time the drug is taken.
- FDE occur repeatedly at the identical skin site (i.e. fixed) within hours of ingestion.
- Anti-inflammatory agents such as salicylates, NSAIDs (including paracetamol), phenylbutazone and phenacetin are important implicated agents.
- Fluoroquinolones and tetracyclines are also implicated.

## Treatment of Drug Reactions

- Management of mild cases is aimed at eliminating the offending drug while treating the symptoms.
- More severe cases require prompt medical attention and treatment with systemic corticosteroids and antihistamines.

## URTICARIA AND ANGIOEDEMA

- The term 'urticaria' is increasingly being used to describe a disease that may present with wheals, angioedema or both.
- Wheals (synonym 'nettle rash', hives) is the descriptive term for transient, well-demarcated, superficial erythematous or pale swellings of the dermis, which are usually very itchy and are associated with a surrounding red flare initially.
- Angioedema (synonym angioneurotic edema, Quincke's edema) swellings affect the deeper dermal, subcutaneous and submucosal tissues. They are usually painful rather than itchy, poorly defined, and pale or normal in color.
- Anaphylaxis is an acute, severe, life-threatening, generalized or systemic hypersensitivity reaction. It consists of a combination of symptoms and signs, including diffuse erythema, pruritus, urticaria and angioedema, hypotension and difficulty in breathing.
- Urticaria is traditionally classified into acute and chronic, with a time division arbitrarily chosen between 6 weeks and 3 months.
- When urticaria is present daily or almost daily for less than 6 weeks, it is called acute. If urticaria occurs continuously on most days for longer than this, it is called chronic.

## Pathophysiology of Urticaria

### Mast Cell Mediated Urticaria

- **Mediators**
  - Histamine
  - Cysteinyl leukotrienes (C4, D4, E4)
  - Prostaglandin D2
  - Platelet activating factor
- **Cytokines**
  - Interleukin –3, –4, –5
  - Granulocyte macrophage colony-stimulating factor
  - Tumor necrosis factor-$\alpha$
- **Releasing stimuli (*in vivo*)**
  - Allergen cross-linking of specific IgE on FcεRI
  - Anti-FcεRI and anti-IgE autoantibodies
  - IgG1 and 3 subclasses for functionality
  - Complement dependence
  - Immune complex deposition (serum sickness and urticarial vasculitis)
  - Neuropeptides (*in vitro* only)

- Cellular response
  - Basophil, eosinophil, neutrophil and lymphocytes.

### Non-Mast Cell Mediated Urticaria (Angioedema Without Wheals)

- Kallikrein-kininogen-kinin-kininase system
  - C1 esterase inhibitor deficiency
  - Angiotensin converting enzyme inhibitors

### Etiology

- The common *physical urticarias* include dermatographism, solar urticaria, cold urticaria, and cholinergic urticaria. Patients with *dermatographism* exhibit linear wheals following minor pressure or scratching of the skin. It is a common disorder, affecting ~5% of the population.
- *Solar urticaria* characteristically occurs within minutes of sun exposure and is a skin sign of one systemic disease—erythropoietic protoporphyria. In addition to the urticaria, these patients have subtle pitted scarring of the nose and hands.
- *Cold urticaria* is precipitated by exposure to the cold, and therefore exposed areas are usually affected. In occasional patients, the disease is associated with abnormal circulating proteins more commonly cryoglobulins and less commonly cryofibrinogens. Additional systemic symptoms include wheezing and syncope, thus explaining the need for these patients to avoid swimming in cold water.
- *Cholinergic urticaria* is precipitated by heat, exercise, or emotion and is characterized by small wheals with relatively large flares. It is occasionally associated with wheezing.
- **Ingestants**
  - Foods—cheese, eggs, nuts, fish
  - Food additives
  - Food preservatives
  - Drugs—penicillin, salicylates
- **Injectants**
  - Insect bites
  - Drugs, sera, blood
- **Inhalants**
  - Pollen
  - Animal dander

- **Infestations**
  - Amoebiasis
  - Giardiasis
  - Ankylostoma
  - Enterobius
- **Infections**
  - Focus in teeth, tonsil, sinuses
- **Contact urticaria**
- **Physical causes**
  - Dermographism—stroking of skin with blunt object
  - Pressure urticaria—pressure
  - Cholinergic urticaria—decrease in core body temperature
  - Cold urticaria—cold air or water
  - Heat urticaria—heated object
  - Solar urticaria—sun
  - Exercise induced urticaria—exercise
  - Aquagenic urticaria—water
  - Vibratory urticaria—vibratory instruments
- **Underlying connective tissue disorder or malignancy**
- **Idiopathic—no cause found.**

## Management

### Investigations

- **Acute urticaria**
  - Usually none, except where suggested by the history
  - Specific IgE (CAP fluoroimmunoassay or skin-prick tests)
  - Tests for upper respiratory viral or bacterial infection
- **Episodic urticaria**
  - Pseudoallergy challenge capsules (if available)
  - Food additives
  - Nonsteroidal anti-inflammatory drugs
- **Chronic urticaria**
  - Physical challenge provocation tests (where suggested by the history)
  - Blood tests (ordinary urticaria, if unresponsive to H1-antihistamines)
    - FBC, ESR, thyroid antibodies, thyroid function tests
    - C4 complement (angioedema without wheals and urticaria vasculitis)
    - Autologous serum skin test (where facilities are available)
    - Basophil histamine release assay (if available)
    - Others: As determined by the history and physical examination

➤ Skin biopsy (12–16 hrs old lesions, if urticarial vasculitis suspected)
➤ Stool examination for parasites (if infection suspected)
➤ Testing for *Helicobacter pylori* infection (if peptic ulcer symptoms)
➤ Testing for celiac disease (primarily symptomatic children)
➤ Imaging: None routinely

**Treatment**

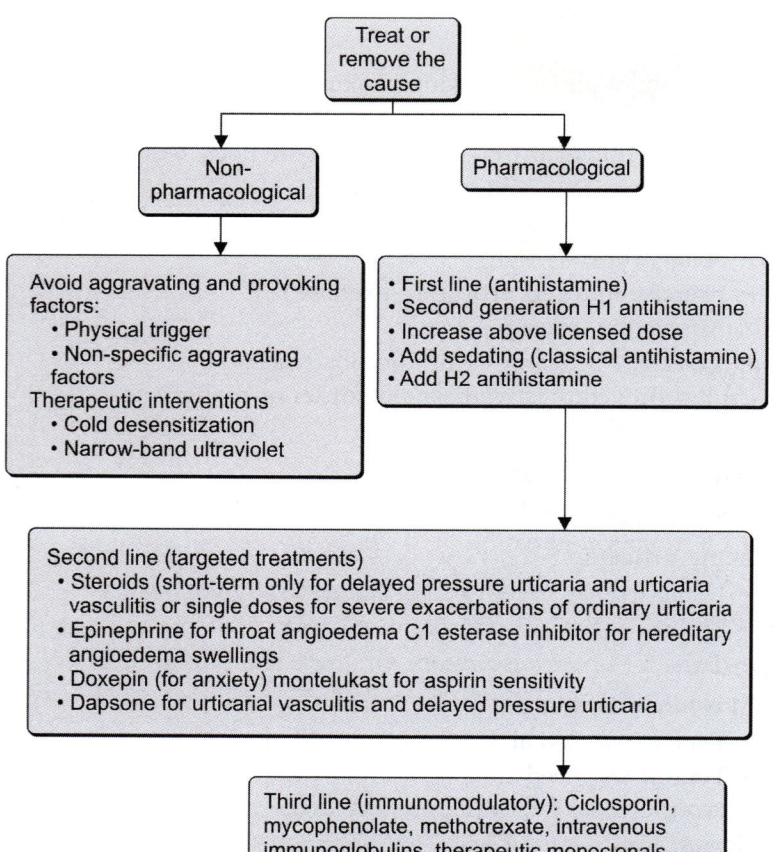

## ANGIOEDEMA

### Acquired

- Idiopathic
- Drug-related, especially:
  ➤ Angiotensin converting enzyme inhibitors
  ➤ Nonsteroidal anti-inflammatory drugs

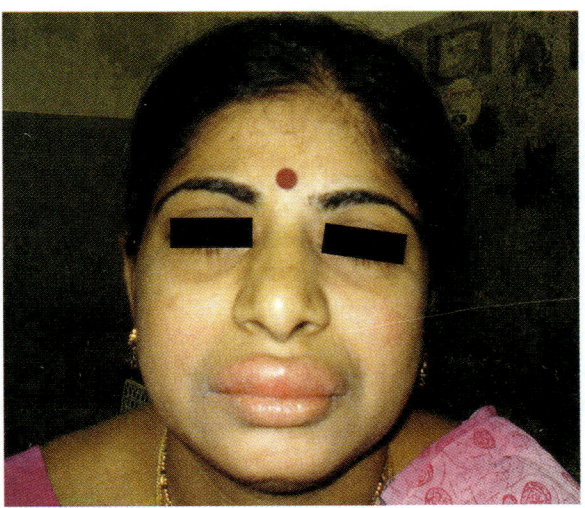

**Fig. 6.1:** Angioedema of lips

- Physical
  - ➤ Exercise-induced angioedema
  - ➤ Vibratory angioedema
- Acquired C1 esterase inhibitor deficiency
  - ➤ Lymphoproliferative disease
  - ➤ C1 inhibitor autoantibody
  - ➤ Others (including systemic lupus erythematosus)
- Episodic angioedema with eosinophilia (Gleich's syndrome) (Fig. 6.1)

## Hereditary

- C1 esterase inhibitor deficiency
  - ➤ Type I (reduced absolute level of C1 esterase inhibitor)
  - ➤ Type II (reduced functional inhibitor but normal or increased level)
- Normal C1 esterase inhibitor
- Type III (estrogen-dependent)

## *Hereditary Angioedema*

- Autosomal dominant disease
- Chromosome 11
- **Types**
  - ➤ Deficiency of C1INH (type 1) in 85% of cases.
  - ➤ Dysfunctional protein (type 2) in 15% of cases.

- Aggravated by administration of an ACE inhibitor (captopril).
- Diagnosis of hereditary angioedema is suggested by:
  - Family history
  - Lack of pruritus and of urticarial lesions
  - Prominence of recurrent gastrointestinal attacks of colic
  - Episodes of laryngeal edema.
- Treatment of inborn C1INH deficiency:
  - Attenuated androgens (Danozol, Stanozolol) (correct the biochemical defect and afford prophylactic protection).
  - Antifibrinolytic agent: Epsilon-aminocaproic acid (for preoperative prophylaxis).
  - Isolated C1INH protein infusion (being assessed for amelioration of attacks).
  - Bradykinin 2 receptor antagonist; SC administration (being assessed for amelioration of attacks).
  - **Ecallantide,** the recombinant peptide plasma kallikrein inhibitor DX-88, reduces the severity of acute hereditary angioedema. C1INH blocks the catalytic function of activated factor XII (Hageman factor) and of kallikrein, as well as the complement components of C1.

## QUESTIONS FROM PREVIOUS EXAMINATIONS

1. Pressure urticaria
2. Chronic urticaria
3. Sweet's syndrome
4. Approach for urticaria
5. Clinical features and Rx of erythema induratum
6. Account on pyoderma gangrenosum
7. Erythema necroticans
8. Poikiloderma atrophic vasculare
9. Leuckocytoclastic vasculitis
10. Syndromes associated with maldevelopement of the blood vessels
11. Erythema multiforme
12. Annular erythemas
13. Erythema nodosum
14. Causes of leg ulcers, etiopathogenesis, and Rx
15. Dermatological purpura
16. Intensive care in dermatology
17. Acute skin failure
18. Mechanism and pathogenesis of the drug reactions

19. Antibiotic in dermatology
20. Jarisch-Herxheimer reaction
21. Steroid addiction
22. FDE
23. Angioedema

## MULTIPLE CHOICE QUESTIONS

1. **"Target lesions" are characteristically seen in:**    *(PGI 08)*
   (a) Pemphigus vulgaris    (b) Psoriasis
   (c) Urticaria pigmentosa    (d) Erythema multiforme
   (e) Atopic dermatitis
2. **Most common cause of erythema multiforme is:**    *(MH 05)*
   (a) Herpes simplex    (b) Mycoplasma
   (c) Varicella zoster    (d) Influenza virus
3. **Exfoliative dermatitis can be due to all of the following *except*:**
   *(AI 02; PGI 06)*
   (a) Drug hypersensitivity    (b) Pityriasis rubra pilaris
   (c) Pityriasis rosea    (d) Psoriasis
4. **Cause(s) of erythroderma is/are:**    *(PGI 05)*
   (a) Pityriasis alba    (b) Pityriasis versicolor
   (c) Psoriasis    (d) Lichen planus
   (e) Eczema
5. **Gold poisoning leading to exfoliative dermatitis is Rx by:**
   (a) Chloroquine    (b) Steroid
   (c) Antibiotics    (d) Antihistaminics
6. **Recurrent erythematous plaques on glans penis in a 19-yr-old sexually active male which heals with residual hyperpigmentation, is suggestive of:**    *(AIIMS Nov 09)*
   (a) Aphthous balanitica    (b) Fixed drug eruption
   (c) Herpes gestationis    (d) Chlamydial infective
7. **Darrier's sign is seen in:**    *(JIPMER 97)*
   (a) Xeroderma pigmentosum (b) Urticaria pigmentosa
   (c) Herpes zoster    (d) Glucagonoma
8. **A 5-year-old male child has multiple hyperpigmented macules over the trunk. On rubbing the lesion with the rounded end of a pen, he developed urticarial wheal confined to the border of the lesion. Most likely diagnosis is:**    *(AI 93)*
   (a) FDE    (b) LP
   (c) Urticaria pigmentosa    (d) Urticarial vsaculitis

9. A circular depigmented patch on center of forehead in a female is mostly due to: *(AIIMS 2008)*
   (a) Hydroquinone
   (b) Ether metabolite of hydroquinone
   (c) Paratertiary butyl phenol
   (d) Paratertiary butyl catechol

10. Most common drug-induced skin reaction: *(MH 06)*
   (a) Maculopapular rash
   (b) Morbilliform rash
   (c) Fixed drug eruption
   (d) Photosensitivity reaction

11. A 45-year-old farmer has itchy erythematous papular lesions on face, neck, 'V' area of chest, dorsum of hands and forearms for 3 years. The lesions are more severe in summers and improve by 75% in winters. Most appropriate test to diagnose condition would be: *(AIIMS 04; AI 06)*
   (a) Skin biopsy
   (b) Estimation of IgE levels in blood
   (c) Patch test
   (d) Intradermal prick test

12. A 26-year-old sexually active male develops vesiculobullous lesion on the glans penis soon after taking paracetamol table for fever. Later, the lesion healed with residual hyperpigmenta-tion. The most likely diagnosis is: *(AI 2007)*
   (a) Behçet's syndrome     (b) Herpes genitalis
   (c) Fixed drug eruption     (d) Pemphigus

13. Features favoring pityriasis rubra pilaris over psoriasis include following *except:* *(JIPMER 08)*
   (a) Furfuraceous scalp scaling
   (b) No salmon patches
   (c) Keratoderma
   (d) Arthropathy

14. Which of the following are photosensitive diseases? *(PGI 01)*
   (a) SLE     (b) Liver spots
   (c) Calcinosis cutis     (d) Morphea
   (e) Porphyria cutanea tarda

15. A patient has history of episodic painful edema of face and larynx. Which of the following is likely to be deficient? *(AI 2009)*
   (a) C3     (b) C1 esterase inhibitor
   (c) C5     (d) Properdin

16. **Not true about angioneurotic edema:**    *(AI 2009)*
    (a) Pitting edema of face, lips and mucous membrane
    (b) C1 esterase inhibitor deficiency can cause it
    (c) Extreme temperature exposure can provoke it
    (d) Known with ACE inhibitors

17. **Drugs that commonly cause Stevens-Johnson syndrome:** *(PGI 08)*
    (a) Sulfonamides          (b) Nevirapine
    (c) Allopurinol           (d) Amitriptyline
    (e) NSAIDs

18. **Which of the following is not a photosensitive disease?**
    *(Kerala 03)*
    (a) Variegate porphyria    (b) Pellagra
    (c) Hydroa estivale        (d) Gaucher's disease
    (e) Dermatomyositis

19. **True about pityriasis rubra pilaris:**    *(PGI 01)*
    (a) Isolated patches of normal skin are found
    (b) Cephalocaudal distribution
    (c) IV cyclosporine effective
    (d) Common in females
    (e) Oral cyclosporine effective

20. **A 9-year-old boy has multiple itchy erythematous wheals all over the body for 2 days. There is no respiratory difficulty. Which is the best treatment?**    *(AIIMS 2004)*
    (a) Antihelminthics
    (b) Systemic corticosteroids
    (c) Antihistaminics
    (d) Adrenaline

21. **Rakesh, a 7-year-old boy had itchy, excoriated papules on the forehead and the exposed parts of the arms and legs for 3 yrs. The disease was most severe in the rainy season and improved completely in winter. The most likely diagnosis is:** *(AIIMS '2004)*
    (a) Insect bite hypersensitivity
    (b) Scabies
    (c) Urticaria
    (d) Atopic dermatitis

22. **A man develops small reddish itchy maculopapular lesions which increases on exposure to heat and sunlight:** *(AIIMS May 2013)*
    (a) Psychogenic  urticaria
    (b) Cholinergic urticaria
    (c) Dermographism
    (d) Solar urticaria

## Answers

1. **Ans. (d)** Erythema multiforme *(Ref. Rook's Textbook of Dermatology, 7th edn/ Vol 4, page 74.6)*

2. **Ans. (a)** Herpes simplex

3. **Ans. (c)** Pityriasis rosea *(Ref. IADVL, 2nd edn/441)*

4. **Ans. (c)** and **(e)** (psoriasis and eczema) *(Ref. IADVL, 2nd edn/ 441; Harrison's Medicine, 17th edn/ Table 54–3)*

5. **Ans. (b)** Steroid *(Ref. IADVL, 2nd edn/441)*

6. **Ans. (b)** Fixed drug eruption *(Ref. Harrison's Internal Medicine, 17th edn, Chapter 56)*

7. **Ans. (b)** Urticaria pigmentosa *(Ref. IADVL, 2nd edn/1142)*

8. **Ans. (c)** Urticaria pigmentosa *(Ref. IADVL, 2nd edn/1142; Harrison's Medicine 17th edn / Table 54–14)*

9. **Ans. (c)** Paratertiary butyl phenol *(Ref.  Rook's Dermatology, 7th edn/21.15)*

10. **Ans. (b)** Morbilliform rash

11. **Ans. (c)** Patch test

12. **Ans. (c)** Fixed drug eruption *(Ref. Fitzpatrick's Colur Atlas and Synopsis of Clinical Dermatology, 5th edn/556; Behl 9th edn/275)*

13. **Ans. (d)** Arthropathy *(Ref. Rook's Dermatology, 7th/ 34.65)*

14. **Ans. (a, b, e)**

15. **Ans. (b)** C1 esterase inhibitor *(Ref: Harrison, 17th edition, Chapter 311, page 2066)*

16. **Ans. (a)** Pitting edema of face, lips and mucous membrane *(Ref: Harrison, 17th edition, Chapter 311, page 2066)*

17. **Ans. (a, b, c, e)** *(Ref. Harrison's Internal Medicine, 17th edn / Chapter 56.)*

18. **Ans. (d)** Gaucher's disease *(Ref. Harrison's Medicine, 17th edn/ Table 57–2)*

19. **Ans. (a)** Isolated patches of normal skin are found *(Ref. Rook, 7th edn/34.67)*

20. **Ans. (c)** Antihistaminics *(Ref: Harrison, 17th edn/Chapter 57)*

21. **Ans. (a)** Insect bite hypersensitivity *(Ref. Harrison's Internal Medicine, 17th edn/Chapter 53).*

22. **Ans. (b)** Cholinergic urticaria.

# 7    Papulosquamous Disorders

## PSORIASIS

- Psoriasis is a common inflammatory scaling dermatosis (well-demarcated erythematous plaques surmounted by characteristic silvery white scaling) with a bilateral symmetric distribution and may be associated with a seronegative spondyloarthropathy.
- Predominantly affects the extensor aspects of the extremities and lumbosacral area of the trunk.
- It affects 1–3% of the world's population with no gender preference. Up to one-third of patients develop psoriatic arthritis (PSA).
- The mean age of onset of psoriasis is about 30 years.
- Etiology is unknown.

### Immunopathogenesis of Psoriasis

Recognition of antigen by antigen-presenting cell (APC)
↓

Maturation of APC and migration to lymph nodes
↓

T cell: APC binding (blocked by alefacept, efalizumab)
↓

Antigen presentation to T cell
↓

T cell activation
↓

Differentiation and expansion of type 1 T cells
↓

Selective trafficking of activated T cells into skin
↓

Secretion of cascade of inflammatory cytokines (GMCSF, EGF, IL-1, IL-6, IL-8, IL-12, interferon-$\alpha$ and TNF-$\alpha$ in the local microenvironment ← (TNF-$\alpha$ blockers etanercept, infliximab, adalimumab, onercept)
↓

Keratinocyte proliferation, angiogenesis and events causing chronic inflammation
↓

Psoriasis

**Known trigger factors for psoriasis**
- Emotional stress
- Local trauma to the skin (*Köebner's phenomenon*)
- Infection especially **streptococcal** (guttate psoriasis)
- Drugs:
  - β-blockers
  - Antimalarials
  - Lithium salts
  - ACE inhibitors
  - NSAIDs
  - Withdrawal of steroids.

## Plaque Psoriasis

- It is the most common variety of psoriasis, characterized by well-defined raised erythematous papules and plaques with silvery white scales (Fig. 7.1).
- *The distribution is typically symmetric, and sites of predilection include*
  - the extensor surfaces of the extremities, particularly the elbows and knees

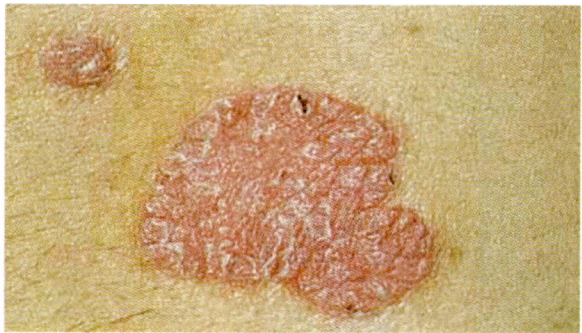

**Fig. 7.1:** Erythematous scaly plaque of psoriasis

> Sacrum
> Scalp
> Nape of the neck, and to a lesser extent
> The remainder of the trunk
> Genitalia
> Face
> Ears
- *Additional features of psoriatic plaques include*
  > Auspitz sign
  > Woronoff 's ring
  > Köebner's phenomenon.

| | |
|---|---|
| **Auspitz sign** | Presence of pinpoint bleeding at the base of a plaque after scale is forcibly removed. The successive removal of **psoriatic** scales usually reveals an underlying smooth, glossy, red **membrane (membrane** of **Bulkeley)** with small bleeding points where the thin suprapapillary epithelium is turn off. The red membrane is known as **Bulkeley's membrane.** |
| **Woronoff 's ring** | Presence of a white ring around erythematous plaques undergoing topical treatment or phototherapy. |
| **Isomorphic or Köebner's phenomenon** | Development of lesions at sites of trauma, including those from sunburn. |

- **Isomorphic response (Köebner's phenomenon)**
  > Psoriasis is one of the several conditions in which various types of trauma may elicit the disease in previously uninvolved skin.
  > It occurs 7–14 days after trauma.
  > Other conditions associated with **isomorphic response/ Köebner's phenomenon** are:
    - **Psoriasis (best known in)**
    - **Vitiligo**
    - **Lichen planus**
    - **Lichen nitidus**
    - **Molluscum contagiosum**
    - **Kaposi's sarcoma**
    - **Pityriasis rubra pilaris**
    - **Warts**
    - **Darier's disease**
    - **DLE**

> Warts, molluscum contagiosum, and eczematous lesions show pseudoisomorphic phenomenon (due to autoinoculation).
> Clearing of psoriasis following injury has been observed and termed the **reverse Köebner's phenomenon**.

## Inverse Psoriasis

- Inverse psoriasis is characterized mainly by its distribution
- It is localized predominantly to intertriginous regions including:
  > Axillae
  > Infra or Submammary regions
  > Gluteal cleft
  > Abdominal folds
  > Inguinal folds (groin)
  > Genitals.
- It also tends to affect the scalp, palms, and soles
- These lesions also differ in morphology from that of typical plaque psoriasis lesions in that they are well-defined shiny erythematous patches or thin plaques without significant scale.
- The presentation may initially be confused for bacterial or candidal intertrigo.

## Guttate (Eruptive) Psoriasis

- Characterized by an acute generalized eruption of smaller round to oval-shaped well-defined erythematous scaly papules and plaques up to 1 cm in size all over the body, particularly on the trunk and proximal limbs and rarely on soles (Fig. 7.2).
- Considered to be more of an eruptive form of psoriasis and is often associated with infection, especially hemolytic streptococcal pharyngitis.
- More common in children and young adults, guttate psoriasis may initially respond well to antibiotics, heliotherapy, or phototherapy and go into remission, only to recur with reinfection.
- Patients with guttate psoriasis may have a higher risk of developing plaque psoriasis later in life.
- Guttate psoriasis can also be easily confused with the papular type of acutely flaring plaque psoriasis.
- Guttate psoriasis may also be confused with pityriasis rosea (PR), but differs in the nature of the scale (psoriatic scale involves the entire lesion and is more coarse, rather than the finer localized trailing ring pattern of the scale in PR), pattern (psoriasis does not

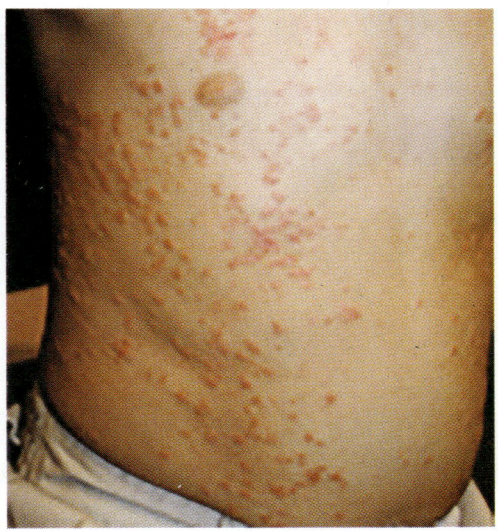

**Fig. 7.2:** Multiple well-defined erythematous scaly plaques and papules over trunk

present in a Christmas tree pattern and is less likely to appear in linear arrangements in the axilla and neck), and course (guttate psoriasis often lasts longer than 8 weeks unless appropriately treated, while PR often resolves within 6–8 weeks without treatment).

- This variety has good prognosis.

## Rupioid, Elephantine and Ostraceous Psoriasis

- These terms describe plaques associated with gross hyperkeratosis.
- Rupioid psoriasis refers to limpet-like coneshaped lesions.
- The term elephantine psoriasis might be used to describe unusual but very persistent, thickly scaling, large plaques that sometimes occur on the back, limbs, hips or elsewhere.
- Ostraceous psoriasis, an infrequently used term, refers to a ring-like hyperkeratotic lesion with a concave surface, resembling an oyster shell.

## Scalp Psoriasis

- Individuals may present with hyperkeratotic scaling disease localized to the scalp only, making it difficult to discriminate from severe seborrheic dermatitis or *tinea capitis*. This presentation has been called *tinea amiantacea* and requires evaluation to distinguish between these 3 entities (Fig. 7.3).

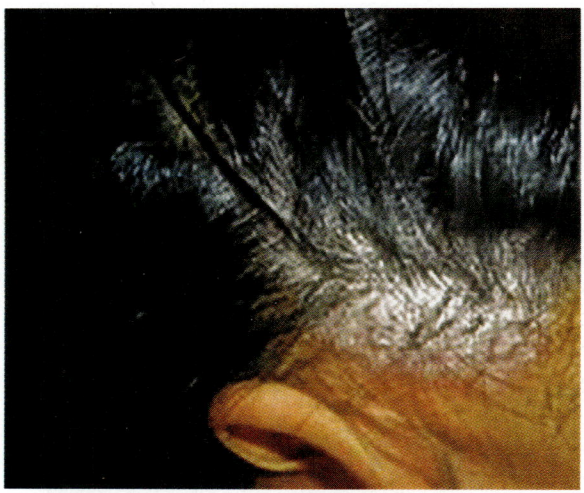

**Fig. 7.3:** Scaly plaque over scalp

## Pustular Psoriasis

- Pustular psoriasis is a form of psoriasis in which macroscopic pustules appear.
- It tends to go in a cycle—reddening of the skin followed by formation of pustules and scaling
- It is of 2 types:
  - ➢ *Localized*
    - Palmoplantar pustulosis
    - Acrodermatitis continua of Hallopeau
  - ➢ *Generalized*
    - Acute (von Zumbusch)
    - Pregnancy (impetigo herpetiformis)
    - Infantile and juvenile
    - Circinate
    - Localized (not hands and feet)
- **Provocative factors**
  - ➢ Injudicious use of coal tar and diathranol
  - ➢ Infection
  - ➢ Pregnancy
  - ➢ Stress
  - ➢ Hypocalcemia (hypoparathyroidism)
  - ➢ Salicylates

- ➢ Iodides
- ➢ Lithium
- ➢ Phenylbutazone
- ➢ Withdrawal of steroids
- **Types of pustular psoriasis**

## von Zumbusch

- von Zumbusch can appear abruptly on the skin.
- It is characterized by widespread areas of reddened skin, which then become painful and tender. Within hours, the pustules appear. Over the next 24 to 48 hours, the pustules dry leaving the skin with a glazed and smooth appearance.
- von Zumbusch is rarely seen in children, although when it does, it is often the first manifestation of psoriasis and may have a better outcome than in adults.
- This form can be life-threatening and medical care must begin immediately. People with von Zumbusch pustular psoriasis often require hospitalization for rehydration and initiation of topical and systemic treatments, which typically included antibiotics.
- von Zumbusch is associated with fever, chills, sever itching, dehydration, a rapid pulse rate, exhaustion, anemia, weight loss and muscle weakness.

## Palmoplantar Pustulosis (PPP)

- Palmoplantar pustulosis, a type of pustular psoriasis that causes pustules on the palms of the hand and soles of the feet.
  The base of the thumb and the sides of the heels are commonly affected sites.
- The pustules initially appear in a studded pattern overlying red plaques of skin, but then turn brown, peel and become crusted.
- The course of PPP is usually cyclical, with new crops of pustules followed by periods of low activity.

## Acropustulosis (Acrodermatitis Continua of Hallopeau)

- Acropustulosis is a rare type of psoriasis characterized by skin lesions on the ends of the fingers and sometimes on the toes.
- The eruption occasionally starts after an injury to the skin or infection.
- Often the lesions are painful and disabling, producing deformity of the nails.
- Occasionally bone changes occur in severe cases.

- **Treatment**
  - ➢ *Generalized pustular psoriasis*: The goal of treatment is to restore the skin's barrier function, prevent further loss of fluid, stabilize the body's temperature and restore the skin's chemical balance. Acitretin, cyclosporine, methotrexate, oral PUVA and TNF-α blockers, such as infliximab, are often prescribed.
  - ➢ *Localized pustular psoriasis:* Topical treatments are usually prescribed first. However, this form often proves stubborn to treat. PUVA, ultraviolet light B (UV B), acitretin, methotrexate or cyclosporine may be used to achieve clearance.

**Rx of pustular psoriasis**
- Retinoids—*drug of 1st choice*
- Methotrexate—*drug of 2nd choice*

**Pustular psoriasis in pregnancy:** Corticosteroids are drug of 1st choice.[Q]

## Erythrodermic Psoriasis

- Two forms exist.
- In the first form, chronic lesions may evolve gradually into an exfoliative phase, and can be regarded as extensive plaque psoriasis involving all, or almost all, the cutaneous surface. There are usually some areas of uninvolved skin. The psoriatic characteristics are retained, mild treatment is well-tolerated and the prognosis is good.
- The second form is part of the spectrum of 'unstable' psoriasis. It may occur at any time, either presenting suddenly and unexpectedly, or be ushered in by a period of increasing intolerance to local applications, UV therapy and loss of control over the disease. The characteristics of the disease are often lost, the whole skin is involved, the patient may be febrile and ill, the course is often prolonged, relapses are frequent and there is an appreciable mortality.
- **Histopathology of psoriasis**
  - ➢ From a histological point of view, psoriasis is a dynamic dermatosis that changes during the evolution of an individual lesion; we can classify it in an:
    - – Early stage
    - – Advanced stage
    - – Later lesions.
  - ➢ Lesions are usually diagnostic only in early stages or near the margin of advancing plaques.
  - ➢ Munro microabscesses and Kogoj micropustules are diagnostic clues of psoriasis, but they are not always present.

### Early changes

➤ The early stage consists in elongation and dilatation of blood vessels of the papillary dermis, with associated edema and lymphocytic infiltrate (perivascular cuffing).

➤ Vessels are dilated and tortuous, with some neutrophils in their lumen.

➤ Lymphocytes and neutrophils emerge from the vessel reaching the epidermis ("squirting" papilla).

➤ Rare erythrocytes extravasated may be found.

➤ Epidermis during this phase, is quite normal.

➤ Shortly after, there is a thickening of epidermis with loss of granular cell layer and formations of mounds of parakeratosis, which is thought to result from a markedly shortened cellular turnover time.

➤ Keratinocytes proliferate and mature rapidly, so that terminal differentiation is incomplete.

➤ Thus, squamous keratinocytes aberrantly retain intact nuclei and release a few extracellular lipids that normally cement adhesion of corneocytes.

### Advanced stage

➤ It is characterized by regular acanthosis (thickening of stratum spinosum) and epidermal **"psoriasiform hyperplasia"** with regular elongation of the rete ridges and thinning of suprapapillary plates.

➤ When subcorneal abscesses are prominent, the disease is designated as pustular psoriasis.

➤ Dermal inflammatory infiltrate is heavier than in early lesions, it is composed by T-lymphocytes, containing a few Langerhan cells with occasional neutrophils.

• Parakeratosis become confluent, with loss of granular layer. There is transmigration of inflammatory cells through epidermis into parakeratotic scale resulting in intracorneal collections of neutrophils, the so-called *Munro microabscesses*.

• Similar accumulation in the stratum spinosum is defined as *spongiform pustule of Kogoj*.

### Later lesions

➤ There is orthokeratosis, an intact granular layer and mild exocytosis of inflammatory cells.

➤ Munro microabscesses and Kogoj micropustules are diagnostic clues of psoriasis, but they are not always present.

## Nail Psoriasis

- Nail involvement is common in patients with psoriasis and psoriatic arthritis, affecting **80–90% of patients** at some time (Table 7.1).

| Psoriasis Sign/Symptom | Site | Features |
|---|---|---|
| **Table 7.1:** Features of nail psoriasis | | |
| 1. Oil drop or salmon patch | Nailbed | Translucent yellow-red discoloration in the nailbed, resembles drop of oil under nail plate |
| 2. Pitting (thimble) | Proximal nail matrix | Loss of parakeratotic cells from surface of nail plate |
| 3. Beau's lines | Proximal nail matrix | Transverse lines in nails due to intermittent inflammation causing growth arrest lines |
| 4. Leukonychia | Mid-matrix disease | Areas of white nail plate due to foci of parakeratosis within the body of the nail plate |
| 5. Subungual hyperkeratosis | Hyponychium and nailbed | Excessive proliferation of the nailbed and hyponychium. May lead to onycholysis. |
| 6. Onycholysis | Nailbed and hyponychium | Nail plate separates from its underlying attachment to nailbed. Nail plate whitens and may detach. Secondary infection may occur. |
| 7. Nail plate crumbling | Nailbed or nail matrix | Nail plate weakens due to disease of underlying structures |

## Treatment of nail psoriasis

- There is no cure for nail psoriasis but it may improve by itself and may even return to a normal appearance.
- Calcipotriol solution applied twice daily to the nail folds is safe to use and may help nail psoriasis if applied over prolonged periods.
- Topical high-potency corticosteroid solution or ointment works best when covered by cellophane wrap at bedtime. Avoid prolonged occlusion (2 weeks at most) or continuous therapy with corticosteroids.
- Intralesional triamcinolone acetonide injected into proximal nail folds is helpful (but painful) in nail matrix psoriasis.

- Topical 5-fluorouracil cream applied to the matrix for 6 months may improve pitting and subungual hyperkeratosis.
- Psoralen and UVA (photochemotherapy or PUVA) may improve nail psoriasis.
- Systemic treatment with oral methotrexate, retinoids and ciclosporin is usually prescribed for generalized psoriasis but may also be helpful for nail disease.
- Antifungal treatment may be prescribed if secondary infection is present.
- Chemical or surgical avulsion therapy, i.e. complete removal of the nail, is rarely recommended.

## Psoriatic Arthritis

- An inflammatory arthritis associated with psoriasis of the skin and/or nails, with usually a negative serological test for rheumatoid factor and the absence of rheumatoid nodules.
- The Moll and Wright classification includes five clinical groups, which often overlap.
  - ➢ Predominantly peripheral mono- or asymmetrical oligoarthritis is the most common form, and often overlooked. Enthesitis— inflammation at the site of tendon insertion into the bone—is common.
  - ➢ Predominantly distal interphalangeal arthritis, the well recognized classical form, but less common than previously emphasized.
  - ➢ Predominantly symmetrical, rheumatoid-like, rheumatoid factor—negative polyarthritis, usually less severe than rheumatoid arthritis.
  - ➢ 'Arthritis mutilans', a relatively uncommon, severely deforming arthritis involving fingers and toes predominantly.
  - ➢ Predominantly axial arthritis: Psoriatic spondylitis and/or sacroiliitis, with or without variable peripheral arthropathy.
- **Treatment**
  - ➢ NSAIDs
  - ➢ Disease modifying antirheumatic drugs: Methotrexate, ciclosporine, gold salts, sulfasalazine.
  - ➢ Biological therapies
  - ➢ Surgery

## Psoriasis: Treatment

- Most patients with localized, plaque-type **psoriasis** can be managed with midpotency topical glucocorticoids, although their long-term use is often accompanied by loss of effectiveness (tachyphylaxis) and atrophy of the skin.

- A topical vitamin D analogue and a retinoid are also efficacious in the treatment of limited **psoriasis** and have largely replaced other topical agents such as coal tar, salicylic acid, and anthralin.

  Ultraviolet light, natural or artificial, is an effective therapy for many patients with widespread **psoriasis**.

  ➢ Ultraviolet B (UV B) light, narrowband UV B, and ultraviolet A (UV A) spectrum with either oral or topical psoralens (PUVA) are also extremely effective.

  ➢ The long-term use of UV light may be associated with an increased incidence of non-melanoma and melanoma skin cancer.

**Table 7.2:** FDA-approved systemic therapy for psoriasis

| Agent | Medication class | Administration | | Adverse events |
|---|---|---|---|---|
| | | Route | frequency | |
| Methotrexate | Antimetabolite | Oral | Weekly | • Hepatotoxicity<br>• Pulmonary toxicity<br>• Pancytopenia<br>• Potential for malignancies<br>• Ulcerative stomatitis<br>• Nausea<br>• Diarrhea<br>• Teratogenicity |
| Acitretin | Retinoid | Oral | Daily | • Teratogenicity<br>• Osteophyte formation<br>• Hyperlipidemia<br>• Flare of inflammatory bowel disease,<br>• Hepatoxicity<br>• Depression |
| Cyclosporine | Calcineurin inhibitor | Oral | Twice daily | • Renal dysfunction<br>Hypertension<br>Hyperkalemia<br>Hyperuricemia<br>Hypomagnesemia<br>Hyperlipidemia<br>• ↑ Risk of malignancies |

**Table 7.3:** Biologics approved for psoriasis or psoriatic arthritis

| Agent | Mechanism of action | Indication | Administration | | Warnings |
| | | | Route | Frequency | |
|---|---|---|---|---|---|
| **Alefacept** | Anti-CD2 (fusion protein against LFA-3) | Ps | IM | Once weekly × 12 weeks; may repeat | Lymphopenia, potential for increased malignancies, serious infections |
| **Etanercept** | Anti-TNF-α | Ps, PsA | SC | Once or twice weekly | Serious infections, neurologic events, hematologic events, potential for increased malignancies |
| **Efalizumab** | Anti-CD11a | Ps | SC | Once weekly | Serious infections, potential for increased malignancies, thrombocytopenia, hemolytic anemia, psoriasis worsening |
| **Adalimumab** | Anti-TNF-α | PsA | SC | Every other week | Serious infections, neurologic events, potential for increased malignancies, hypersensitivity reactions, hematologic events |
| **Infliximab** | Anti-TNF-α | PsA | IV | Initial infusion followed by infusions at weeks 2, 6, then every 8 weeks | Serious infections, hepatotoxicity, hematologic events, hypersensitivity reactions, neurologic events, potential for increased malignancies |

➤ UV light therapy is contraindicated in patients receiving cyclosporine and should be used with great care in all immunocompromised patients due to an increased risk of developing skin cancers.

- Various systemic agents can be used for severe, widespread psoriatic disease (Tables 7.2 and 7.3).
  ➤ Oral glucocorticoids should not be used for the treatment of **psoriasis** due to the potential for developing life-threatening pustular **psoriasis** when therapy is discontinued.
  ➤ Methotrexate is an effective agent, especially in patients with psoriatic arthritis.
  ➤ The synthetic retinoid, acitretin, is useful, especially when immunosuppression must be avoided; however, teratogenicity limits its use.

- **PUVA/ Photochemotherapy**
  ➤ It is valuable in Rx of:
    - Chronic plaque psoriasis
    - Generalized pustular psoriasis
    - Erythrodermic psoriasis
    - Palmoplantar pustulosis
    - Nail psoriasis.

**Psoralen and UVA (photochemotherapy or PUVA)**

| *Oral* | *Topical* |
|---|---|
| 8 methoxypsoralen tab (0.6 mg/kg) given 2 hrs before irradiation. | High intensity fluorescent UVA tubes used. Rx given 2–4 times weekly. UVA dosage is $\uparrow$ by 0.5–1.5 J/cm$^2$ according to response |

**Eye protection**

During irradiation UVA-opaque goggles must be worn and for reminder of the day of photochemotherapy UVA blocking sunglasses should be worn.

- **Contraindications**
  ➤ Renal, hepatic, or CVS disease
  ➤ Cataract
  ➤ Pre-existing light aggravated diseases like SLE, porphyria, and multiple melanocytic naevi.
  ➤ Family history of malignant melanoma
  ➤ Pregnancy
  ➤ Children <19 years.

- **Note:** See below

| Nail changes | Associated clinical condition |
|---|---|
| 1. Pin-point pitting of nails | Psoriasis |
| 2. Periungual or nail-fold telangiectasia | Dermatomyositis |
| 3. 'Half-and-half nail' | Uraemia |
| 4. White nails with loss of demarcation of the lunulae (leukonychia, Terry's nails) | Cirrhosis |
| 5. 'Mee's lines' on the nails | Chronic arsenic poisoning |
| 6. 'Splinter hemorrhages' under the finger and toe nails | Infective endocarditis |
| 7. Flattened, spoon-shaped nails, koilonychias | Iron deficiency anemia |
| 8. Transverse ridges (Beau's lines) | Serious preceding illness |
| 9. Shedding of finger and toenails (onycholysis) | Hemodialysis patients who received large doses of cephaloridine or cloxacillin. |

## LICHEN PLANUS (LP)

- Papulosquamous disease of unknown etiology
  The classical cutaneous lesions of LP are:
  - ➢ **Purplish** (faintly erythematous or violaceous)
  - ➢ Pruritic
  - ➢ Polygonal
  - ➢ Planar (flat topped)
  - ➢ Papules.
- The size is from pinpoint to a cm or more.
- Network of fine lines is present in many papules (**Wickham's striae**). These can be magnified by a drop of mineral oil.
- LP involves flexural areas preferentially, commonly wrist, lumbar region, and around the ankles.
- Face and scalp are spared in classical LP.
- Köebner's phenomenon is a common occurrence.
- LP affects all age groups.
- LP also affects mucous membrane and nails.
- **LP** (both cutaneous and oral) has been reported to be associated with chronic liver disease, primarily secondary to hepatitis C viral infection.

- LP is associated with many other autoimmune conditions like:
  - ➤ Vitiligo
  - ➤ Thymoma
  - ➤ MG
- **Variants of LP**
  - ➤ Actinic LP: Seen in young. Affects sun-exposed areas. Common in middle east, east Africa and India.
  - ➤ Lichen planopilaris—hair follicles are affected
  - ➤ Atrophic LP
  - ➤ Hypertrophic LP
  - ➤ Lichen planus pigmentosus
  - ➤ Lichen planus pemphigoides
  - ➤ Bullous LP
  - ➤ Linear LP
  - ➤ Annular LP
  - ➤ LP of palms and soles
  - ➤ Guttate LP
- Graham Little–Piccardi–Lasseur syndrome comprises the triad of multifocal scalp cicatricial alopecia, non-scarring alopecia of the axillae and/or groin, and keratotic lichenoid follicular papules.
- **Histology of lichen planus** (Fig. 7.4)
  - ➤ Lichen planus can usually be diagnosed clinically and histology is not often required. Skin biopsy is characteristic:

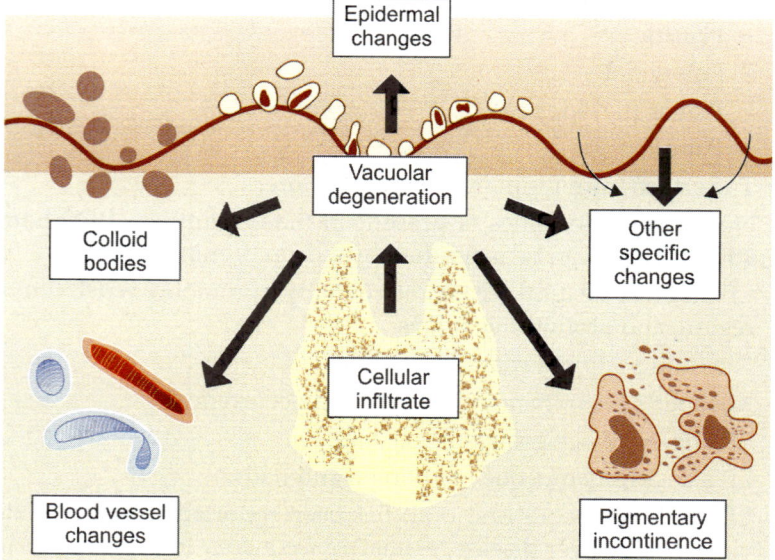

**Fig. 7.4:** Pathology of LP

> The *earliest finding* is an increase in epidermal Langerhans' cells, associated with a superficial perivascular infiltrate of lymphocytes and histiocytes, impinging on the dermal–epidermal junction (DEJ).
> A focal increase in thickness of the granular layer and infiltrate corresponds to the presence of **Wickham's striae**.
> Degenerating basal epidermal cells are transformed into **colloid bodies** (15–20 μm diameter) which appear singly or in clumps.
> The rete ridges may appear flattened or effaced (**'saw-tooth' appearance**).
> Focal separation from the dermis may lead **Max Joseph spaces**.
> In older or hypertrophic lesions, the number of colloid bodies is considerably reduced.
> In 'active' LP, a band-like infiltrate of lymphocytes and histiocytes, rarely admixed with plasma cells, obliterates the DEJ.
> Epidermal melanocytes are absent or considerably decreased in number, while pigmentary incontinence with dermal melanophages is characteristic.
> Direct immunofluorescence shows globular deposits of IgM (occasionally IgG and IgA).

- **Colloid body/Civatte body**
  > Describes the homogeneous eosinophilic rounded body which is 20 microns in diameter, PAS positive and diastase resistant resulting from degeneration and death of keratinocytes, particularly in the lower layers of the epidermis. This structure is found in various lichenoid tissue reactions and is involved in the process of apoptosis.
  > Colloid, hyaline, cytoid or Civatte bodies are seen in routinely stained sections in 37%.
  > On direct immunofluorescence staining with IgM, they can be seen in 87% of cases of LP.

## Mucosal LP

- Mucosal lesions occur in oral cavity, esophagus, conjunctiva, bladder, nose, larynx, vulva, vagina, glans, and stomach.
- **Oral LP**
  > 4–12%
  > Posterior buccal mucosa frequently involved.
  > Reticulate (lacy pattern), erosive, and atrophic most commonly reported.
  > Plaque type—smokers.

- **Genital LP**
  - ➤ Usually involved in 25% of cases, most commonly glans. Lesions may be annular, linear white striae or ulcerated plaques.

## Nails in LP

- Nail involvement occurs in up to 10% of cases, but is usually a minor feature of the disease.
- The majority of cases present during the fifth or sixth decades; long-term permanent damage to the nails is rare.
- Fingernails are more frequently affected than toenails.
- The most common changes are exaggeration of the longitudinal lines and linear depressions, due to slight thinning of the nail plate.
- Elevated ridges may be seen on the nail.
- Adhesion between the epidermis of the dorsal nail fold and the nailbed may cause partial destruction of the nail (**pterygium unguis**).
- Subungual hyperkeratosis
- Rarely, the nail is completely shed

> √  **Inverse pterygium** is seen in *systemic sclerosis.*

### Lichen planus treatment

- **LP** is essentially benign and **self-limiting disease**.
- Rx is largely symptomatic.
- For limited cutaneous involvement, topical corticosteroids may suffice.
- Oral steroids:
  - ➤ Extensive LP
  - ➤ Bullous LP
  - ➤ Follicular LP of scalp
  - ➤ Extensive ulcerative lesions on oral or vaginal mucosa
  - ➤ Nail atrophy and pterygium

### Other treatments

- Retinoids
- Dapsone
- Cyclosporine
- PUVA

## LICHEN NITIDUS

- Characterized by the presence of pinpoint to **pinhead-sized papules**, which are usually asymptomatic, flesh colored, with a flat, shiny surface.

- Most cases occur in children or young adults.
- They are found on any part of the body but the sites of predilection are the forearms, penis, abdomen, chest and buttocks.
- Usually asymptomatic.
- Nails are involved. Occasionally mucous membranes may be involved.
- May coexist with LP
- Köebner's phenomenon is seen.
- *DD:* Lichen scrofulosorum and keratosis pilaris
- *Treatment:* It is usually selflimiting. Topical steroids can be used.

## PITYRIASIS RUBRA PILARIS

**Definition:** Pityriasis rubra pilaris (PRP) is a heterogeneous group of disorders that have in common circumscribed follicular keratoses, branny scale and an orange-red erythema, and PPK.

**Age and sex:** There is a bimodal age of onset, but juvenile and adult forms of PRP, and indeed their variant forms, may be unrelated disorders.

### Type I

- Adult onset, classical.
- The most common and recognizable form, classical adult PRP affects the sexes equally with highest incidence between 40 and 60 years of age.
- Cephalocaudal progression is seen.
- Erythroderma is common. In many cases, islands of normal skin persist in the erythrodermic regions, and horny plugs may be evident around their margins.
- These normal pale 'islands' are very suggestive of the diagnosis, and the skin on the palms and soles often has an orange discoloration.
- Spontaneous resolution within 1–3 yrs

### Type II

- Adult onset, atypical.
- This uncommon variety affects 5% of patients.
- Follicular hyperkeratosis is prominent in some areas, while more lamellar scaling may be seen elsewhere, especially on the legs.
- Erythroderma is less common.
- Cephalocaudal progression is not seen.

### Type III

- Juvenile onset, classical.
- The onset is between the ages of 5 and 18.
- It resembles type I PRP and spontaneous clearing is usual within 1–2 years.

### Type IV

- Juvenile onset, circumscribed.
- This usually occurs below the age of 12 years.
- Well-demarcated plaques of follicular plugging with variable degrees of erythema appear on the knees and elbows.
- A few scattered scaly erythematous macules are often found on the trunk or in the scalp.
- Some cases also show marked keratoderma.

### Type V

- Juvenile onset, atypical.
- Familial PRP is often of this type, which overlaps clinically with ichthyoses and erythrokeratoderma.
- Patients show erythema and hyperkeratosis at birth or in the first few years of life.
- Follicular plugging and erythema suggest a diagnosis of PRP, but keratoderma is common and several patients have shown a scleroderma-like change of the digits.

## Histopathology

- Affected follicles are filled with dense horny plugs and there are foci of parakeratosis in the perifollicular shoulder and interfollicular epidermis.
- At other sites, basket-weave hyperkeratosis overlies a prominent granular layer and there is a little parakeratosis.

## Associated Disorders

- Leukemia
- Metastatic carcinoma
- Sézary syndrome.

## Treatment

- Intensive topical and supportive treatment is needed for the erythrodermic state.
- Topical and systemic corticosteroids are ineffective. Oral retinoids are widely used. In the erythrodermic phase, acitretin or isotretinoin are used.

- Topical vitamin D analogues are reported to be beneficial.
- Methotrexate has been effective as an alternative or adjunct to oral retinoids.

## PITYRIASIS ROSEA

- It is a rash that primarily affects young adults, the origin of which is unknown, but is thought to be caused by an infective agent.
- Numerous viruses have been investigated, thus far with no conclusive evidence.
- The incidence is highest in **winter**.
- Cases occur in clusters and among persons who are in close contact with each other, indicating an infectious spread. However, there are no data to support communicability. It may be an immune response to  number of agents.
- The characteristic lesion is an oval macule or papule with surrounding erythema. The lesion spreads with central clearing, much like *tinea corporis.* This initial lesion is a solitary lesion called the **herald patch** and is usually on the trunk or neck.
- As the lesion enlarges and begins to fade away (2 to 10 days), successive crops of lesions appear on the trunk and neck. The lesions on the back have a characteristic **"Christmas tree" pattern**. The extremities, the face, and scalp may be involved. Mild to severe pruritus may occur.
- Plaques are covered with scales that are attached to the periphery of the lesion and free on the inner side—*collarette scales.*
- The disease is self-limited and usually disappears within 6 to 8 weeks. Relapse occurs in hardly 2% cases.
- HPE similar to subacute or chronic eczema. Dyskeratotic keratinocytes and extravasated RBCs in dermal papillae may be seen.
- **Treatment** measures are palliative and include topical steroids, antihistamines, and colloid baths. Systemic corticosteroids may be indicated in severe cases.

### QUESTIONS FROM PREVIOUS EXAMINATIONS

1. Clinical variants + treatment of chronic hypertrophic LP
2. Lichenoid eruptions
3. Civatte bodies
4. HPE of LP
5. Lichen nitidus

6. Oral LP
7. Tropical LP
8. Lichen amyloidosis
9. Wickham's striae
10. Graham–Little–Piccardi syndrome
11. LPP
12. Pustular psoriasis
13. Guttate psoriasis
14. Treatment of psoriasis
15. Pityriasis rubra pilaris
16. Pityriasis rosea
17. Erythrodermic psoriasis
18. Psoriatic arthritis
19. Nail changes in psoriasis
20. Biologicals in psoriasis
21. Phototherapy in psoriasis

## MULTIPLE CHOICE QUESTIONS

1. **Psoriasis is precipitated by:**            *(AP 97; AI 98)*
   (a)  β-blockers            (b)  OC pills
   (c)  Steroids            (d)  All of the above
2. **Guttate psoriasis is associated with:**       *(AP 2000)*
   (a)  Drug allergy            (b)  Streptococcal infection
   (c)  Autoimmunity            (d)  Trauma
3. **Most important feature of psoriasis:**        *(AMC 99)*
   (a)  Crusting            (b)  Scaling
   (c)  Oozing            (d)  Erythema
4. **Bulkeley membrane is seen in:**           *(DNB 90)*
   (a)  Psoriasis            (b)  Pemphigus
   (c)   Tinea            (d)  Pityriasis rubra
5. **"Oil drop sign" is seen in:**            *(AP 96)*
   (a)  Psoriasis            (b)  Lichen planus
   (c)  Clubbing            (d)  *T. unguium*
6. **Auspitz sign is seen in:**            *(PGI 93)*
   (a)  Psoriasis            (b)  Acanthosis nigricans
   (c)  Seborrheic dermatitis            (d)  Impetigo
7. **Pitting of nails is seen in:**            *(PGI 98)*
   (a)  Lichen planus            (b)  Psoriasis
   (c)  Pemphigus            (d)  Arsenic poisoning

8. **In psoriasis following are seen** *except:*
   - (a) Nail changes
   - (b) Arthritis
   - (c) CNS involvement
   - (d) Skin involvement

9. **Micro-Munro abscess is a feature of:** *(Kar 92)*
   - (a) Lichen planus
   - (b) Psoriasis
   - (c) Impetigo contagiosa
   - (d) Carbuncle

10. **A patient with psoriasis was on systemic steroid therapy. After stopping the Rx, he developed generalized pustules all over the body. The most likely cause:**
    - (a) Drug-induced reaction
    - (b) Pustular psoriasis
    - (c) Bacterial infection
    - (d) Septicemia

11. **Pustular psoriasis is most successfully managed using:**
    - (a) Coal tar with UV rays
    - (b) Corticosteroids
    - (c) Methotrexate
    - (d) Psoralen

12. **Calcipotriol is used in Rx of:** *(Manipal 01)*
    - (a) Lichen planus
    - (b) Psoriasis
    - (c) Acne vulgaris
    - (d) Erythema multiforme

13. **Psoralen UVA is used in Rx of:** *(AP 91)*
    - (a) Porphyria
    - (b) Psoriasis
    - (c) Pemphigus
    - (d) *Tinea versicolor*

14. **Photochemotherapy is used in Rx of:** *(AI 92)*
    - (a) Porphyria
    - (b) Psoriasis
    - (c) Pemphigus
    - (d) *Tinea versicolor*

15. **Nail changes are present in_____cases of psoriasis.** *(TN 2008)*
    - (a) All
    - (b) One-third
    - (c) One-half
    - (d) Two-thirds

16. **Köebner's phenomenon is seen in:** *(AI 90, SGPG 2002)*
    - (a) Lupus erythematosus
    - (b) Syphilis
    - (c) Lupus vulgaris
    - (d) Psoriasis

17. **Which of the following biologic agents approved for treatment of psoriasis or psoriatic arthritis is not anti-TNF-α?** *(JIPMER 2009)*
    - (a) Etanercept
    - (b) Alefacept
    - (c) Infliximab
    - (d) Adalimumab

18. **Micro-Munro abscess is:** *(PGI 99)*
    - (a) Dermal tissue
    - (b) Stratum basale
    - (c) Stratum corneum
    - (d) Stratum malpighi

19. **HPR findings seen in psoriasis are:** *(PGI 06)*
    - (a) Micro-Munro abscess
    - (b) Suprapapillary thinning
    - (c) Grenz zone
    - (d) Pautrier's abscess
    - (e) Hyperkeratosis

20. **DOC for pustular psoriasis is:**                    *(AIIMS 02)*
    (a) Thalidomide            (b) Retinoids
    (c) Hydroxyurea            (d) Methotrexate

21. **DOC for psoriatic arthropathy is:**              *(AIIMS 93)*
    (a) Methotrexate           (b) 5FU
    (c) PUVA                   (d) Steroid

22. **A 30-year-old male presented with silvery scales on elbow and knee, that bleed on removal. The probable diagnosis is:**
                                                        *(Orissa 08)*
    (a) Pityriasis             (b) Seborrheic dermatitis
    (c) Psoriasis              (d) Secondary syphilis

23. **Auspitz sign is seen in:**                  *(AIIMS May 2008)*
    (a) Plaque psoriasis       (b) Guttate psoriasis
    (c) Pustular psoriasis     (d) Erythrodermic psoriasis

24. **"Isomorphic response" can be a feature of the following diseases except:**                                    *(MH 2002)*
    (a) Warts                  (b) Tinea
    (c) Psoriasis              (d) Molluscum contagiosum

25. **Arthritis mutilans is a feature of:**              *(MH 2002)*
    (a) Lichen planus
    (b) Psoriasis
    (c) Staphylococcal scalded skin syndrome
    (d) Eczema

26. **Köebner's phenomenon is seen in the following except:** *(MH 2003)*
    (a) Psoriasis              (b) Warts
    (c) *Tinea corporis*       (d) Molluscum contagiosum

27. **Treatment of psoriasis includes the following except:** *(MH 2003)*
    (a) Retinoids              (b) Methotrexate
    (c) Cyclosporine           (d) Oral corticosteroids

28. **Psoriasis associated with β-hemolytic streptococcal infection:**
                                                        *(MH 2009)*
    (a) Psoriasis vulgaris     (b) Erythrodermic psoriasis
    (c) Pustular psoriasis     (d) Guttate psoriasis

29. **Which of the following is seen in psoriasis?**     *(PGI Dec 07)*
    (a) Pautrier's microabscess
    (b) Fused rete ridges
    (c) Grenz zone
    (d) Hyperkeratosis
    (e) Suprapapillary epidermal thinning

30. **HPR findings in psoriasis are:**                          *(PGI 06)*
    (a) Spongiform pustules of Kogoj
    (b) Parakeratosis
    (c) Max-Joseph's space
    (d) Koilocytosis
    (e) Hyperkeratosis
31. **Munro microabscess is noted in:**                         *(AI 91)*
    (a) Stratum malpighian          (b) Stratum granulosum
    (c) Stratum corneum             (d) Stratum basale
32. **Isomorphic response may be seen in:**                     *(DNB 09)*
    (a) Darier's disease            (b) Cutis mormorata
    (c) Pemphigus foliaceous        (d) Behçet's disease
33. **Following are causes of papulosquamous lesions** *except:*
                                      *(PGI 2000; SGPGI 02)*
    (a) Psoriasis                   (b) Parapsoriasis
    (c) Squamous cell carcinoma (d) Mycosis fungoides
    (e) Congenital syphilis
34. **An 8-year-old boy presents with multipe discrete, shiny, pinhead-sized papules/lesions on dorsal aspect of hand, forearm and penis. Likely diagnosis:**                      *(AIIMS May 2013)*
    (a) Scabies                     (b) Lichen planus
    (c) Lichen nitidus              (d) Molluscum contagiosum
35. **The first biologic agent approved by US FDA for the treatment of psoriasis is:**
    (a) Alefacept                   (b) Efalizumab
    (c) Etanercept                  (d) Infliximab
36. **Efalizumab disrupts the interaction between which of the following adhesion molecules?**
    (a) LFA-3 and ICAM-1            (b) LFA-1 and ICAM-1
    (c) LFA-3 and ICAM-3            (d) LFA-3 and CD2
37. **Which of the following biologic agents used for the treatment of psoriasis is not a TNF-α blocker?**
    (a) Etanercept                  (b) Infliximab
    (c) Adalimumab                  (d) Efalizumab
38. **The exclusion criteria for biologic therapy include all** *except:*
    (a) Active tuberculosis
    (b) Chronic hepatitis B and C
    (c) History of demyelinating disease
    (d) 50 treatments with PUV A

39. **CD4 count should be monitored weekly during therapy with:**
    - (a) Efalizumab
    - (b) Onercept
    - (c) Infliximab
    - (d) Alefacept

40. **Which of the following biologic agents is likely to cause thrombocytopenia during treatment?**
    - (a) Basiliximab
    - (b) Silplizumab
    - (c) Efalizumab
    - (d) Etanercept

41. **The adult dose of etanercept for psoriasis is:**
    - (a) 25 mg/week SC
    - (b) 50 mg/week SC
    - (c) 50 mg/week IM
    - (d) 100 mg/week SC

42. **Which of the following anti-TNF-α agents binds to both soluble and transmembrane bound forms of TNF-α?**
    - (a) Etanercept
    - (b) Infliximab
    - (c) Adalimumab
    - (d) Onercept

43. **Dissemination of the following fungal infection has been observed with etanercept:**
    - (a) Candidiasis
    - (b) Histoplasmosis
    - (c) Blastomycosis
    - (d) Sporotrichosis

44. **Max-Joseph's space is a histopathological feature of:**

    *(AIIMS May 2006)*
    - (a) Psoriasis
    - (b) Lichen planus
    - (c) Pityriasis rosea
    - (d) Parapsoriasis

45. **Degeneration of basal cells occurs in:**    *(PGI 2002)*
    - (a) Lichen planus
    - (b) Pemphigus
    - (c) Psoriasis
    - (d) DLE

46. **Koebner's phenomenon is seen in:**    *(AI 92)*
    - (a) Pemphigus
    - (b) Darrier's disease
    - (c) Lichen planus
    - (d) Psoriasis

47. **Köebner's phenomenon is seen in:**    *(PGI 04)*
    - (a) Lichen planus
    - (b) Warts
    - (c) Behçet's disease
    - (d) Psoriasis
    - (e) Vitiligo

48. **Itchy polygonal violaceous papules are seen in:**    *(AI 98)*
    - (a) Pemphigus
    - (b) Pityriasis rosea
    - (c) Lichen planus
    - (d) Psoriasis

49. **Wickham's striae are seen in:**    *(AI 02)*
    - (a) Bullous pemphigoid
    - (b) Pemphigus vulgaris
    - (c) Lichen planus
    - (d) Psoriasis

50. **Characteristic nail finding in lichen planus:**
(*AIIMS 01; AI 06; NEET 2012*)
(a) Thimble pitting          (b) Pterygium
(c) Beau's lines             (d) Hyperpigmentation of nails

51. **A 10-year-old child has violaceous papules and pterygium of nails. Diagnosis is:** (*AIIMS 99*)
(a) Pemphigus               (b) Pityriasis rosea
(c) Psoriasis               (d) Lichen planus

52. **Rx of choice for lichen planus:** (*AIIMS 01*)
(a) Topical salicylic acid   (b) UV rays
(c) Systemic steroids        (d) Erythromycin

53. **Oral lesions are seen in:** (*AI 94*)
(a) Psoriasis               (b) Lichen planus
(c) Basal cell carcinoma     (d) Ichthyosis vulgaris

54. **Lichen planus is associated with:**
(a) Hepatitis A              (b) Hepatitis B
(c) Hepatitis C              (d) Hepatitis D

55. **True about *lichen planus* is:** (*PGI 04*)
(a) Basal cell degeneration
(b) Colloid bodies
(c) Epidermal hyperplasia in chronic cases
(d) Wickham's striae
(e) Autoimmune disease

56. **True about *lichen planus* is:** (*PGI 04*)
(a) Thinning of nail plate is most common
(b) Nonscarring alopecia
(c) Violaceous lesions on skin and mucous membrane
(d) Wickham's striae

57. **A patient presented with scarring alopecia, thinned nails, hypopigmented macular lesions over the trunk and oral mucosa. Diagnosis is:** (*AIIMS 01*)
(a) Psoriasis               (b) Leprosy
(c) Lichen planus           (d) Pemphigus

58. **Civatte bodies are found in:** (*Kerala 98*)
(a) Lichen planus           (b) Psoriasis
(c) Dermatophytosis         (d) Vitiligo

59. **Lacy-White lesions in mouth with pterygium are seen in:**
(*SGPGI 01*)
(a) Psoriasis               (b) Pityriasis alba
(c) Lichen planus           (d) Leprosy

60. **All of the following regarding** *lichen planus* **is true** *except:*
    *(MP 05)*
    (a) Does not involve mucous membrane
    (b) Associated with hepatitis C
    (c) Topical steroids are mainstay of Rx
    (d) Spontaneous remissions occur in 6 months–2 yrs

61. **All the following are true about lichen planus** *except*: *(AI 2000)*
    (a) Hypopigmentation is residual disease
    (b) Lymphatic infiltration in supradermal layer
    (c) Itchy polygonal purple papules
    (d) Skin, hair, and oral mucosa commonly involved

62. **PUVA therapy is useful in** *Rx* **of:**    *(Kar 94)*
    (a) Lichen planus          (b) Pemphighus
    (c) Leprosy               (d) All of the above

63. **Lichenoid drug eruption can be caused by the following** *except:*    *(Bihar 07)*
    (a) Frusemide             (b) Gold
    (c) Antimalarials         (d) Captopril

64. **The most characteristic feature of lichen planus is:**    *(PGI 08)*
    (a) Civatte bodies        (b) Basal cell degeneration
    (c) Thinning of nail plate (d) Violaceous lesions

65. **The earliest histological finding in lichen planus is:**    *(PGI 09)*
    (a) Colloid bodies
    (b) Max-Joseph's spaces
    (c) Flattened rete ridges
    (d) Focal increase in thickness of the granular layer
    (e) Increase in epidermal Langerhans' cells with perivascular infiltrate.

## Answers

1. **Ans. (a)** β-blockers *(Ref. Rook's Textbook of Dermatology, 7th edn/35.3)*
2. **Ans. (b)** Streptococcal infection *(Ref. Rook's Textbook of Dermatology, 7th edn/35.11)*
3. **Ans. (b)** Scaling. *(Ref. Rook's Textbook of Dermatology, 7th edn/35.10; Harrison, 17th edn / Table 53–2)*
4. **Ans. (a)** Psoriasis *(Ref. Rook's Textbook of Dermatology, 7th edn/35.10)*
5. **Ans. (a)** Psoriasis *(Ref. Rook's Textbook of Dermatology, 7th edn/35.15)*
6. **Ans. (a)** Psoriasis *(Ref. IDVL Textbook of Dermatology, 2nd edn/ 817)*
7. **Ans. (b)** Psoriasis *(Ref. Rook's Textbook of Dermatology, 7th edn/ 35.15)*

8. **Ans. (c)** CNS involvement *(Ref. Rook's Textbook of Dermatology, 7th edn/35.51, 56; 35.60)*

9. **Ans. (b)** Psoriasis *(Ref. Rook's Textbook of Dermatology, 7th edn/35.8; 35.9)*

10. **Ans. (b)** Pustular psoriasis *(Ref. Rook's Textbook of Dermatology, 7th edn/35.51, 56; 35.60)*

11. **Ans. (c)** Methotrexate *(Ref. Rook's Textbook of Dermatology, 7th edn/ 35.51, 35.56, 35.60)*

12. **Ans. (b)** Psoriasis *(Ref. Rook's Textbook of Dermatology, 7th edn/35.26)*

13. **Ans. (b)** Psoriasis *(Ref. Rook's tTextbook of Dermatology, 7th edn/35.31)*

14. **Ans. (b)** Psoriasis *(Ref. Rook's Textbook of Dermatology, 7th edn/35.31)*

15. **Ans. (c)** One half cases *(Ref. Rook's Textbook of Dermatology, 7th edn/35.15)*

16. **Ans. (d)** Psoriasis *(Ref. Rook's Textbook of Dermatology, 7th edn/35.8)*

17. **Ans. (b)** Alefacept *(Ref. Harrison's Medicine, 17th edn / Table 53–4)*

18. **Ans. (c)** Stratum corneum *(Ref. Rook's Textbook of Dermatology, 7th edn/35.8–35.9)*

19. **Ans. (a, b, e)** *(Ref. Rook's Textbook of Dermatology, 7th edn/35.8–35.9)*

20. **Ans. (b)** Retinoids *(Ref. Rook's Textbook of Dermatology, 7th edn/35. 48–35.63)*

21. **Ans. (a)** Methotrexate *(Ref. Rook's Textbook of Dermatology, 7th edn/35.1–35.63)*

22. **Ans. (c)** Psoriasis *(Ref. Pasricha, 3rd edn/ 97–99)*

23. **Ans. (a)** Plaque psoriasis

24. **Ans. (b)** Tinea

25. **Ans. (b)** Psoriasis

26. **Ans. (c)** *Tinea corporis (Ref. Harrison's Principles of Internal Medicine, 17th edn, 311)*

27. **Ans. (d)** Oral corticosteroids

28. **Ans. (d)** Guttate psoriasis *(Ref. IADVL Dermatology, 2nd edn/818; Harrison's Medicine, 17th edn/Ch 53)*

29. **Ans. (b, d, e)** *(Ref. Rook's Dermatology, 7th edn/35.8)*

30. **Ans. (a, b, c)** *(Ref. Rook's Dermatology 7th edn/35.8)*

31. **Ans. (c)** Stratum corneum *(Ref. Roxburgh's Dermatology, 17th edn/ 136)*

32. **Ans. (a)** Darier's disease *(Ref. Rook's Dermatology, 7th edn/22.3; Table 22.1)*

33. **Ans. (e)** Congenital syphilis *(Ref. Rook's Textbook of Dermatology, 7th edn/35.10; Table 53–2)*

34. **Ans. (c)** Lichen nitidus *(Ref. Rook's Textbook of Dermatology, 8th edn/41.21; IADVL, 3rd edn/pg. 1081)*
35. **Ans. (a)** Alefacept
36. **Ans. (b)** LFA-1 and ICAM-1
37. **Ans. (d)** Efalizumab
38. **Ans. (d)** 50 treatments with PUVA
39. **Ans. (d)** Alefacept
40. **Ans. (c)** Efalizumab
41. **Ans. (b)** 50 mg/week SC
42. **Ans. (b)** Infliximab
43. **Ans. (b)** Histoplasmosis
44. **Ans. (b)** Lichen planus *(Ref. IADVL, 2nd edn/850)*
45. **Ans. (a)** Lichen planus *(Ref. IADVL, 2nd edn/850; 955)*
46. **Ans. (c)** Lichen planus *(Ref. Pasricha, 4th edn/184–189)*
47. **Ans. (a, b, d, e)** *(Ref. Pasricha, 4th edn/184–189)*
48. **Ans. (c)** Lichen planus *(Ref. IADVL, 2nd edn/847)*
49. **Ans. (c)** Lichen planus *(Ref. IADVL, 2nd edn/847)*
50. **Ans. (b)** Pterygium *(Ref. IADVL, 2nd edn/849)*
51. **Ans. (d)** Lichen planus *(Ref. Rook's Dermatology, 7th edn/ 41.13)*
52. **Ans. (c)** Systemic steroids *(Ref. IADVL, 2nd edn/852)*
53. **Ans. (b)** Lichen planus *(Ref. IADVL, 2nd edn/848)*
54. **Ans. (c)** Hepatitis C *(Ref. IADVL, 2nd edn/849)*
55. **Ans. (a, b, c, d, e)** *(Ref. IADVL, 2nd edn/850)*
56. **Ans. (d)** Wickham's striae *(Ref. IADVL, 2nd edn/850; 955)*
57. **Ans. (c)** Lichen planus *(Ref. Roxburgh's Common Skin Diseases, 17th edn/274–278)*
58. **Ans. (c)** Dermatophytosis *(Ref. Rook's Dermatology, 7th edn/42. 1–42.14)*
59. **Ans. (a)** Psoriasis *(Ref. Rook's Dermatology, 7th edn/42. 1–42.14)*
60. **Ans. (a)** Does not involve mucous membrane *(Ref. Rook's Dermatology, 7th edn/42. 1–42.14)*
61. **Ans. (a)** Hypopigmentation in residual disease *(Ref. Rook's Dermatology, 7th edn/42. 1–42.14)*
62. **Ans. (a)** Lichen planus and **(b)** pemphighus *(Ref. Rook's Dermatology, 7th edn/35. 1–35.63)*
63. **Ans. (a)** Frusemide
64. **Ans. (b)** Basal cell degeneration *(Ref. Rook's Dermatology, 7th edn/7.40)*
65. **Ans. (e)** Increase in epidermal Langerhans' cells with perivascular infiltrate *(Ref. Rook's Dermatology, 7th edn/ 42.3)*.

# 8 Ichthyosis and Other Disorders of Keratinization

## ICHTHYOSIS

- Ichthyosis describes dry, rough skin with scaling over much of the body (Greek ichthys/ikhthus, fishosis).
- Congenital and acquired ichthyoses.
  - ➤ **Congenital ichthyoses**
    - Ichthyosis vulgaris (syn. autosomal dominant ichthyosis)
    - X-linked recessive ichthyosis (steroid sulphatase deficiency)
    - Non-bullous ichthyosiform erythroderma
    - Lamellar ichthyosis
    - Harlequin ichthyosis
    - Bullous ichthyosiform erythroderma (syn. epidermolytic hyperkeratosis)
    - Ichthyosis bullosa of Siemens
    - Ichthyosis hystrix
  - ➤ **Ichthyosiform syndromes**
    - Netherton's syndrome (syn. ichthyosis linearis circumflexa)
    - Sjögren-Larsson syndrome
    - Neutral lipid storage disease (syn. Chanarin–Dorfman syndrome)
    - Refsum's disease
    - Kallmann's syndrome
    - Multiple sulphatase deficiency syndrome
    - X-linked dominant ichthyosis (syn. Conradi-Hünermann-Happle syndrome)
    - IBIDS (syn. Tay syndrome, trichothiodystrophy, PIBIDS)
    - KID syndrome (keratitis, ichthyosis, deafness)
    - CHILD syndrome (congenital hemidysplasia, ichthyosiform erythroderma, unilateral limb defects)

- – Ichthyosis follicularis with alopecia and photophobia (IFAP)
- – Neu-Laxova syndrome
> **Acquired ichthyosis**

## Ichthyosis Vulgaris

- Most common
- Autosomal dominant
- At birth skin may appear normal
- Skin gradually becomes dry, rough and scaly, with most signs and symptoms appearing by the age of 5
- The scale is white or grey, small, flaky or branny, and semi-adherent with turned-up edges
- Most pronounced on the extensor surfaces of arms and lower legs (Fig. 8.1)
- Flexures are  usually spared
- Hyperlinearity of palms and soles
- Associated with atopic dermatitis and keratosis pilaris
- Improvement with warm and sunny weather
- Gradually improves by adolescence
- Filaggrin synthesis is defective.

## Lamellar Ichthyosis

- Collodion baby  at birth—baby is covered by a thickened collodion-like membrane which is then shed.
- Scaling occurs over the whole body, including creases and bends.
- The scale in LI is typically large, dark brown or grey and firmly adherent.

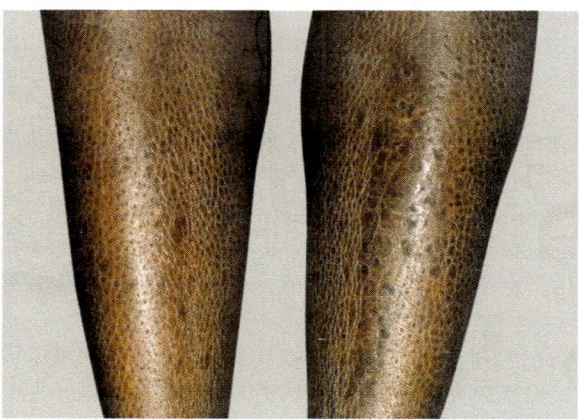

**Fig. 8.1:** Dry scaly skin over anterior aspect of legs

- Drooping of lower eyelids (ectropion), palmoplantar keratoderma and scarring alopecia may be seen.
- Limitation of joint movement, flexion contractures and digital sclerodactyly may result.
- Nails may be small but hair shaft, mucous membranes and teeth are not affected.
- May be associated with mutation in transglutaminase 1 gene.

## Epidermolytic Hyperkeratosis

- Autosomal dominant
- Previously called 'Bullous ichthyosiform erythroderma'
- Skin is moist, red, and tender at birth
- Fluid filled flaccid blisters, peeling, superficial erosions at the sites of trauma and friction may be seen within a few hours of life.
- Increasing hyperkeratosis is obvious from early childhood and is most prominent around the anterior neck, flexures, abdominal wall, infragluteal folds and scalp.
- Yellow–brown, waxy, ridged or corrugated scale builds up in skin creases, sometimes forming spiny (hystrix) outgrowths.
- Palmoplantar hyperkeratosis may be seen which results in painful fissures, contractures and sclerodactyly.
- Pathology shows epidermolytic hyperkeratosis.

## Nonbullous Congenital Ichthyosiform Erythroderma

- Severe autosomal recessive inflammatory ichthyosis.
- Presents at birth with collodion baby appearance.
- Generalized scaly erythroderma is apparent after shedding of collodion membrane.
- Typically, scaling affects all areas including the scalp, ears, face, flexures, palms and soles. The scale of NBIE is white or grey, thin superficial and semi-adherent (Fig. 8.2).
- It appears feathery on the face, arms and trunk but may become lamellar or plate-like on the lower legs.
- Palmoplantar keratoderma occurs in up to 70% of patients, and can cause recurrent painful fissures, digital contractures and sclerodactyly.
- Scalp involvement may lead to *tinea amiantacea* and patchy cicatricial alopecia, especially on the temporal scalp.
- Ectropion and dystrophy of nails is common
- Hair, teeth and mucous membranes are normal

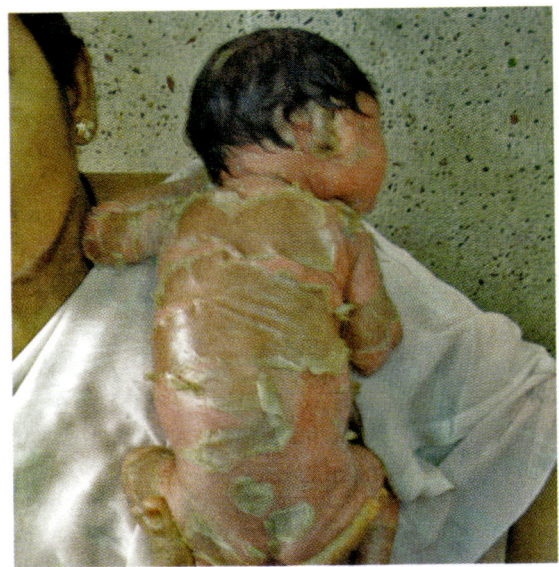

**Fig. 8.2:** Generalized erythematous scaling of skin with involvement of scalp

### X-linked Ichthyosis

- X-linked recessive
- Occurs in males. Females may be heterozygotes
- Generalized scaling is present at or shortly after birth
- Scaling is most prominent over the extremities, neck, trunk, and buttocks
- Typically, the scale is medium to large, polygonal, adherent, dull and light to dark brown, depending on skin type
- Flexures are involved
- Associated with steroid sulphatase deficiency in fibroblasts and elevated plasma cholesterol sulphate
- May be associated with testicular disease (cryptorchidism and testicular cancer)
- Corneal opacities detected by slit-lamp examination are seen/can be seen in female carriers also.

### *Ichthyosis Treatment*

- Liberal use of emollients (containing urea and lactic acid)
- Avoid excess use of soap
- Keratolytics
- Oral retinoids in severe cases.

## Acquired Ichthyosis

- Sudden onset of ichthyosis similar to the pattern of ichthyosis vulgaris in adult life.
- Does appear to be associated with internal malignancy and particularly lymphoreticular tumors?
- The most commonly reported malignancy that produces ichthyosis is Hodgkin's disease. Ichthyosis has also been reported in association with non-Hodgkin's lymphoma, mycosis fungoides, multiple myeloma, carcinoma of breast, lung, cervix and liver, leiomyosarcoma and Kaposi's sarcoma.
- The acquired change should not be confused with asteatosis, which of course is a common problem in elderly people.
- Acquired ichthyosiform changes can be a manifestation of other systemic disorders, including:
  - ➢ Nutritional deficiencies
  - ➢ Sarcoidosis
  - ➢ Leprosy
  - ➢ Lupus erythematosus
  - ➢ Drugs (e.g. nicotinic acid, hypocholesterolemic agents, maprotiline)
  - ➢ Chronic hepatic disease, renal failure, thyroid and parathyroid disease
  - ➢ Acquired immune deficiency syndrome

## Ichthyosiform Syndromes

- Ichthyosis may be part of a more widespread congenital abnormality (all very rare) as in the following syndromes:
  - ➢ KID (keratitis, ichthyosis, and deafness)
  - ➢ CHIME (colobomas of the eye, heart defects, ichthyosiform dermatosis, mental retardation, and ear defects)
  - ➢ Netherton sydrome (ichthyosis, erythroderma, hair shaft defects, atopic features)
  - ➢ Sjögren-Larsson (ichthyosis, spastic diplegia, pigmentary retinopathy, and mental retardation)
  - ➢ Refsum's disease (ichthyosis and pigmentary retinopathy).

## *Pityriasis Rotunda*

A fixed, annular, scaling, dry-skin change more often seen in the African and Asian races It has been associated with neoplasia, particularly hepatocellular carcinoma. However, it may also be seen in other systemic diseases and in leprosy.

## DARIER'S DISEASE/KERATOSIS FOLLICULARIS

- Autosomal dominant
- Mutations in the gene which encodes sarco-/endoplasmic reticulum calcium ATPase type 2.
- The distinctive lesion of Darier's disease is a firm, rough papule, which is skin-colored, yellow–brown or brown.
- Seborrheic areas of the trunk and face, particularly the scalp margins, temples, ears and scalp, are most often involved (Fig. 8.3).
- On the dorsa of the hands and feet, discrete papules are clinically indistinguishable from acrokeratosis verruciformis of Hopf .
- In Darier's disease, characteristic nail changes include red or white longitudinal bands of varying width, often ending in a patho-gnomonic notch at the free margin of the nail.
- Palms and soles show minute pits
- Mucous membranes may be involved. Cobblestone papules are seen on the palate.
- Rash is exacerbated by heat and light
- Increased incidence of infections. Kaposi's varicelliform eruption is common.
- **HPE:** Suprabasal clefting with acantholytic dyskeratotic keratinocytes termed corps ronds are seen.
- **Treatment:** Topical and oral retinoids.

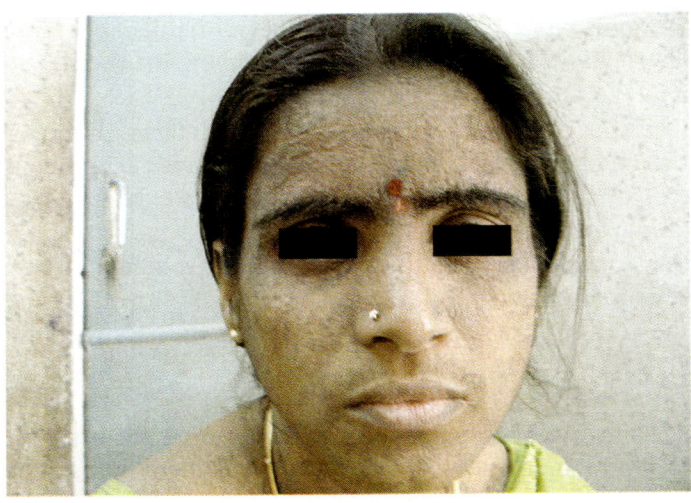

**Fig. 8.3:** Involvement of seborrheic areas of face in Darier's disease

## POROKERATOSES

- Autosomal dominant
- **Disseminated forms**
  - ➢ *Disseminated superficial actinic porokeratosis* (DSAP) is the most common presentation, with many lesions of up to 10 mm predominantly in sun-exposed sites in middle-aged individuals, especially those with sun-sensitive skin.
  - ➢ *Disseminated superficial porokeratoses of immunosuppression* are recognized after renal, hepatic, cardiac and bone marrow transplantation, and in AIDS.
  - ➢ *Disseminated superficial porokeratosis of childhood* may be inherited as an autosomal dominant condition, but sporadic cases are seen. Widely disseminated, flat lesions usually begin in childhood, the majority between the ages of 5 and 10 years, but may be present at birth or may first appear at puberty or later.
- **Porokeratosis of Mibelli:** Refers only to the form with single or scanty and larger lesions. These develop as annular dry plaques surrounded by a raised, fine keratotic wall and sometimes also a furrow (Fig. 8.4). Lesions are most common on the limbs. The center is usually atrophic but may be hyperkeratotic.
- **Giant porokeratoses:** Up to 20 cm in diameter with a surrounding wall of 1 cm.
- **Linear porokeratosis:** Linear porokeratoses showing typical cornoid lamellae and following the lines of Blaschko usually appear in childhood.
- **HPE:** Cornoid lamella is the characteristic feature.
- **Treatment:** Cryotherapy, $CO_2$ laser, pulsed dye laser, photodynamic therapy, topical 5-fluorouracil and imiquimod, oral etretinate.

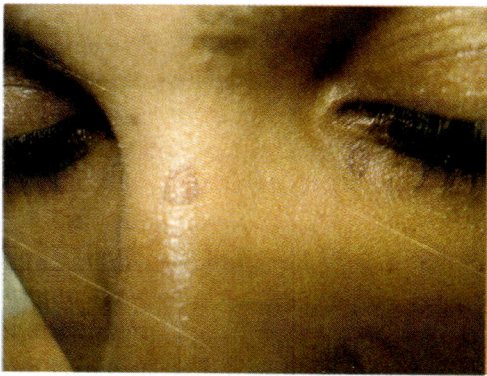

**Fig. 8.4:** Annular plaque over face of young female

## ACANTHOSIS NIGRICANS

- Acanthosis nigricans is characterized by asymptomatic brown to black, poorly defined, velvety hyperpigmentation of the skin. It is usually found in body folds, such as the posterior and lateral folds of the neck, the axilla, groin, umbilicus, forehead, and other areas.

- **Causes**
  - ➤ *Inherited forms of acanthosis nigricans*
    - – In isolation may be inherited as autosomal dominant trait.
    - – Also seen in leprachaunism, lipodystrophies, Rabson-Mendenhall syndrome
  - ➤ *Benign acquired acanthosis nigricans*
    - – Seen in obesity, diabetes mellitus and other conditions with insulin resistance like polycystic ovarian syndrome
  - ➤ *Associated with endocrinopathies*
    - – Acromegaly
    - – Cushing's syndrome
  - ➤ *Malignant*
    - – When seen in individuals older than age 40, this disorder is commonly associated with an internal malignancy, usually adenocarcinoma, and most commonly of the GI tract or uterus; less commonly of the lung, prostate, breast, or ovary. Acanthosis nigricans of the oral mucosa or tongue is highly suggestive of a neoplasm, especially of the GI tract.
  - ➤ *Drug induced*
    - – Triazinate, oral contraceptives, nicotinic acid, and fusidic acid.
  - ➤ *HPE*
    - – Typically demonstrates papillomatosis and hyperkeratosis.
    - – Despite the term "acanthosis," the actual amount of acanthosis is typically mild.
    - – The dark color of AN is likely due to hyperkeratosis rather than to a mild increase in melanin pigmentation.
    - – A subtle infiltrate composed of lymphocytes, plasma cells, or neutrophils may be present, as well as horn pseudocyst formation.

- **Management**
  - ➤ Underlying cause should be treated. Topical retinoids, dermabrasion and lasers may be used.

## QUESTIONS FROM PREVIOUS EXAMINATIONS

1. Harlequin fetus
2. Darier's disease
3. Acanthosis nigricans
4. Porokeratosis
5. Icthyosiform syndromes
6. Icthyosis vulgaris
7. Lamellar icthyosis

## MULTIPLE CHOICE QUESTIONS

1. **Disorder of hyperkeratinization:**           *(WB 2009)*
   (a) Icthyosis vulgaris        (b) Psoriasis
   (c) Atopic dermatitis         (d) Seborrheic dermatitis
2. **Parakeratosis involves in which layer?**     *(Kerala 2008)*
   (a) Stratum basale            (b) Stratum spinosum
   (c) Stratum granulosum        (d) Stratum lucidum
   (e) Startum corneum
3. **In which of the following conditions parakeratosis most frequently occurs?**     *(AI 2006)*
   (a) Actinic keratoses         (b) Seborrheic keratoses
   (c) Molluscum contagiosum     (d) Basal cell carcinoma
4. **The most common malignancy that produces ichthyosis:**
   *(AMU 2007)*
   (a) Hodgkin's disease         (b) Mycosis fungoides
   (c) Kaposi's sarcoma          (d) Carcinoma breast
5. **Ichthyosis is caused by:**                   *(NIMHANS 01)*
   (a) Hemosiderosis             (b) Refsum's disease
   (c) Niacin deficiency         (d) Stevens-Johnson syndrome

### Answers

1. **Ans. (a)** Icthyosis vulgaris *(Ref. Robbin's Pathology, 8th edn, 838; Rook's Dermatology, 4th edn, 34.52)*
2. **Ans. (e)** Startum corneum *(Ref. Robbin's Pathology, 8th edn, 838; Rook's Dermatology, 4th edn, 34.52)*
3. **Ans. (a)** Actinic keratoses *(Ref. Roxburgh's Dermatology, 17th edn, 136; Robbin's Pathology, 7th edn, 791, 794, 800)*
4. **Ans. (a)** Hodgkin's disease *(Ref. Rook's Dermatology, 7th end, 34.52)*
5. **Ans. (b)** Refsum's disease.

# 9    Pigmentary Disorders

- Disorders of melanin pigmentation can be divided on morphological grounds into two types:
  - *The first type* is hypermelanosis, where there is an increased amount of melanin in the skin. This excess may be confined to the epidermis, when the skin appears browner than normal, or it may be present in the dermis, producing a slaty grey or blue appearance.
  - *The second type* is hypomelanosis, where there is a lack of pigment in the skin, which therefore appears white or lighter than the normal color.
- Amelanosis is the term applied when there is a total lack of melanin in the skin.
- Hypermelanosis and hypomelanosis can be generalized and diffuse, or may be localized and circumscribed.

## CAUSES OF HYPOPIGMENTATION IN A PIGMENTED SKIN

- Congenital or genetic
  - Albinism, piebaldism
- Infections
  - Leprosy, onchocerciasis, pinta, pityriasis versicolor, herpes zoster
- Papulosquamous disorders
  - Pityriasis alba, pityriasis rosea, pityriasis lichenoides chronica, psoriasis, seborrheic dermatitis
- Physical or chemical agents
  - Burns, cryotherapy, ammoniated mercury, hydroquinone products, fluorinated corticosteroids
- Postinflammatory
  - Discoid lupus erythematosus, systemic sclerosis, sarcoidosis, some eczematous eruptions
- Miscellaneous
  - Vitiligo, idiopathic guttate hypomelanosis

## Vitiligo

- An acquired depigmentary disorder of skin.
- Derived from Greek word *vitelius,* meaning calf.
- Worldwide, it affects people of all races regardless of gender with an incidence rate of 1 to 2%.
- Appears at any age; roughly half of cases begin before the age of 20.
- **Etiology**
  - ➤ The cause is unknown; however, several hypotheses have been postulated.
  - ➤ A hereditary predisposition because up to 38% of people with vitiligo report a family history.
  - ➤ An autoimmune process in which there is immunologic destruction of the melanocytes because the disorder often accompanies other autoimmune diseases, such as diabetes mellitus and pernicious anemia.
  - ➤ Neural mechanisms in which the melanocytes are destroyed by a cytotoxic chemical secreted by nearby nerve endings.
  - ➤ A self-destruct phenomenon in which the melanocytes are preprogrammed for self-destruction.
  - ➤ A lack of melanocyte growth factors
- In some cases, vitiligo has been reportedly precipitated by emotional stress or physical trauma, such as sunburn.
- **HPE:** There is a marked absence of melanocytes and melanin in the epidermis. Histochemical studies show a lack of dopa positive melanocytes in the basal layer of the epidermis.
- Hypomelanotic macules are usually first noted on the sun-exposed areas of skin, on the face or on the dorsa of hands.
- Damage to the 'normal' skin frequently results in an area of depigmentation—an isomorphic or Köebner's phenomenon.
- The pigment loss may be partial or complete, or both may occur in the same areas (trichrome vitiligo).
- The macules are round or oval, milky white and of variable size. The macules have a convex outline, increase irregularly in size and fuse with neighboring lesions to form complex patterns. The hairs in the patches frequently remain normally pigmented, but in older lesions the hairs too are often amelanotic.
- The margins of the lesion may be hyperpigmented.

  Spontaneous repigmentation may be seen in 20% of patients. It is perifollicular.

- **Classification**
  - ➤ *Localized vitiligo*
    - Focal vitiligo—one or two lesions
    - Segmental vitiligo—distributed along the dermatome
  - ➤ *Generalized vitiligo*
    - *Vitiligo vulgaris:* Common type. Symmetrical widespread macules over limbs and trunk
    - *Acrofacial vitiligo:* Face and acral areas are affected.
    - *Lip-tip vitiligo:* Tips of fingers and toes are involved along with mucosal surface of lips.
    - *Universal vitiligo:* A few areas are spared, almost whole of the body is involved.
- Diagnosis of vitiligo is mainly clinical.
- **Diseases associated with vitiligo**
  - ➤ Thyroid disease
    - Hyperthyroidism
    - Hypothyroidism
  - ➤ Pernicious anemia
  - ➤ Addison's disease
  - ➤ Diabetes mellitus
  - ➤ Hypoparathyroidism
  - ➤ Myasthenia gravis
  - ➤ Alopecia areata
  - ➤ Morphea and lichen sclerosus
  - ➤ Halo nevus
  - ➤ Malignant melanoma
- **Treatment**
  - ➤ Corticosteroids administered topically, intralesionally, and orally have been used successfully.
  - ➤ Broad (large area) and narrow band (focused) UV B has also been used successfully in the treatment of vitiligo.
  - ➤ The combination of psoralens like 8 methoxy psoralen, 5 methoxy psoralen and trimethyl psoralen and UVA (PUVA) treatment has also been successful in some people with large areas of skin involvement. PUVA can be used topically or systemically.
  - ➤ A variety of skin-grafting techniques have been used in persons unresponsive to other therapies. Successful skin-grafting techniques include punch grafting, suction blister grafting, partial split thickness grafting or cultured melanocyte grafting.

➤ Micropigmentation (tattooing) has been done on smaller, recalcitrant areas, but it is often difficult to attain a correct color match.

➤ If extensive skin surfaces are involved, the treatment may be reversed and the pigmented areas bleached to match the remainder of the skin color using 20% monobenzyl ether of hydroquinone.

## Piebaldism

- It is a rare autosomal dominant disorder of melanocyte development.
- Affects both the sexes and all races.
- Piebaldism is due to an absence of melanocytes in affected skin and hair follicles as a result of mutations of the KIT proto-oncogene.
- Patches of skin totally devoid of pigment are present at birth and usually remain unchanged throughout life.
- Most common is a frontal median or paramedian patch, associated with a mesh of white hair (white forelock).
- White patches occur on the upper chest, abdomen and limbs, bilaterally but not necessarily symmetrically.
- Islands of normal or hypermelanotic skin occur in the white areas, or less often on normal skin.
- **Treatment:** Photoprotective preparations should be prescribed. Cosmetic camouflage can be used. Surgical techniques like punch grafts and autologous cultured melanocytes can be tried.

## Albinism

- Oculocutaneous albinism—partial or complete failure to produce melanin in the skin and eyes.
- Melanocytes are present in normal distribution but fail to synthesize melanin adequately.
- **AR inheritance**
    - ➤ *Tyrosinase positive:* The most frequent variant; complete at first, later small amount of melanin is formed.
    - ➤ *Tyrosinase negative:* Complete albinism
- There is marked dilution of the pigmentation of the skin, hair and eyes. In tyrosinase negative OCA, the skin is pink in color, the hair is white and the patients show a prominent red reflex. This is the most severe variant of OCA.
- In tyrosinase positive OCA, some pigment is formed and with increasing age is to be found in the iris, skin and hair, the latter often developing a flaxen-yellow color.

- In both types, patients have photophobia; often they have a characteristic facial expression due to apparent squinting. Errors of refraction are common, especially in the tyrosinase negative. Nystagmus is seen.
- Actinic keratoses, squamous cell carcinomas and occasionally melanomas appear on sun-exposed areas of the body. This may lead to early deaths.
- **Treatment:** Strict photoprotection. Regular screening for malignancies.

## Waardenburg's Syndrome

- Autosomal dominant
- Global disorder of neural crest development.
- Characterized by lateral displacement of the inner canthi and the lacrimal puncta, prominent nasal root and medial eyebrows, congenital deafness and heterochromic irides.
- Other pigmentary changes are a 'dappled' appearance of the skin, a white forelock, and premature greying of hair, eyebrows and cilia.
- A few patients show piebaldism.

## Nevus Achromicus

- This circumscribed area of depigmentation is congenital, but may not be apparent at birth.
- There are three clinical variants; the commonest is the single, circumscribed, rounded lesion.
- Segmental and systematized forms are very rare, and may resemble hypomelanosis of Ito.
- Lesions occur most commonly on the trunk. Hair within the depigmented macules are usually depigmented.
- Histology may show either normal or reduced numbers of melanocytes.
- A functional defect in melanocytes, with morphological abnormalities of melanosomes, has been identified.

## Nevus Anemicus (NA)

- Naevus anaemicus is a congenital anomaly of the skin, characterized by macular areas of pallor having a normal texture and normal melanin pigmentation, due to reduced blood flow.
- It is a congenital localized cutaneous anomaly most often seen on the trunk.
- It represents a pale-colored irregularly shaped patch of histologically normal-appearing skin in which the pharmacological

response to certain mediators may be aberrant, with sympathetic vasoconstriction likely responsible for the pallor.

- Hence, it has been called a **pharmacological nevus**.
- It may be linked with certain genodermatoses, including neurofibromatosis and phakomatosis pigmentovascularis.
- Treatment is generally not required.

## CAUSES OF HYPERPIGMENTATION

### I. Primary cutaneous disorders

A. *Localized*

1. Epidermal alteration
   a. Seborrheic keratosis
   b. Acanthosis nigricans (obesity)
   c. Pigmented actinic keratosis
2. Proliferation of melanocytes
   a. Lentigo
   b. Nevus
   c. Melanoma
3. Increased pigment production
   a. Ephelides (freckles)
   b. Café au lait macule
   c. Post-inflammatory hyperpigmentation

B. *Localized and diffuse*
   Drugs

### II. Systemic diseases

A. *Localized*

1. Epidermal alteration
   a. Seborrheic keratoses (sign of Leser-Trélat)
   b. Acanthosis nigricans (endocrine disorders, paraneoplastic)
2. Proliferation of melanocytes
   a. Lentigines (Peutz-Jeghers and LEOPARD syndromes; xeroderma pigmentosum)
   b. Nevi [Carney complex (LAMB and NAME syndromes)]
3. Increased pigment production
   a. Café au lait macules (neurofibromatosis, McCune-Albright syndrome)
   b. Urticaria pigmentosa
4. Dermal pigmentation
   a. Incontinentia pigmenti (stage III)
   b. Dyskeratosis congenital

**B. Diffuse**
1. Endocrinopathies
   a. Addison's disease
   b. Nelson syndrome
   c. Ectopic ACTH syndrome
2. Metabolic
   a. Porphyria cutanea tarda
   b. Hemochromatosis
   c. Vitamin $B_{12}$, folate deficiency
   d. Pellagra
   e. Malabsorption, Whipple's disease
3. Melanosis secondary to metastatic melanoma
4. Autoimmune
   a. Biliary cirrhosis
   b. Scleroderma
   c. POEMS syndrome
   d. Eosinophilia—myalgia syndrome
5. Drugs and metals

### Freckles/Ephelides

Autosomal dominant
Common in individuals with red or blonde hair and blue eyes.
- Freckles are small macules of hyperpigmentation, usually measuring 2–4 mm in size.
- They first appear at about the age of 5 years as light-brown pigmented macules on light-exposed skin.
- They are most numerous on the face, upper back, and dorsal forearms and hands.
- They increase in number, size and depth of pigmentation during the summer months and are smaller, lighter and fewer in number in the winter.
- **HPE:** No increase in number of melanocytes but melanosomes are long and rod shaped.
- Cosmetic concern
- Also seen in xeroderma pigmentosum, neurofibromatosis, Moynahan's syndrome and progeria.
  **Treatment:** 2–4% hydroquinone. Regular use of sunscreens.

### Lentigo
- Macular hyperpigmented lesions as a result of proliferation of melanocytes at the dermoepidermal junction without evidence of proliferation downwards into the dermis.

- Common in fairskinned individuals.
- A lentigo is a macular area of brown or brownblack pigmentation, usually circular or oval, although several individual lentigines may coalesce. There may be slight scaling of the surface, but the skin markings are unaltered.
- Mucosae may be involved.
- Do not darken or increase in number on sun exposure.
- Do not disappear during the winter months.
- Lentigines usually start to appear in childhood and increase in number in the second and third decades.
- Rarely, they may erupt in large numbers, sometimes after inflammation, or related to use of immunosuppressive agents.
- They are commonly subclassified, but excessive exposure to natural or artificial UV radiation is the major etiological factor for all of the following: Simple lentigines, actinic (or solar) lentigines, psoralen UVA (PUVA) lentigines and the ink-spot lentigo.
- Familial lentigines: Peutz-Jeghers syndrome, LEOPARD syndrome, Carney complex.
- Generalized lentiginosis: Lentigines are commonly multiple but appear singly or in small crops at irregular intervals from infancy onwards.
- Unilateral lentiginosis (zosteriform lentiginosis): Lentigines may occur on one side of the body.
- Eruptive lentiginosis: Widespread occurrence of very large numbers of lentigines that develop rapidly over the course of a few months to years. The condition usually occurs in adolescents and young adults who show no evidence of systemic abnormalities.
- Centrofacial lentiginosis: It is characterized by a triad of clinical features: Lentigines limited to the medial face, neuropsychiatric problems and dysraphic anomalies.

## Incontinentia Pigmenti

- Incontinentia pigmenti (IP) is an **X-linked dominant neuro-cutaneous** syndrome with cutaneous, neurologic, ophthalmologic, and dental manifestations.
- **Ectodermal changes**
  - ➢ Skin features occur in 4 stages:
    - – *Stage 1 (vesicular)* is characterized by the development of red papules and vesicles on an erythematous base that follow Blaschko lines. Lesions are seen predominantly on the extremities but may also occur on the trunk or on the head

and neck. The vesicular stage has been reported to occur in 90–95% of patients. In most patients (>90%), lesions are present at birth or develop within the first 2 weeks of life. They resolve within several months.

- *Stage 2 (verrucous)* is characterized by thickened, warty-appearing linear and whorled plaques on an erythematous base that follow Blaschko lines. In general, lesions develop on the extremities and trunk but may also be seen on the head and neck. Verrucous lesions have been reported to occur in 70–80% of IP patients. In most patients, verrucous lesions develop in the first few weeks to months of life and subsequently resolve over weeks to months.

- *Stage 3 (hyperpigmented)* is characterized by the development of streaks and whorls of brown or slate-gray pigmentation along Blaschko lines; this occurs in 90–98% of IP patients. Hyperpigmented lesions usually involve the trunk but may also involve the extremities, the skin folds, or the head and neck. The location of the hyperpigmented lesions does not appear to correlate with areas of prior skin involvement during the earlier vesicular and verrucous stages. Hyperpigmented lesions generally develop within the first few months of life and resolve slowly by adolescence.

- *Stage 4 (atrophic/hypopigmented)* is characterized by hypopigmented, atrophic, and reticulate or linear patches observed on the lower extremities, usually involving the calves. Atrophic lesions usually develop during adolescence and persist into adulthood. Atrophic lesions have been reported to occur in 30–75% of IP patients.

➢ Hair changes include scarring alopecia and are seen in 28–38% of patients.

➢ Nail features include nail dystrophy, which ranges from mild pitting or ridging of the nail plate to hyperkeratosis and onycholysis.

➢ Dental abnormalities are seen in 80% of patients and can involve both deciduous and permanent teeth. Dental anomalies are permanent and thus serve as a very useful diagnostic finding in older patients. Delayed dentition, partial anodontia, and conical or pegged teeth are the most common dental findings.

- **Ophthalmologic findings**
  ➢ Ophthalmologic findings occur in 20–35% of patients, and asymmetric involvement is common. Loss of visual acuity and blindness are significant complications.

➤ Retinal manifestations include retinal detachment, proliferative retinopathy, fibrovascular retrolental membranes, foveal hypoplasia, vitreous hemorrhages, and atrophy of the ciliary body.

➤ Nonretinal manifestations include strabismus, optic nerve atrophy, conjunctival pigmentation, microphthalmia, keratitis, cataracts, iris hypoplasia, nystagmus, and uveitis.

- **Neurologic abnormalities**
  ➤ Neurologic complications occur in 30% of IP patients and often manifest within the neonatal period.

  ➤ Seizures are the most common neurologic complication and usually develop within the first few weeks of life.

  ➤ Other neurodevelopmental manifestations include developmental delay, mental retardation, ataxia, spastic paralysis, microcephaly, cerebral atrophy, porencephaly, hypoplasia of the corpus callosum, and periventricular cerebral edema.

  ➤ IP is caused by mutations in the **NEMO/IKK** gamma gene

- **Differential diagnosis**
  ➤ Infantile pemphigoid
  ➤ Epidermolysis bullosa

- **Treatment**
  ➤ Family counseling may prevent occurrence of new cases
  ➤ Skin lesions subside in adulthood spontaneously

## Melasma/Chloasma/Mask of Pregnancy

- This common acquired hypermelanosis is seen mainly in women, and occurs mainly on sun-exposed skin on the face, only occasionally affecting the forearms.
- Hypermelanosis affects the upper lip, cheeks, forehead and chin and is more apparent following sun exposure.
- Affected skin is brown in color. The pigmentary changes are usually bilateral and are frequently symmetrical.
- **Etiology:** Exact etiology is not known
  ➤ Genetic
  ➤ Idiopathic
  ➤ Hormonal—seen in pregnancy
  ➤ Sun induced
  ➤ Drug induced—phenytoin and OC pills

- **Classification**
  - ➤ Based on distribution
    - – Centrofacial pattern
    - – Malar pattern
    - – Mandibular pattern
  - ➤ Based on pigment distribution on Wood's lamp examination
    - – Epidermal
    - – Dermal
    - – Mixed
- **Treatment:** Difficult usually persistent. Various methods tried are:
  - ➤ Topical hydroquinone, azelaic acid or kojic acid
  - ➤ Chemical peels
  - ➤ Photoprotection

## Nevus of Ota

- The hyperpigmentation affects one side of the face in the area supplied by the ophthalmic and maxillary divisions of the trigeminal nerve. Occasionally, it is bilateral (Fig. 9.1).
- It is usually congenital but may appear later in life.
- It is more prevalent in the Japanese but is observed in other races.
- The color is variable, but is usually either slate-brown or blue.
- The sclera is involved and there may be hyperpigmentation of the cornea, iris, retina, ocular muscles and orbit. Sometimes, there is pigmentation of the hard palate.

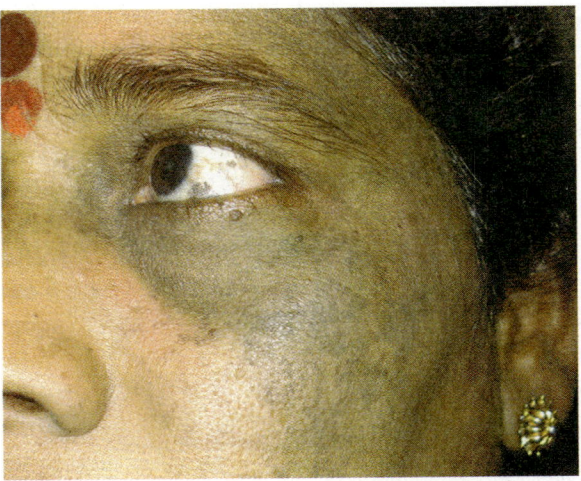

**Fig. 9.1:** Involvement of one side of face and sclera in nevus of Ota

## Naevus of Ito

- In this condition, the increased pigmentation affects the area supplied by the posterior supraclavicular and lateral brachial cutaneous nerves.
- It is relatively common in the Japanese.

## Drug-induced Pigmentation

- Chronic arsenic poisoning — Rain drop pigmentation
- Mepacrine — Bright-yellow or greenish-yellow color
- Clofazimine — Redness of the skin
- Hydroxyurea — Skin + nail pigmentation
- Minocycline and chlorpromazine — Blue–black pigmentation (slate-like)
- Amiodarone — Grey–blue pigmentation

### QUESTIONS FROM PREVIOUS EXAMINATIONS

1. Incontinentia pigmenti
2. Nevus of Ota
3. Melasma
4. Nevus anemicus
5. Piebaldism
6. Vitiligo, etiopathogenesis
7. Management of vitiligo
8. Surgeries in vitiligo
9. Vitiligo, clinical features
10. Albinism
11. Freckles
12. Lentigines

### MULTIPLE CHOICE QUESTIONS

1. **True about vitiligo are all** *except:*          *(AIIMS Nov 07)*
    (a) Genetic predisposition is known
    (b) Leucotrichia is associated with good prognosis
    (c) PUVA-B is used for treatment
    (d) Topical steroids give good results

2. **Piebaldism refers to:** *(Kar 07)*
   - (a) Androgenetic alopecia
   - (b) Cicatricial alopecia
   - (c) Association of vitiligo with white forelock
   - (d) None of the above

3. **Diffuse form of hyperpigmentation is seen in:** *(MH 2006)*
   - (a) Vitamin $B_{12}$ deficiency
   - (b) Ectopic ACTH secretion
   - (c) Whipple's disease
   - (d) All of the above

4. **Pigmentation due to increased melanin production but no melanin proliferation is seen in:** *(MH 08)*
   - (a) Nevus
   - (b) Ephelides
   - (c) Lentigo
   - (d) Melanoma

5. **A 38-year-old Bengali man presents with complains of multiple papular lesions over the body especially involving the palms and soles. The lesions are not painful. He has pigmentation of skin over the abdomen. He also has vertical white ridges over the nails. Which of the following is the most likely diagnosis?** *(AI 08)*
   - (a) Xeroderma pigmentosa
   - (b) Chronic arsenic poisoning
   - (c) Lichen planus
   - (d) Erythrodermoplasia verruciformis

6. **True about incontinentia pigmenti includes the following *except:*** *(AI 09)*
   - (a) X-linked dominant
   - (b) Primary skin abnormality
   - (c) Avascularity of peripheral retina
   - (d) Ocular involvement is seen in almost 100% cases and is typically unilateral

7. **A otherwise healthy young adult male presents with multiple, irregular, painless, non-itchy spots of brownish pigmentation on right lower leg since almost a year. There is no history of trauma. His physical examination is otherwise normal and the routine lab results are normal. What is the diagnosis?** *(AMC 2005)*
   - (a) Lichen purpuricus
   - (b) Henoch Schönlein purpura
   - (c) Schamberg's disease
   - (d) *Tinea pedis*

8. **A child is brought by parents with complain of a solitary well-defined whitish patch on the child's thigh. Which of the following would be the most likely diagnosis?** *(AIIMS 2000)*
   - (a) Piebaldism
   - (b) Albinism
   - (c) Nevus achromicus
   - (d) Acral vitiligo

9. **Hypopigmented patches may be seen in:**    *(PGI 2005)*
   - (a) Becker's nevus
   - (b) Freckles
   - (c) Nevus of Ota
   - (d) Nevus of Ito
   - (e) Nevus anemicus

10. **The mode of inheritance of incontinentia pigmenti:**    *(PGI 2005)*
    - (a) Autosomal dominant
    - (b) Autosomal recessive
    - (c) X-linked dominant
    - (d) X-linked recessive

11. **Causes of hypopigmentation in a pigmented skin include the following** *except:*    *(Kar 99)*
    - (a) Pityriasis alba
    - (b) Pityriasis rosea
    - (c) Pityriasis versicolor
    - (d) Pityriasis rubra pilaris

12. **Disorders associated with vitiligo:**    *(PGI 08)*
    - (a) Hyperthyroidism
    - (b) Hypothyroidism
    - (c) Addison's disease
    - (d) Diabetes mellitus
    - (e) Androgentic alopecia

13. **In a patch of vitiligo:**    *(PGI 90)*
    - (a) Melanin synthesis is inhibited
    - (b) Melanosomes are absent
    - (c) Melanocytes are absent
    - (d) Melanocytes are reduced

14. **Slate-like discoloration of skin:**    *(AIIMS 80)*
    - (a) Amiodarone
    - (b) Minocycline
    - (c) Hydroxyurea
    - (d) Clofazimine
    - (e) Mepacrine

15. **Hyperpigmentation is not seen in:**    *(AI 93)*
    - (a) Addison's disease
    - (b) Cushing's disease
    - (c) Graves' disease
    - (d) Hypothyroidism

16. **Fine reticular skin pigmentation with palmar pits is seen in:**
    - (a) Dowling-Degos' disease
    - (b) Bloom's syndrome
    - (c) Cockyane syndrome
    - (d) Rothmund-Thomson disease

## Answers

1. **Ans. (b)** Leucotrichia is associated with good prognosis *(Ref. Rook's Dermatology, 7th edn/39.54)*
2. **Ans. (c)** Association of vitiligo with white forelock *(Ref. Genetic Disorders of the Skiný by Joseph C. Alper, page 146)*
3. **Ans. (d)** All of the above *(Ref. Harrison's Principles of Internal Medicine, 17th edn/ Table 54–11)*
4. **Ans. (b)** Ephelides *(Ref. Robbin's Pathology, 7th edn, page 1231)*
5. **Ans. (b)** Chronic arsenic poisoning

6. **Ans. (d)** Ocular involvement is seen in almost 100% cases and is typically unilateral *(Ref. Rook's Textbook of Dermatology, 7th edition, 39.20 to 63.22)*

7. **Ans. (c)** Schamberg's disease *(Ref. Rook's Dermatology, 7th edition, 48.10)*

8. **Ans. (c)** Nevus achromicus *(Ref. Harrison, 17th edn/324; Rook, 7th edn/38–12, 39.53)*

9. **Ans. (e)** Nevus anemicus *(Ref. Rook's Dermatology, 7th edn/15.76)*

10. **Ans. (c)** X-linked dominant *(Ref. IADVL Textbook of Dermatology, 2nd edn/634)*

11. **Ans.** (d) Pityriasis rubra pilaris *(Ref. Rook's Dermatology, 7th edition, **Table 69.1**)*

12. **Ans. (a, b, c, d)** *(Ref. Rook's Dermatology, 7th edn / Table 39.6)*

13. **Ans. (c)** Melanocytes are absent *(Ref. Rook's Dermatology, 7th edition, Table 39.54)*

14. **Ans. (b)** Minocycline *(Ref. Rook's Dermatology, 7th edn/39.63)*

15. **Ans. (d)** Hypothyroidism *(Ref. Harrison's Medicine, 17th edn / Table 54–11)*

16. **Ans. (a)** Dowling-Degos' disease. *Dowling-Degos' disease is reticulate pigmented anomaly.*

# 10    Disorders of Hair

- Histologically, the hair follicle consists of three parts: The lower portion, which extends from the base of the follicle to the insertion of the arrector pili muscle; the isthmus, which extends from the insertion of the arrector pili muscle to the entrance of the sebaceous duct; and the infundibulum, which extends from the entrance of the sebaceous duct to the follicular orifice.

- Hair grows at different rates in different regions of the body (Fig. 10.1).

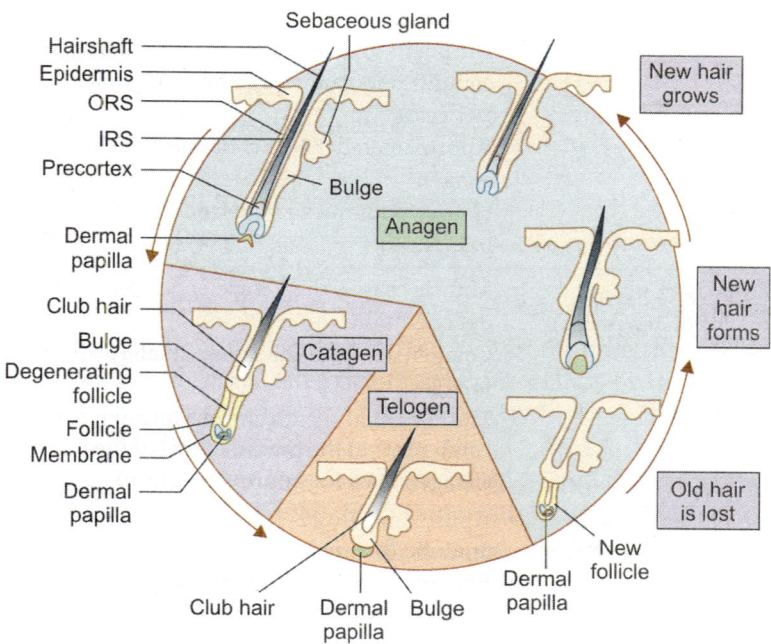

**Fig. 10.1:** Hair growth cycle

On the human scalp, the daily growth rate is around 0.3 mm. In women, scalp and body hair grows faster and slower, respectively, than in men. The activity of hair follicles is intermittent.

➢ Anagen is the active period, which may last for 3 or more years.
➢ Telogen is the resting phase, usually lasting about 3 months.
➢ Catagen is the transition or regression phase, usually approximately 3 weeks in duration.

• In the human scalp, at any one point in time, approximately 84% of hair is in anagen, 14% in telogen, and 2% in catagen.
• Assuming that the scalp contains about 100,000 hairs, it can reasonably be expected that 100 hairs will be shed daily.

## Hair Growth Cycle (Fig. 10.2)

• Scalp hair follicles have a four phase cycle (Table 10.1).
• Anagen (growth), catagen (transition), telogen (resting) and exogen (hairshaft evacuation).

| Table 10.1: Hair growth cycle | |
|---|---|
| The anagen phase (growing phase) | • During the process of folliculo-regenesis, the follicle + epithelial sheath + new hairshaft is recreated<br>• During its growth (anagen) phase the hair shaft continues to gain length for a period of 2–7 years<br>• Approximately 80–85% of hair follicles are in anagen<br>• Hair growth rates range from 0.5 to 1.45 cm per month |
| The catagen phase (involutionary phase) | • Mitosis ceases, the follicle enters a period of degeneration<br>• Catagen accounts for approximately 3% of hair follicles.<br>• The epithelial sheath shrinks forming a minute "club root" at the proximal end of the hairshaft<br>• Catagen lasts for approximately 10–20 days |
| The telogen phase (resting or dying phase) | • Approximately 12–20% of hairshafts are in the amitotic (resting) phase<br>• Eventually (up to 3 months) the hairshaft vacates the follicle |
| The exogen phase | • In which the hair-shaft is evacuated |

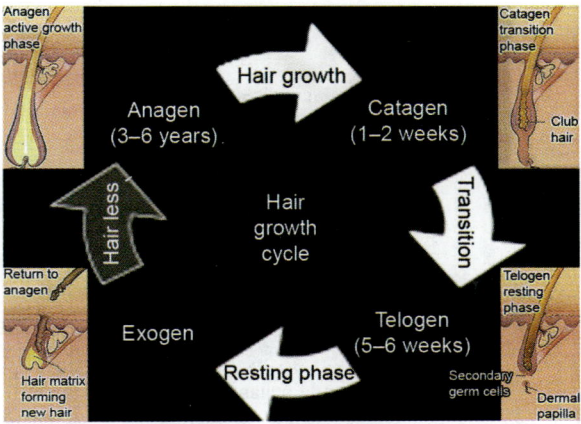

**Fig. 10.2:** Hair growth cycle

## ALOPECIA

- Defined as loss of hair.
- It may be diffuse or patchy; scarring or nonscarring.

### Nonscarring Alopecia (Table 10.2)

- The most common form of **nonscarring alopecia** is male pattern alopecia, which appears to be related to androgen levels and to aging. Genetic predisposition commonly influences the time of onset, degree of baldness, speed with which it spreads, and pattern of hairloss.
- Other forms of nonscarring alopecia include:
  - ➢ Physiologic alopecia (usually temporary): Sudden hairloss in infants, loss of straight hairline in adolescents, and diffuse hair loss after childbirth.
  - ➢ Alopecia areata (idiopathic form): Generally reversible and self-limiting; occurs most frequently in young and middle age adults of both sexes.
  - ➢ Trichotillomania: Compulsive pulling out of one's own hair; most common in children.
  - ➢ Traction alopecia: Localized areas of hair loss due to chronic use of tight braids (such as cornrows) or other hair styles. This condition may also result in scarring alopecia.
- Predisposing factors of nonscarring alopecia also include radiation, many types of drug therapies and drug reactions, bacterial and fungal infections, psoriasis, seborrhea, and endocrine disorders, such as thyroid, parathyroid, and pituitary dysfunctions.

**Table 10.2:** Nonscarring alopecia (primary cutaneous disorders)

| | | | |
|---|---|---|---|
| *Telogen effluvium* | Diffuse shedding of normal hairs. Follows either major stress (high fever, severe infection) or change in hormones (post-partum) Reversible without treatment | Stress causes the normally asynchronous growth cycles of individual hairs to become synchronous; therefore, large numbers of growing (anagen) hairs simultaneously enter the dying (telogen) phase | Observation; discontinue any drugs that have alopecia as a side effect; must exclude underlying metabolic causes, e.g. hypothyroidism and hyperthyroidism |
| *Androgenetic alopecia (male pattern; female pattern)* | Miniaturization of hairs along the midline of the scalp Recession of the anterior scalp line in men and some women | Increased sensitivity of affected hairs to the effects of testosterone. Increased levels of circulating androgens (ovarian or adrenal source in women) | If no evidence of hyperandrogen state, then topical minoxidil; finasteride; hair transplant |
| *Alopecia areata* | Well-circumscribed, circular areas of hairloss, 2–5 cm in diameter. In extensive cases, coalescence of lesions and/or involvement of other hair-bearing surfaces of the body pitting of the nails | The germinative zones of the hair follicles are surrounded by T lymphocytes. Occasional associated diseases: Hyperthyroidism Hypothyroidism Vitiligo, Down syndrome | Topical anthralin; intralesional glucocorticoids; topical contact sensitizers |

*Contd.*

**Table 10.2:** Nonscarring alopecia (primary cutaneous disorders) *Contd.*

| | | |
|---|---|---|
| *Tinea* | Varies from scaling with minimal hairloss to discrete patches with "black dots" (broken hairs) to boggy plaque with pustules (kerion) | Invasion of hairs by dermatophytes, most commonly *Trichophyton tonsurans* | Oral griseofulvin or terbinafine plus 2.5% selenium sulfide or ketoconazole shampoo; examine family members |
| *Traumatic alopecia* | Broken hairs, irregular outline | Traction with curlers, rubber bands, braiding. Exposure to heat or chemicals (e.g. hair straighteners), mechanical pulling (trichotillomania) | Discontinuation of offending hair style or chemical treatments; trichotillomania may require hair clipping and observation of shaved hairs or biopsy for diagnosis, possibly followed by psychotherapy |

## Telogen Effluvium

- Acute telogen effluvium relates to a specific **form of diffuse alopecia**—eviction of hairshafts that have prematurely entered the telogen phase (telogen hair increase to 25%, normal—13%).
- Excessive loss of hair can occur.
- Telogen effluvium tends to become apparent 6–12 weeks following the cause.
- Such a hairloss can result in 1–2 cm stubble in extreme cases within weeks.
- **Causes include**
  - Pyrexia (body temperature reaching 103.5°C +)
  - Childbirth (rare)
  - Telogen gravidarum
  - Severe infection (especially toxemia)
  - Major surgery
  - Protein deficiency due to unsupervised diets
  - Drugs including:
    - Beta blockers
    - Antidepressants
    - Minoxidil
  - Severe psychological stress.
- Spontaneous regrowth occurs in 3–6 months.

## Anagen Effluvium

- Hairloss during anagen
- The onset may be rapid (within 2–4 weeks of the cause).
- Hairloss may be severe.
- Causes include: Chemotherapy drugs (antimitotic agents), radiotherapy, malnutrition, seborrheic dermatitis, oral contraceptives, vitamin A poisoning, thallium, mercury and arsenic poisoning, iron deficiency, chronic infections and some drugs.
- The insult to the hair follicle is sufficiently severe to cause an immediate metabolic arrest with complete cessation of hair production.
- The hair may come out by the root, or if the insult is brief, the hair shaft will narrow, providing a point of weakness that subsequently snaps off.
- The follicle may remain in anagen, in which case recovery is quick, or move into telogen, in which case regrowth will be delayed by about 3 months.

## *Androgenetic Alopecia*

- Androgenetic alopecia (male pattern baldness/female pattern baldness/patterned hairloss) is **the most common type of non-scarring hairloss.**
- Progressive patterned hair loss that occurs in genetically predisposed individuals when exposed to androgens.
- The process involves androgen-mediated miniaturization of terminal hair follicles.
- Pigmented terminal hairs are progressively replaced by finer hair, which are short and virtually non-pigmented.
- Hamilton and Norwood scale is used for grading male pattern hair loss. The posterior and lateral scalp margins are relatively spared, and only affected in the most advanced cases and with old age.
- Patterned balding occurs in women, but the susceptibility, age of onset, rate of progression and pattern are different from men.
- The age of onset of FPHL is later than that seen in men.
- Fewer than 1% of women progress to Hamilton–Norwood stage IV or above (equivalent to Ludwig stage III). Severe bitemporal recession (Hamilton–Norwood III) is uncommon.
- Ludwig described the earliest change (Ludwig grade I) as rarefaction of the hair on the crown . This produces an oval area of alopecia encircled by a band of variable breadth with normal hair density. Frontally the fringe is narrow (1–3 cm) and at the sides the margin is 4–5 cm wide. Progression to Ludwig grade II results in further rarefaction of the crown, with preservation of the fringe. Grade III is near-complete baldness of the crown.
- Olsen observed the so-called **Christmas-tree pattern**, with widening of the central parting line most noticeably in the mid-frontal scalp in females (Fig. 10.3).

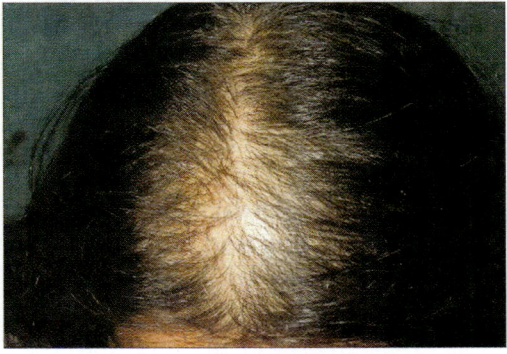

**Fig. 10.3:** Androgenetic alopecia in female

- **Treatment of androgenetic alopecia**
  - ➤ Medical management
  - ➤ Surgical management
  - ➤ Cosmetic camouflage and wigs

*Medical management*

- ➤ Topical 5% **minoxidil** lotion or oral **finasteride** (1 mg daily) can help arrest progression and may cause a small amount of regrowth, providing it is used early in disease but the treatment needs to be continued possibly lifelong.
- ➤ Approximately one-third of patients will not respond to either therapy.
- ➤ Finasteride is a selective inhibitor of $5\alpha$-reductase type II and it can cause side-effects in 1% of patients such as loss of libido. It should not be used in females as it can affect the sexual development of a male fetus.
- ➤ However, antiandrogen therapy (e.g. cyproterone acetate or spironolactone) helps some women.

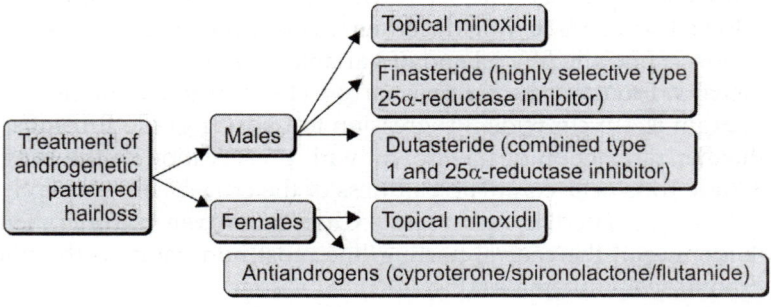

**Alopecia Areata**

- It is an autoimmune, nonscarring disorder of hair growth affecting genetically predisposed individuals.
- It is associated with other organ-specific autoimmune diseases.
- Peaks in second to fourth decades.
- Sex incidence is equal.
- May be associated with atopy.
- It is characterized by circular bald areas and occur on any hair-bearing area of the body. These may regrow to be followed by new patches of hair loss. Regrowth may initially be with white hairs and often occurs slowly over months (Fig. 10.4).

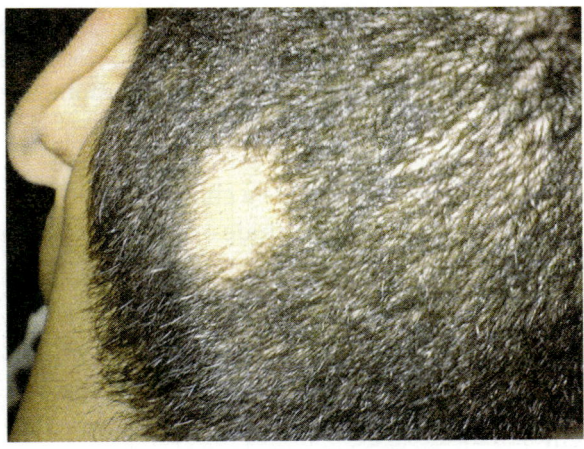

**Fig. 10.4:** Patchy hairloss over scalp

- The extension of alopecia along the scalp margin is known as ophiasis. It has bad prognosis (Table 10.3).
- Severe disease may produce total loss of scalp hair (alopecia totalis) or universal loss of body hair (alopecia universalis).
- The presence of broken **exclamation mark hairs** (narrow at the scalp/wider and more pigmented at the tip) at the edge of a bald area is diagnostic.

| **Table 10.3:** Alopecia | | | |
|---|---|---|---|
| *Alopecia aerata* | *Androgenic alopecia* | *Telogen effluvium* | *Alopecia mucinosa* |
| • Sharply defined noninflamed patches of baldness.<br>• Exclamation mark +<br>• Causes: Autoimmunity<br>• MC on scalp, but involves eyebrows, lashers, beard.<br>• RX: Topical anthralin + intralesional | • MC type<br>• Bitemporal recession then crown involvement<br>• Causes: ↑ sensitivity to testosterone<br>• Rx: Minoxidil + tretinoin | • Asynchronous growth cycle of hair becomes synchronous, so large number of growing hair enter dying phase, i.e. telogen<br>• Cause: Stress (high fever), hormonal changes (post-partum)<br>• Rx: Observation and Rx of underliving | • Non-scarring alopecia with mucin deposition in hair follicles and sebaceous glands causing epithelial reticular degeneration<br>• MC sites: Face and scalp<br>• Associated with folicular plaques and papules, and with mycosis fungoides (15–30% cases) |

MC: Most common

- Exclamation mark hair sign refers to the proximal tapering of hair occasionally seen in alopecia areata, where the dot represents the remains of the bulb. The sign is not pathognomonic for alopecia areata, and its presence may lead to misdiagnosis.
- Sparing of white hair is seen.
- The diagnosis of alopecia areata is a clinical one.
- Rarely, a biopsy is required to exclude other forms of hair loss. The hallmarks of an active lesion are a dense lymphocytic infiltrate around the anagen hair bulbs (swarm of bees appearance).
- The nails may be pitted or roughened. Pits are uniformly arranged to give a scotch blaid pattern.
- **DD**: Trichotillomania, *tinea capitis.*
- **Treatment**
  - ➢ Has no effect on the long-term progression.
  - ➢ Potent topical or injected steroids (triamcinolone acetonide)
  - ➢ Contact immunotherapy with diphencyprone, PUVA or topical 5% minoxidil are occasionally tried but often do not help.
  - ➢ Wigs can be provided for severe cases and patient support groups are often beneficial.

### Trichotillomania

- Behavioral disorder characterized by compulsive hair pulling. Compulsive hair rubbing (trichoteiromania) and hair cutting (trichotemnomania ) fall into the same general category.
- Trichotillomania occurs in two main forms.
  - ➢ In infants and young children, it is usually a habit akin to thumb-sucking and nail biting. It seems slightly more common in boys and usually resolves spontaneously or with minimal treatment.
  - ➢ In older age groups, adolescents and adults, trichotillomania is seen predominantly in females and some form of psychological or behavioral stress is often apparent.
- Hair is plucked most frequently from one frontoparietal region. This results in a patch of hair loss, often in a bizarre or angular pattern, in which the hairs are twisted and broken at various distances from the clinically normal scalp (Fig. 10.5).
- In **trichotillomania**, characteristically the plucked area covers the entire scalp apart from the margins, which is known as **tonsure alopecia** or **orentriech sign.**
- **Treatment:** Habit reversal therapy, SSRIs and clomipramine.

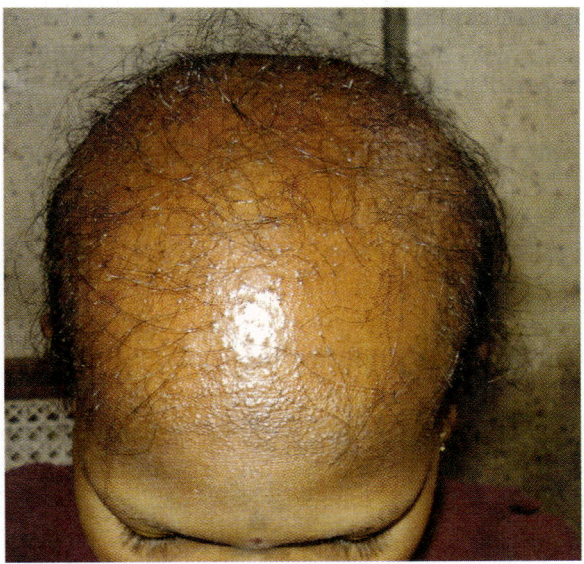

**Fig. 10.5:** Frontoparietal hair loss in a young female with trichotillomania

## Scarring Alopecia

- **Scarring alopecia** results from serious damage to hair follicles which is permanent and replaced by scar tissue.
- **Differentiated from non-scarring alopecia by**
  - ➤ Absence of follicular opening.
  - ➤ Increased wrinkling.
  - ➤ Thin, shiny, dry, depressed skin covered with telangiectases.
  - ➤ Hair may be twisted and standing on end due to fibrotic process in dermis.
- **Causes**
  - ➤ *Developmental*
    - Aplasia cutis
    - Incontinentia pigmenti
    - Focal dermal hypoplasia
    - Darier's disease
    - Porokeratosis of Mibelli
  - ➤ *Traumatic*
    - Thermal, mechanical, chemical injuries
    - Traction alopecia, trichotillomania
  - ➤ *Neoplastic*
    - Basal cell carcinoma
    - Squmous cell carcinoma

- Metastasis
- Lymphomas

➢ *Follicular inflammation*
- *Tinea capitis*
- Bacterial folliculitis
- Folliculitis decalvans
- Pseudopelade of Brocq
- Follicular lichen planus
- Graham-Little syndrome
- Discoid lupus erythematosus
- Lichen sclerosus et atrophicus

➢ *Dermal inflammation leading to secondary follicular damage*
- TB
- Syphilis
- Sarcoidosis
- Morphea
- Cicatricial pemphigoid

## Pseudopelade of Brocq

- Pseudopelade of Brocq is an idiopathic, chronic, slowly progressive, patchy cicatricial alopecia that occurs without any evidence of inflammation. It is primarily an atrophy rather than an inflammatory folliculitis (Fig. 10.6).

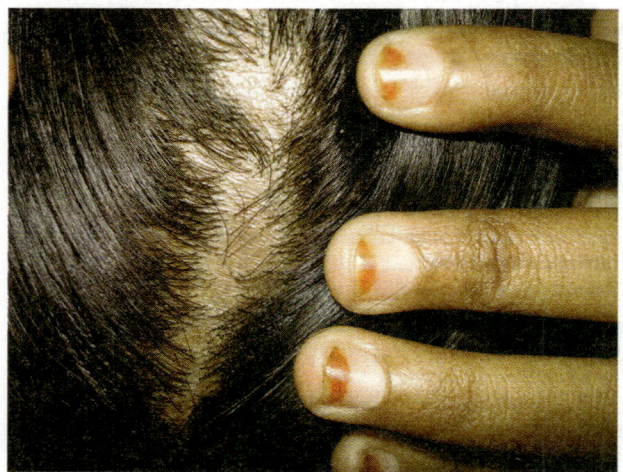

**Fig. 10.6:** "Footprints in the snow" appearance in pseudopelade of Brocq

- More common in women over 40 yrs of age.
- Etiology and pathogenesis are not known.
- Confined to scalp. Initial patch is often on the vertex.
- Irregular bald patches may be formed by confluence of lesions (footprints in the snow).
- Alopecia is irreversible and does not respond to treatment.
- In recent times, the term pseudopelade has been used to describe a generic scarring alopecia, the end result of any number of different pathological processes.

## HIRSUTISM

- Defined as occurrence in women and children of growth of coarse terminal hairs in male sexual pattern.
- It affects the androgen dependent hairs.
- Face is commonest site of affection specially upper lip and chin
- **Causes**
  - ➢ *Without virilization*
    - Pituitary: Cushing's disease, ectopic ACTH
    - Combined ovarian and adrenal cause—puberty
    - Ovarian—pregnancy menopause, ovarian luteoma, thyroid dysfunction (hypo/hyper)
    - Idiopathic
    - Drugs—systemic steroids, ACTH
  - ➢ *With or without virilization*
    - *Pituitary:* Hyperprolactinemia, acromegaly
    - *Adrenal:* Cushing's syndrome, adrenal adenoma, carcinoma, adult onset adrenal hyperplasia
    - *Ovarian:* PCOD, theca/granulosa cell tumor, hilar cell tumor, arrhenoblastoma, gynandroblastoma, Krukenberg's tumor
    - *Drugs:* Anabolic steroids, progestins
  - ➢ *With virilization*
    - *Adrenal:* Congenital and childhood onset adrenal hyperplasia, adrenal rest tumor
    - *Ovarian:* Ovarian hyperthecosis, hilar cell hyperplasia
    - *Drugs:* Testosterone synthetic androgens
- **Investigations**
  - ➢ Serum testosterone levels
  - ➢ LH/FSH level
  - ➢ Serum prolactin levels

- ➢ Dehydroepiandrosterone level
- ➢ USG
- ➢ CT
- ➢ MRI
- • **Treatment**
  - ➢ Cosmetic correction
  - ➢ Temporary—waxing, shaving, plucking
  - ➢ Permanent—electrolysis, laser, epilation
  - ➢ Hormonal correction

## QUESTIONS FROM PREVIOUS EXAMINATIONS

1. Hypertrichosis
2. Hirsutism
3. Non-cicatricial alopecia
4. Alopecia areata
5. Diffuse alopecia
6. Telogen effluvium
7. Cicatricial alopecia
8. Monilithrix
9. Trichonodosis
10. Piedra
11. Pigment of hair
12. Pili torti
13. Premature canities
14. Dissecting folliculitis of the scalp
15. Plica polonica
16. Trichoepithelioma
17. Trichostasis spinulosa
18. Trichotillomania

## MULTIPLE CHOICE QUESTIONS

1. **Growth phase of hair:**                    (AI 98; PGI 99)
   - (a) Anagen
   - (b) Metagen
   - (c) Catagen
   - (d) Telogen
2. **A female patient presents with diffuse alopecia. There is no other significant past or present complain except that she had**

suffered from typhoid fever 4 months back. What would be the most probable diagnosis? *(AIIMS Nov 07)*
- (a) Androgenetic alopecia
- (b) Telogen effluvium
- (c) Anagen effluvium
- (d) Alopecia areata

3. All of the following are causes of cicatrizing alopecia *except:*
                                        *(AIIMS Nov 07)*
- (a) Lichen planus
- (b) Discoid lupus erythematosus
- (c) Alopecia areata
- (d) Lupus vulgaris

4. Most common type of alopecia is:    *(TN 08)*
- (a) Alopecia aerata
- (b) Alpoecia mucinosa
- (c) Telogen effluvium
- (d) Androgenic alopecia

5. Loss of hair from whole body is called:
- (a) Alopecia totalis
- (b) Alopecia globalis
- (c) Alopecia universalis
- (d) Telogen effluvium

6. Inflammation, itching and scales are absent in:    *(Delhi 08)*
- (a) Alopecia areata
- (b) *Tinea capitis*
- (c) Atopic dermatitis
- (d) Lichen planus

7. A 30-year-old male complains of sudden loss of hair of head, beard, and of the eyebrows. On examination, graying of hair is seen with multiple patchy areas of hairloss without scarring are seen involving the head, beard, as well as the eyebrows. What is the most likely diagnosis?    *(AI 08)*
- (a) Androgenetic alopecia
- (b) Telogen effluvium
- (c) Anagen effluvium
- (d) Alopecia areata

8. Orentriech sign is seen in:    *(Rajasthan 07)*
- (a) Telogen effluvium
- (b) Trichotillomania
- (c) Dystrophic epidermolysis bullosa
- (d) Fogo selvagum

9. Hirsutism can be caused by the following *except:*    *(AI 09)*
- (a) Cushing's syndrome
- (b) Acromegaly
- (c) Hyperthyroidism
- (d) Hyperprolactinemia

10. Scarring alopecia is seen in:    *(AI 09)*
- (a) *T. capitis*
- (b) Androgenic alopecia
- (c) Alopecia areata
- (d) Lichen planus

11. Terry's nail is seen in:    *(DNB 07)*
- (a) Hepatic failure
- (b) Sideroblastic anemia
- (c) Arsenic poisoning
- (d) Minimata's disease

12. **Cicatricial alopecia is seen in:**                    *(AI 99)*
    (a) *Tenia capitis*              (b) Psoriasis
    (c) DLE                          (d) Alopecia areata

13. **A 30-year-old female developed diffuse hairloss 3 months after delivery of her first child. The most likely cause is:**
                                               *(SGPGI 03)*
    (a) Androgenic alopecia          (b) Endocrine disease
    (c) SLE                          (d) Telogen effluvium

14. **Diagnosis of a man with diffuse hairloss involving crown and frontal scalp with maintenance of frontal hair line:**
                                               *(JIPMER 98)*
    (a) Alopecia areata              (b) Anagen effluvium
    (c) Male pattern baldness        (d) Female pattern baldness

15. **"Exclamation mark" alopecia is a feature of:**
                                       *(AIIMS Nov 05; Bihar 06)*
    (a) Androgenic alopecia          (b) Alopecia mucinosa
    (c) Alopecia areata              (d) Telogen effluvium

16. **Contraindicated in androgenic alopecia is:**    *(SGPGI 03)*
    (a) Testosterone                 (b) Minoxidil
    (c) Cyproterone                  (d) Finasteride

17. **Causes of cicatrizing alopecia include the following *except:***
                                               *(UP 09)*

    (a) Morphea                      (b) Lichen planus
    (c) Burns                        (d) Post-partum alopecia

18. **Pseudopelade is synonymous with:**           *(Manipal 2009)*
    (a) Alopecia steatoides          (b) Alopecia mucinosa
    (c) Traction alopecia            (d) Cicatricial alopecia

19. **Anagen phase of the hair indicates:**        *(AIIMS 06; UP 09)*
    (a) The phase of activity and growth
    (b) The phase of transition
    (c) The phase of resting
    (d) The phase of degeneration

## Answers

1. **Ans. (a)** Anagen *(Ref. IDVL Textbook of Dearmatology, page 730; Table 26.13)*

2. **Ans. (b)** Telogen effluvium *(Ref. IDVL Textbook of Dearmatology, page 730; Table 26.13)*

3. **Ans. (c)** Alopecia areata *(Ref. IDVL Textbook of Dearmatology, page 739; Table 26.16)*

4. **Ans. (d)** Androgenic alopecia *(Ref. Davidson's Medicine, 18th edn/895)*
5. **Ans. (c)** Alopecia universalis *(Ref. Rook's Textbook of Dermatology, 7th edn/63.20)*
6. **Ans. (a)** Alopecia areata *(Ref. Fizpatrick's Dermatology, 6th edn/634)*
7. **Ans. (d)** Alopecia areata
8. **Ans. (b)** Trichotillomania
9. **Ans. (c)** Hyperthyroidism (amongst given causes hyperthyroidism is least common cause) *(Ref. IADVL Textbook of Dermatology, 2nd edn 722; Rook's Textbook of Dermatology, 7th edn, 63.98 to 63.107)*
10. **Ans. (d)** Lichen planus *(Ref. IADVL Textbook of Dermatology, 2nd edition, 738–739.)*
11. **Ans. (a)** Hepatic failure
12. **Ans. (c)** DLE *(Ref. Harrison's Medicine, 17th edn/ Table 54–4)*
13. **Ans. (d)** Telogen effluvium *(Ref. Harrison's Medicine, 17th edn/ Table 54–5)*
14. **Ans. (d)** Female pattern baldness *(Ref. Rook, 7th edn/ 63.20)*
15. **Ans. (c)** Alopecia aerata *(Ref. Harrison's Medicine, 17th edn/ Table 54–5)*
16. **Ans. (a)** Testosterone *(Ref. Fitzpatrick's Dermatology in General Medicine, 7th edn, 634–52; Rook, 7th edn/63.20)*
17. **Ans. (d)** Post-partum alopecia *(Ref. Fitzpatrick's Dermatology in General Medicine, 7th edn, 634–52; Rook, 7th edn/63.20)*
18. **Ans. (d)** Cicatricial alopecia *(Ref. Rook, 7th edn/ 63.53)*
19. **Ans. (a)** The phase of activity and growth *(Ref. Rook, 7th edn/3.11).*

# 11 Disorders of Nail

## CLUBBING

- There is increased transverse and longitudinal nail curvature with hypertrophy of the soft tissue components of the digit pulp.
- Lovibond's angle is found at the junction between the nail plate and the proximal nail fold, and is normally less than 160°. This is altered to over 180° in clubbing.
- Curth's angle at the distal interphalangeal joint is normally about 180°. This is diminished to less than 160° in clubbing.
- Schamroth's window is seen when the dorsal aspects of two fingers from opposite hands are apposed, revealing a window of light, bordered laterally by the **Lovibond angles**. As this angle is obliterated in clubbing, the window closes.
- Pathological associations of clubbing include:
  - ➢ Inflammatory bowel disease
  - ➢ Carcinoma of the bronchus
  - ➢ Hemiplegic limbs
  - ➢ Congenital heart disease
  - ➢ Bronchiectasis
  - ➢ Cirrhosis
  - ➢ Subungual tumor when in a single digit.

## KOILONYCHIA (NAIL SPOONING)

- In koilonychia (Greek: *koilos,* hollow; *onyx,* nail), there is reverse curvature in the transverse and longitudinal axes giving a concave dorsal aspect to the nail.
- Koilonychia is common in:
  - ➢ Infancy as a benign feature of the great toenail
  - ➢ Trichothiodystrophy.

- Iron deficiency
- Hemochromatosis
- Familial pattern which may be autosomal dominant
- In dermatoses such as psoriasis and dermatophyte infection, nailbed hyperkeratosis may push the nail up distally to produce a spoon-shaped nail.
- Mechanics and hairdressers
- Rickshaw pullers

## TRANSVERSE GROOVES AND BEAU'S LINES

- Transverse grooves may be full or partial thickness through the nail. When they are endogenous they have an arcuate margin matching the lunula. If exogenous, such as those due to manicure, the margin may match the proximal nail fold.
- Transverse grooves may occur on isolated diseased digits (trauma, inflammation or neurological events) or may be generalized, reflecting a systemic event such as drug reaction, coronary thrombosis, measles, mumps or pneumonia.
- If endogenous, they are usually referred to as Beau's lines.
- They arise through temporary interference with nail formation and become visible on the nail surface some weeks after the precipitant.
- The distance of the groove from the nail fold is related to the time since the onset of growth disturbance.

## PITTING

- Pitting presents as punctate erosions in the nail surface.
- Individual pits may be shallow or deep, with a regular or irregular outline.
- When numerous, they appear randomly distributed upon the nail surface or have a geometric pattern. The latter may cause rippling or create a grid of pits.
- Extensive pitting combined with other surface irregularities results in the appearance of trachyonychia.
- Pits are seen in psoriasis, alopecia areata, and eczema.
- An isolated large pit may produce a localized full thickness defect in the nail plate termed elkonyxis, which is found in Reiter's disease, psoriasis and following trauma.
- Histologically, pits represent foci of parakeratosis, reflecting isolated nail malformation.

## TRACHYONYCHIA

- Trachyonychia presents as a rough surface affecting all of the nail plates and up to 20 nails (20-nail dystrophy).
- It is mainly associated with alopecia areata, psoriasis and lichen planus, although the most common presentation is as an isolated nail abnormality.
- In the isolated form, histology shows spongiosis and a lymphocytic infiltrate of the nail matrix.
- It may present as a self-limiting condition in childhood or as a more chronic problem in adulthood.
- There is some response to potent topical, locally injected and systemic steroids, but this may be temporary. Topical 5-fluorouracil has also been used.
- Childhood forms normally resolve spontaneously.

## ONYCHOSCHIZIA

Onychoschizia is also known as lamellar dystrophy and is characterized by transverse splitting into layers at or near the free edge in fingers and toes, especially in infants.

## LEUKONYCHIA

### True Leukonychia

- White discoloration of the nail attributable to matrix dysfunction.
- There is the rare, inherited form called total leukonychia, in which all nails are milky porcelain white.
- In subtotal leukonychia, the proximal two-thirds are white, becoming pink distally. This is attributed to a delay in keratin maturation, and the nail may still appear white at the distal overhang.
- Transverse leukonychia (Mees' line) reflects a systemic disorder, such as chemotherapy or poisoning, or systemic infection affecting matrix function. 1 to 2 mm wide transverse band is in the arcuate form of the lunula and is analogous to a Beau's line, with which it is occasionally found.
- Punctate leukonychia comprises white spots of 1–3 mm diameter attributed to minor matrix trauma (e.g. manicure) and is also seen in alopecia areata.
- With longitudinal leukonychia, there is a parakeratotic focus in the matrix, sometimes attributable to Darier's disease or a small tumor.

## Apparent Leukonychia

In apparent leukonychia, changes in the nailbed are responsible for the white appearance. Nailbed pallor may be a non-specific sign of anemia, edema or vascular impairment.

## TERRY'S NAIL

This is white proximally and normal distally and is attributed to cirrhosis, congestive cardiac failure and adult onset diabetes mellitus.

## HALF-AND-HALF NAILS

- There is a proximal white zone and distal (20–60%) brownish sharp demarcation, the histology of which suggests an increase of vessel wall thickness and melanin deposition.
- It is seen in 9–50% of patients with chronic renal failure and after chemotherapy.

## NEAPOLITAN NAILS

Where there are bands of white, brown and red—a feature of old age.

## MUEHRCKE'S PAIRED WHITE BANDS

- These bands are parallel to the lunula in the nailbed, with pink between two white lines.
- They are commonly associated with hypoalbuminemia, the correction of which by albumin infusion can reverse the sign.
- They have also been reported following placement of a left ventricular assist device in a patient with congestive heart failure.

## BACTERIAL PARONYCHIA

### Acute Paronychia

- It is a common complaint usually due to staphylococcal infection.
- It may result from local injuries, splits, splinters or nail biting.
- It also occurs frequently as a complication of chronic paronychia, when other organisms may be involved, including streptococci, *Pseudomonas pyocyanea,* coliform organisms and proteus vulgaris.
- The condition presents as a painful swelling of the nail fold.
- If superficial it may point close to the nail and can easily be drained by incision with a size 11 scalpel, without anesthesia.
- Deeper lesions are best treated by antibiotics initially, but if they do not improve within 2 days, incision under local anesthesia is required, particularly in childhood.

## Chronic Paronychia

- This is an inflammatory dermatosis of the nail folds, with secondary effects on the nail matrix, nail growth and soft tissue attachments.
- It may be associated with infection on the background of the dermatosis.
- The dermatosis may be directly due to an irritant associated with wet work or caustic materials. Alternatively, it may be on the background of atopy or psoriasis.
- It is predominantly a disease of domestic workers, bar staff, canteen workers and fishmongers.
- The majority of cases are in patients between 30 and 60 years of age.
- The condition begins as a slight swelling at the base of one or more nails, which is tender but much less so than in acute paronychia.
- The cuticle is soon lost and pus may form below the nail fold.
- Inflammation adjacent to the matrix disturbs nail growth, resulting in irregular transverse ridges and other surface irregularities, which may be combined with discoloration.
- Candidial and superadded bacterial infection may be seen.
- **Treatment**
  - ➢ Treatment is a combination of avoidance of precipitants, hand care and medication.
  - ➢ For all wet work the patient should be advised to wear cotton gloves under rubber or plastic gloves and avoid manicure of the proximal nail folds.
  - ➢ Topical therapy requires a combination of steroid and antimicrobial.
  - ➢ More potent topical antibacterials may be needed.
  - ➢ In severe cases systemic antibiotics may be needed. Topical imidazoles should be used in case of candidial superinfection.
  - ➢ Surgical removal of the proximal nail fold and adjacent part of the lateral nail folds may cure recalcitrant cases.

## Pseudomonas Infection

- This is almost always a complication of onycholysis or chronic paronychia and is usually restricted to one or two nails.
- The nail plate has a characteristic bluish-black or green color due to accumulation of debris beneath the nail and the pigment pyocyanin adhering to the undersurface of the nail plate.

## NAIL PSORIASIS

Nail involvement is common in patients with psoriasis and psoriatic arthritis, affecting 80–90% of patients at some time (Table 11.1).

## Treatment

- There is no cure for nail psoriasis but it may improve by itself and may even return to a normal appearance.
- Calcipotriol solution applied twice daily to the nail folds is safe to use and may help nail psoriasis if applied over prolonged periods.
- Topical high-potency corticosteroid solution or ointment works best when covered by cellophane wrap at bedtime. Avoid prolonged occlusion (2 weeks at most) or continuous therapy with corticosteroids.

| Table 11.1: Features of nail psoriasis | | |
|---|---|---|
| Psoriasis sign/ symptom | Site | Features |
| 1. Oil drop or salmon patch | Nailbed | Translucent yellow–red discoloration in the nailbed, resembles drop of oil under nail plate |
| 2. Pitting (thimble) | Proximal nail matrix | Loss of parakeratotic cells from surface of nail plate (Fig. 11.1) |
| 3. Beau's lines | Proximal nail matrix | Transverse lines in nails due to intermittent inflammation causing growth arrest lines |
| 4. Leukonychia | Midmatrix disease | Areas of white nail plate due to foci of parakeratosis within the body of the nail plate |
| 5. Subungual hyperkeratosis | Hyponychium and nailbed | Excessive proliferation of the nailbed and hyponychium. May lead to onycholysis (Figs 11.1 and 11.2) |
| 6. Onycholysis | Nailbed and hyponychium | Nail plate separates from its underlying attachment to nailbed. Nail plate whitens and may detach. Secondary infection may occur |
| 7 Nail plate crumbling | Nailbed or nail matrix | Nail plate weakens due to disease of underlying structures |

- Intralesional triamcinolone acetonide injected into proximal nail folds is helpful (but painful) in nail matrix psoriasis.
- Topical 5-fluorouracil cream applied to the matrix for 6 months may improve pitting and subungual hyperkeratosis.
- Psoralen and UVA (photochemotherapy or PUVA) may improve nail psoriasis.
- Systemic treatment with oral methotrexate, retinoids and ciclosporin is usually prescribed for generalized psoriasis but may also be helpful for nail disease.
- Antifungal treatment may be prescribed if secondary infection is present.
- Chemical or surgical avulsion therapy, i.e. complete removal of the nail, is rarely recommended.

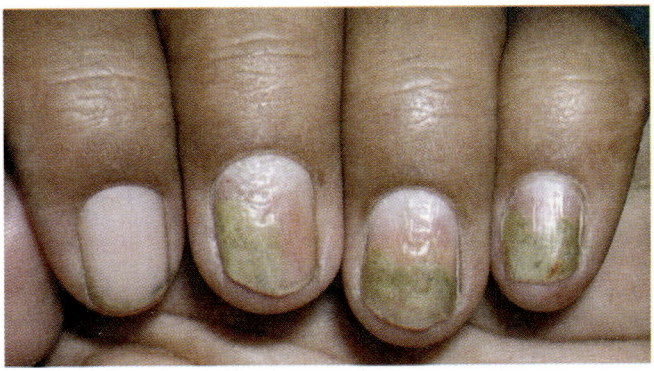

**Fig. 11.1:** Pitting and subungual hyperkeratosis in nail psoriasis

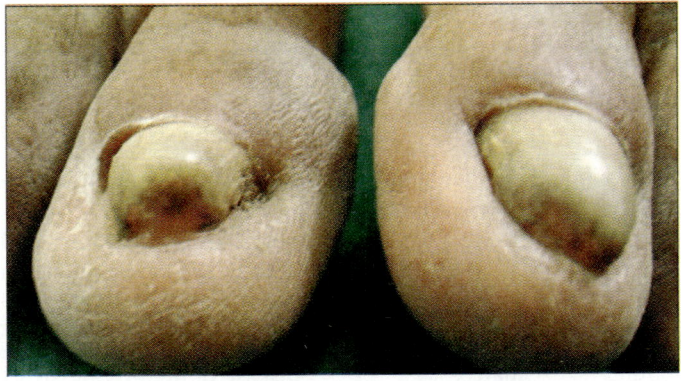

**Fig. 11.2:** Subungual hyperkeratosis of great toes

## NAILS IN LICHEN PLANUS

- Nail involvement occurs in up to 10% of cases, but is usually a minor feature of the disease.
- The majority of cases present during the fifth or sixth decades; long-term permanent damage to the nails is rare.
- Fingernails are more frequently affected than toe nails.
- The most common changes are exaggeration of the longitudinal lines and linear depressions, due to slight thinning of the nail plate.
- Elevated ridges may be seen on the nail.
- Adhesion between the epidermis of the dorsal nail fold and the nailbed may cause partial destruction of the nail (**pterygium unguis**) (Fig. 11.3).
- Subungual hyperkeratosis
- Rarely, the nail is completely shed (onycholysis)

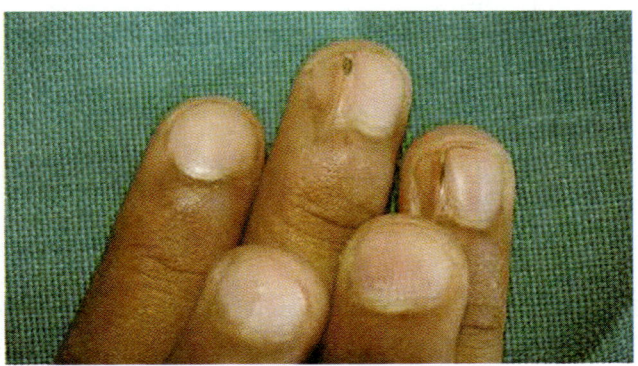

**Fig. 11.3:** Pterygium unguis in LP

### QUESTIONS FROM PREVIOUS EXAMINATIONS

1. Nail changes in systemic disorders
2. Onychomycosis
3. Mees lines
4. Shore like nails
5. Beau's lines
6. Leukonychia
7. Yellow nail syndrome
8. Ainhum
9. Nail—appearance and therapy

## MULTIPLE CHOICE QUESTIONS

1. A young female presented with lacy linear lesions on tongue since a month with elongation of nail fold beyond the nailbed. What is the most likely diagnosis?    *(AI 2010)*
   (a) Psoriasis
   (b) Geographic tongue
   (c) Lichen planus
   (d) Candidiasis

2. A 38-year-old Bengali man presents with complains of multiple papular lesions over the body especially involving the palms and soles. The lesions are not painful. He has pigmentation of skin over the abdomen. He also has vertical white ridges over the nails. Which of the following is the most likely diagnosis?    *(AI 2010)*
   (a) Xeroderma pigmentosum
   (b) Chronic arsenic poisoning
   (c) Lichen planus
   (d) Erythrodermoplasia verruciformis

3. Nail infection is caused by which fungus?    *(AI 2013)*
   (a) *Trichophyton rubrum*
   (b) *Microsporum canis*
   (c) *Candida albicans*
   (d) *Trichophyton verrucosum*

4. For treatment of fungal nail infection griseofulvin should be given for a period of:    *(DNB 2012)*
   (a) 4 weeks
   (b) 6 weeks
   (c) 2 months
   (d) 3 months

5. A 30-year-old female presents with nonscarring alopecia, papular skin lesions and thining of nail plate. Diagnosis is:
   (a) Lichen planus
   (b) Psoriasis
   (c) Dermatophyte infection
   (d) Syphilis

## Answers

1. **Ans. (c)** Lichen planus
2. **Ans. (b)** Chronic arsenic poisoning
3. **Ans. (a)** *Trichophyton rubrum*
4. **Ans. (d)** 3 months
5. **Ans. (a)** Lichen planus

# 12 Disorders of Sebaceous and Sweat Glands

## ROSACEA (ACNE ROSACEA)

- **Rosacea** is a chronic inflammatory disorder of the skin of the facial convexities characterized by persistent erythema and telangiectasias punctated by acute episodes of swelling, papules and pustules.
- Rosacea affects women more commonly than men.
- 30–50 yrs of age.
- Comedones are absent.
- Aggravated by heat, alcohol, emotional stimuli, spicy food and hotdrinks.
- Rosacea of very long-standing may lead to connective tissue overgrowth, particularly of the nose (rhinophyma).
- Rosacea may also be complicated by various inflammatory disorders of the eye, including keratitis, blepharitis, iritis, and recurrent chalazion.
- **Differential diagnosis**
  - ➢ Flushing, autonomic mediated
    - – Exercise
    - – Spicy food
    - – Emotions
    - – Horner syndrome
  - ➢ Atopic dermatitis
  - ➢ Seborrheic dermatitis
  - ➢ Systemic lupus erythematosus
  - ➢ Dermatomyositis
  - ➢ Acne vulgaris and steroid-induced acne
  - ➢ Perioral dermatitis
  - ➢ Physical erythema
    - – Mechanical
    - – Thermal
    - – Electromagnetic

➤ Contact and photocontact dermatitis
➤ Medications
➤ Sarcoidosis

- **Treatment**
  ➤ Oral tetracyclines are **drug of choice**.
  ➤ Topical erythromycin (2%), clindamycin (0.5%) and benzoyl-peroxide are also helpful.
  ➤ Topical metronidazole (0.75%) is also effective.
  ➤ Oral doxycycline, erythromycin and minocycline can also be given.
  ➤ Isotretinoin (0.5 mg/kg body wt) or metronidazole (500 mg twice daily) can be used if no response to above drugs.
  ➤ Lasers have been used to treat erythema and telangiectasia.
  ➤ Rhinophyma may need surgery.

## ACNE VULGARIS

- Chronic inflammatory disease of pilosebaceous units.
- Occurs most commonly during adolescence and frequently continues into adulthood.
- Four major factors are involved in the pathogenesis:
  ➤ Increased sebum production
  ➤ Hypercornification of the pilosebaceous duct
  ➤ Abnormality of the microbial flora especially colonization of the duct with *Propionibacterium acnes*
  ➤ Inflammation.
- It is characterized by noninflammatory follicular papules or comedones and by inflammatory papules, pustules, cysts and nodules in its more severe forms (Fig. 12.1).

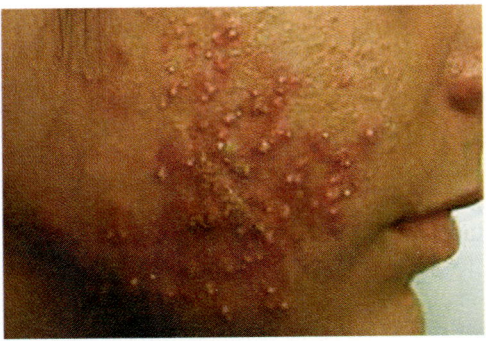

**Fig. 12.1:** Multiple papules and pustules in a young female with acne vulgaris

- Open comedones represent dome-shaped papules in which there are dilated follicular outlets filled with keratin. The apparent black color is thought to be due to melanin deposited within the cellular debris.
- Closed comedones or whiteheads are generally 1 mm in diameter, skin colored and have no visible follicular opening.
- The activity of bacteria *Propionibacterium acnes* within the comedones releases free fatty acids from sebum, causes inflammation within the cyst, and results in rupture of the cyst.
- Acne vulgaris affects the areas of skin with the densest population of sebaceous follicles; these areas include the face, the upper part of the chest, and the back.

*Earliest lesions* *seen in adolescence are generally mildly inflamed or noninflammatory comedones on the forehead.*

- Scarring may be seen in severe acne.
- Scars may show increased collagen (hypertrophic scars and keloids) or be associated with loss of collagen (i.e. ice-pick scars, depressed fibrotic scars, atrophic macules and perifollicular elastolysis).
- **Treatment**
  - ➤ *Directed towards:* Elimination of comedones by normalization of follicular keratinization, decreasing sebaceous gland activity, decreasing the population of *P. acnes*, and decreasing inflammation.
  - ➤ *Topical therapy for acne*
    - This is designed to produce peeling of the skin, restore normal keratinization and produce a bactericidal action.
    - Common peeling agents are sulfur (3.5%), resorcinol (3.5%), benzyl peroxide (2.5–10%) and retinoic acid (0.025–0.1%).
    - Topical antibiotics include erythromycin (1–2%), clindamycin (1–2%) and benzyl peroxide (5–10%).
    - Benzyl peroxide has bacteriostatic properties in addition to its action as a peeling agent.
  - ➤ *Systemic therapy*
    - Antibiotics like tetracycline, doxycycline, minocycline and erythromycin
    - Dapsone
    - Hormonal therapy: Ethinyl estradiol, cyproterone acetate and spironolactone
    - Oral retinoids

- Oral zinc, oral vit A
- Oral corticosteroids are used in severe inflammatory acne.

> **Depending on severity of acne**
  - *Minimal to moderate,* pauci-inflammatory disease may respond adequately to local therapy alone.
  - *Topical agents,* such as retinoic acid, benzoyl peroxide, or salicylic acid may alter the pattern of epidermal desquamation, preventing the formation of comedones and aiding in the resolution of pre-existing cysts.
  - Topical antibacterial agents such as azelaic acid, topical erythromycin (with or without zinc), or clindamycin are also useful adjuncts to therapy.

> **Moderate to severe acne**
  - If will benefit from the addition of systemic therapy, such as tetracycline in doses of 250–500 mg bid, or doxycycline, 100 mg bid.
  - Female patients who do not respond to oral antibiotics may benefit from hormonal therapy.
  - Women placed on oral contraceptives containing ethinyl estradiol and norgestimate have demonstrated improvement in their acne.

> **Patients with severe nodulocystic acne**
  - Unresponsive to the therapies may benefit from treatment with the synthetic retinoid, isotretinoin.
  - Its dose is based on the patient's weight, and it is given once daily for 5 months.
  - 0.5–1 mg/kg/day
  - Its use is highly regulated due to its potential for severe adverse events, primarily teratogenicity. It causes birth defects (deformed babies), loss of baby before birth (miscarriage), death of baby, and early (premature) births. Female patients who are pregnant or who plan to become pregnant must not take isotretinoin.

> **Female patients must not get pregnant**
  - For 1 month before starting isotretinoin
  - While taking isotretinoin
  - For 1 month after stopping isotretinoin.

> Additionally, patients receiving this medication develop:
  - Extremely dry skin
  - Cheilitis
  - Hypertriglyceridemia.

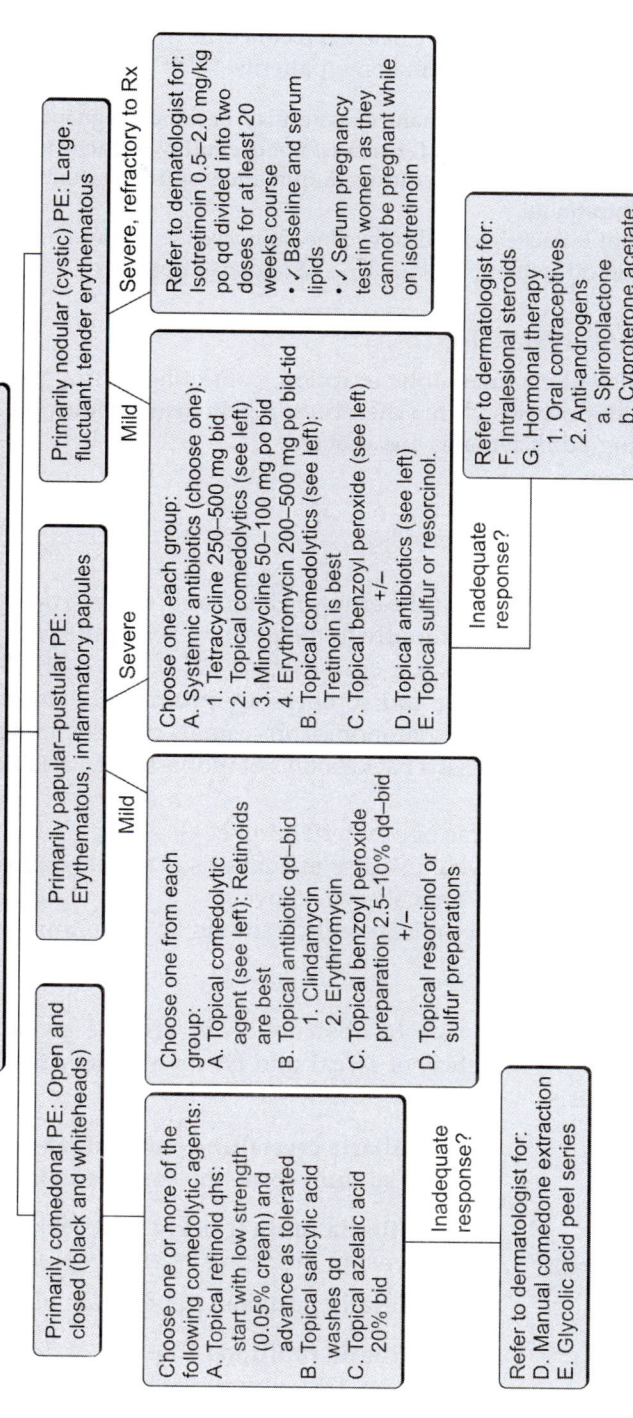

**Fig. 12.2:** Approach to a patient with acne

> ➤ Recently there have also been concerns that it is associated with severe depression in some patients.

**Women who are pregnant or who may become pregnant because of the potential harm to a fetus must not use following acne medications:**
1. Hormonal therapy—estrogen, flutamide, spironolactone
2. Isotretinoin
3. Oral tetracyclines—doxycycline, minocycline, tetracycline
4. Topical retinoids—adapalene, tazarotene, tretinoin

## PERIORAL DERMATITIS

- Persistent erythematous eruption, consisting of tiny papules and papulopustules with a distribution primarily around the mouth.
- Young adult females are affected.
- **Etiology**
  - ➤ Cosmetic products
  - ➤ Potent topical steroids
- **Clinical features**
  - ➤ Characteristically, the eruption begins abruptly in the nasolabial areas spreading rapidly to the perioral zone but sparing the lip margins
  - ➤ Pruritus, burning and soreness are prominent symptoms. The lesions consist of monomorphic small papules and pustules occurring against a background of redness and variable scaling.
- **Treatment**
  - ➤ A 4-week course of oral tetracycline.
  - ➤ Topical tetracycline is also effective as is topical metronidazole cream 1% and topical erythromycin.
  - ➤ Cosmetics and topical steroids should be discontinued.

## MILIARIA

- **Miliaria** occurs due to obstruction of **eccrine sweat glands,** resulting in secretion of sweat into layers of epidermis and focal anhidrosis.

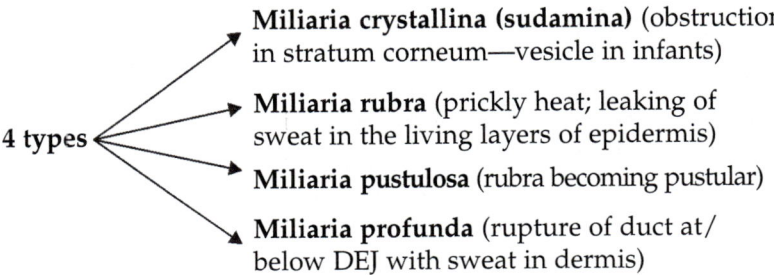

**4 types**
- **Miliaria crystallina (sudamina)** (obstruction in stratum corneum—vesicle in infants)
- **Miliaria rubra** (prickly heat; leaking of sweat in the living layers of epidermis)
- **Miliaria pustulosa** (rubra becoming pustular)
- **Miliaria profunda** (rupture of duct at/below DEJ with sweat in dermis)

- **Clinical features**
  - ➢ *Miliaria crystallina*
    - Clear, thin-walled vesicles, 1–2 mm in diameter, without an inflammatory areola are usually symptomless and develop in crops, mainly on the trunk.
    - In persistent febrile illnesses, recurrent crops may occur.
    - The vesicles soon rupture, and are followed by superficial, branny desquamation.
  - ➢ *Miliaria rubra*
    - The typical lesions develop on the body, especially in areas of friction with clothing, and in flexures.
    - The lesions are uniformly minute erythematous papules, which may be present in very large numbers.
    - They produce intense pricking sensation.
  - ➢ *Miliaria profunda*
    - This nearly always follows repeated attacks of miliaria rubra, and is uncommon except in the tropics.
    - The affected skin is covered with pale, firm papules 1–3 mm across, especially on the body, but sometimes also on the limbs.
    - There is no itching or discomfort from the lesions.
- **Complications**
  - ➢ Secondary infection
  - ➢ Disturbance of heat regulation
- **Treatment**
  - ➢ Avoidance of further sweating
  - ➢ Calamine lotion

## HIDRADENITIS SUPPURATIVA

- This is a rare condition characterized by chronic inflammation and scarring of the skin at sites rich in apocrine glands (axillae, groins, natal cleft).
- The cause is unknown but it is commoner in females, and within some families it appears to be inherited in an autosomal dominant fashion.
- Clinically it presents after puberty with papules, nodules and abscesses which often progress to cysts and sinus formation. With time, scarring may arise.
- The condition follows a chronic relapsing/remitting course and is often worse in obese individuals.

- **Treatment** is very difficult but weight loss, antibiotics, oral retinoids and co-cyprindiol ('2 mg cyproterone acetate + 35 µg ethinylestradiol' in females only) have been tried. Severe recalcitrant cases have been treated occasionally with surgery and skin grafting and more recently intravenous infliximab, a monoclonal antibody.

## FOX-FORDYCE DISEASE

- Fox-Fordyce disease is a disorder of the apocrine glands comparable with prickly heat of the eccrine glands.
- The etiology is unknown.
- Obliteration of the apocrine duct at the infundibulum is felt to be the cause.
- Occurs mainly in women soon after puberty.
- Dome-shaped skin-colored follicular papules are seen in axillae, pubic area, labia, perineum, areola and other apocrine gland bearing areas (Fig. 12.3).
- Itching is prominent.
- **Treatment:** Unsatisfactory; topical steroids, clindamycin, pimecrolimus and retinoids have been tried.

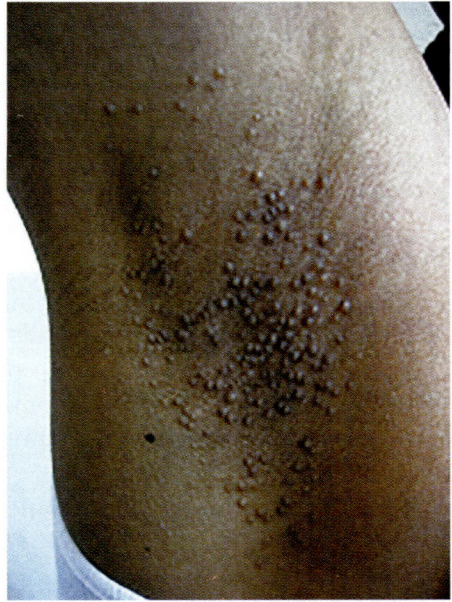

**Fig. 12.3:** Multiple skin-colored follicular papules in axilla

- *Modes of secretion* of exocrine glands can be classified as:
  - ➢ Merocrine
  - ➢ Apocrine
  - ➢ Holocrine.

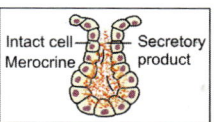 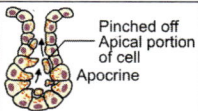 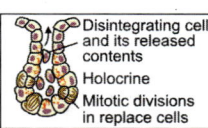

| MEROCRINE METHOD | APOCRINE METHOD | HOLOCRINE METHOD |
|---|---|---|
| • Cells that secrete products via the **merocrine** method form membrane-bound secretory vesicles internal to the cell.<br>• These are moved to the apical surface where the vesicles coalesce with the membrane on the apical surface to release the product.<br>• Most glands release their products in way. | • In those glands that release product via the **apocrine** method, the apical portions of cells are pinched off and lost during the secretory process.<br>• This results in a secretory product that contains a variety of molecular components including those of the membrane.<br>• Mammary glands release their products in this manner.<br>• Others, e.g. axilla, eyelid (Moll's glands), nipple, areola, perianal, external genitalia | • The third type of secretory release, **holocrine**, involves death of the cell.<br>• The secretory cell is released and as it breaks apart, the contents of the cell product.<br>• This mode of secretion results in the most complex secretory product<br>• Some sweat glands located in the axillae, pubic areas, and around the areola of the breasts release their products in this manner.<br>• Sebaceous glands also are of this type |

| | |
|---|---|
| Eccrine glands | • Abundant<br>• Almost present in every part of skin<br>• Most numerous in every part of skin<br>• Least in neck and back<br>• Merocrine (watery) secretion |
| Ceruminous glands | These are modified apocrine sweat glands of external acoustic meatus. |
| Sebaceous glands | These are present all throughout the skin (dermis) except palms and soles. |

## ACNEIFORM ERUPTIONS

- Glucocorticoids, topical or systemic, may also elicit acne.
- Other systemic medications such as oral contraceptive pills, lithium, isoniazid, androgenic steroids, halogens, phenytoin, and phenobarbital may produce acneiform eruptions or aggravate pre-existing acne.

## QUESTIONS FROM PREVIOUS EXAMINATIONS

1. Acne vulgaris—pathogenesis and etiogenesis
2. Treatment of palmar hyperhidrosis
3. Miliaria
4. Hypohydrosis
5. Drug excretion in sweat
6. Chromo-onychosis
7. Sebum
8. Severity of acne
9. Rosacea
10. Topical therapy in acne
11. Flushing and blushing reactions

## MULTIPLE CHOICE QUESTIONS

1. **All the following diseases have to be considered in the differential diagnosis of rosacea** *except:*          *(Kar 07)*
   - (a) Seborrheic dermatitis
   - (b) Discoid lupus erythematosus
   - (c) Carcinoid syndrome
   - (d) Pityriasis versicolor

2. **A 40-year-old female presents with a 2-year history of erythematous papulopustular lesions on the convexities of face. There is background of erythema and telangiectasia. The most probable diagnosis would be:**          *(AI 07)*
   - (a) Acne vulagris
   - (b) Rosacea
   - (c) SLE
   - (d) Polymorphic light eruptions

3. **Hidradenitis suppurativa is a disease of:**          *(AI 13)*
   - (a) Eccrine sweat glands
   - (b) Apocrine sweat glands
   - (c) Kaposi sarcoma
   - (d) Hair follicles

4. **Fordyce spots are:**  *(UPSC 99)*
   (a) Ectopic sebaceous glands  (b) Ectopic eccrine
   (c) Ectopic apocrine  (d) Ectopic mucosal glands

5. **The clinical hallmark of acne vulgaris is:**  *(Bihar 07)*
   (a) Papules  (b) Nodules
   (c) Pustules  (d) Comedones

6. **Which of the following should not be used in the topical treatment of rosacea?**  *(MH 09)*
   (a) Isotretin  (b) Metronidazole
   (c) Steroids  (d) Benzyol peroxide

7. **A 24-year-old unmarried woman has multiple nodular, cystic, pustular and comedonic lesions on face, upper back and shoulders for 2 years. The drug of choice for treatment:**  *(AI 06)*
   (a) Acitretin  (b) Isotretinoin
   (c) Doxycycline  (d) Azithromycin

8. **Benzyl peroxide acts in acne vulgaris by:**  *(TN 08)*
   (a) Decreased sebum production
   (b) Acts as oxidizing agent
   (c) Reduces epithelial proliferation
   (d) Decreasing bacterial count

9. **Most appropriate Rx for nodulocystic acne:**  *(AI 94; AIIMS 95)*
   (a) Erythromycin  (b) Tetracycline
   (c) Corticosteroids  (d) Isotretinoin

10. **Recalcitrant pustular acne is best treated by:**  *(AIIMS 92)*
    (a) Erythromycin  (b) Benzyol peroxide
    (c) Corticosteroids  (d) Retinoid

11. **Which of the following should be avoided in treatment of acne rosacea?**  *(AMU 09)*
    (a) Topical glucocorticoids  (b) Topical metronidazole
    (c) Doxycycline  (d) Laser therapy

12. **Miliaria is disorder of:**  *(PGI 07)*
    (a) Eccrine sweat glands  (b) Apocrine sweat glands
    (c) Sebaceous glands  (d) Hair follicles
    (e) Merocrine glands

13. **Apocrine mode of secretion is classically seen in _____ gland.**
    (a) Mammary gland  (b) Sebaceous gland
    (c) Parotid gland  (d) All of the above

14. **Drugs that may aggravate pre-existing acne include the following** *except:*
    (a) Paracetamol  (b) Glucocorticoid
    (c) Lithium  (d) Phenytoin

## Answers

1. **Ans. (d)** Pityriasis versicolor *(Ref. Differential Diagnosis in Dermatology by Richard Ashton, page 105)*
2. **Ans. (b)** Rosacea *(Ref. Roxburgh, 17th edn/162)*
3. **Ans. (b)** Apocrine sweat glands
4. **Ans. (a)** Ectopic sebaceous glands *(Ref. Harrison's Medicine, 17th edn/ 128; 218f)*
5. **Ans. (d)** Comedones
6. **Ans. (c)** Steroids *(Ref. IADVL, 2nd edition, 702, 703)*
7. **Ans. (b)** Isotretinoin
8. **Ans. (d)** Decreasing bacterial count *(Ref. Behl, 9th edn/408)*
9. **Ans. (d)** Isotretinoin *(Ref. Roxburgh's Common Skin Diseases, 17th edn/149)*
10. **Ans. (d)** Retinoid *(Ref. Fitzpatrick's Dermatology in General Medicine, 7th edn, 685)*
11. **Ans. (a)** Topical glucocorticoids *(Ref. Fitzpatrick's Dermatology in General Medicine, 7th edn, 685)*
12. **Ans. (a)** Eccrine sweat glands *(Ref. Rook's Dermatology, 7th edn, 45.23, 36.49, 66.23)*
13. **Ans. (a)** Mammary gland *(Ref. Handbook of General Anatomy by Chaurasia, 3rd edition, page 129)*
14. **Ans. (a)** Paracetamol *(Ref. Harrison, 17th edn/Chapter 53; Behl, 9th edn/408)*

# 13 Immunological Mediated Skin Diseases

## Causes of Vesicles/Bullae

- **Primary cutaneous diseases**
  - ➤ Primary blistering diseases (autoimmune)
  - ➤ Pemphigus
  - ➤ Bullous pemphigoid
  - ➤ Gestational pemphigoid
  - ➤ Cicatricial pemphigoid
  - ➤ Dermatitis herpetiformis
  - ➤ Linear IgA disease
  - ➤ Epidermolysis bullosa acquisita
  - ➤ Secondary blistering diseases
  - ➤ Contact dermatitis
  - ➤ Erythema multiforme
  - ➤ Toxic epidermal necrolysis
  - ➤ Infections
  - ➤ Varicella-zoster virus
  - ➤ Herpes simplex virus
  - ➤ Enteroviruses, e.g. hand-foot-mouth disease
  - ➤ Staphylococcal scalded skin syndrome
  - ➤ Bullous impetigo
- **Systemic diseases**
  - ➤ Autoimmune
  - ➤ Paraneoplastic pemphigus
  - ➤ Infections
  - ➤ Cutaneous emboli
  - ➤ Metabolic
  - ➤ Diabetic bullae
  - ➤ Porphyria cutanea tarda
  - ➤ Porphyria variegata
  - ➤ Pseudoporphyria

> Bullous dermatosis of hemodialysis
> Ischemia
> Coma bullae

## Classification of Vesiculobullous Diseases (Table 13.1)

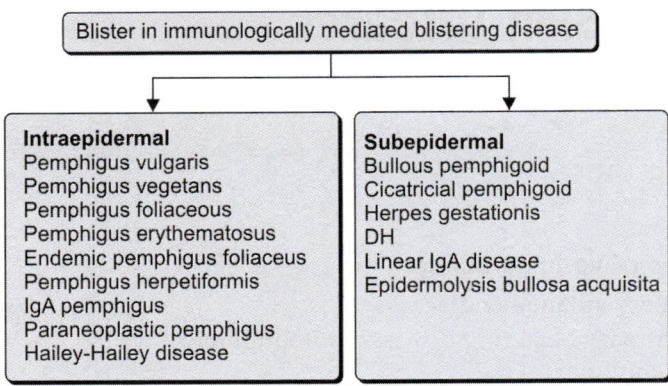

Blister in immunologically mediated blistering disease

**Intraepidermal**
Pemphigus vulgaris
Pemphigus vegetans
Pemphigus foliaceous
Pemphigus erythematosus
Endemic pemphigus foliaceus
Pemphigus herpetiformis
IgA pemphigus
Paraneoplastic pemphigus
Hailey-Hailey disease

**Subepidermal**
Bullous pemphigoid
Cicatricial pemphigoid
Herpes gestationis
DH
Linear IgA disease
Epidermolysis bullosa acquisita

## DERMATITIS HERPETIFORMIS

- Genetic factors are believed to play a role in the pathogenesis of DH because the HLA antigens B8, DRw17 and DQw2 have been separately found in 80–100% of patients.
- These antigens are coded by genes that are present on chromosome 6.
- Associated with celiac sprue.
- Presents most often in 2nd or 3rd decade.
- Slight male predominance.
- Eruption is characteristically polymorphous. The primary lesion is an erythematous papule or urticarial plaque or classically small vesicle on erythematous, edematous base (Fig. 13.1).

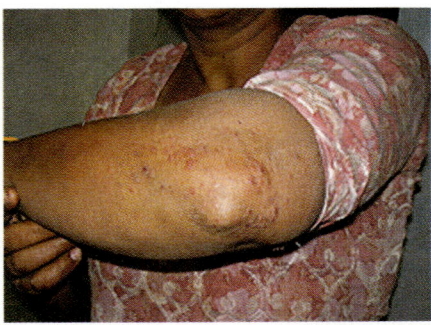

**Fig. 13.1:** Multiple erythematous papules and plaques over elbow and extensor aspect of left upper limb

**Table 13.1:** Immunologically mediated blistering diseases

| Disease | Clinical features | Histology | Immunopathology | Autoantigens |
|---|---|---|---|---|
| **Pemphigus foliaceus** | Crusts and shallow erosions on scalp, central face, upper chest, and back | Acantholytic blister formed in superficial layer of epidermis | Cell surface deposits of IgG on keratinocytes | Dsg1 |
| **Pemphigus vulgaris** | Flaccid blisters, denuded skin, oromucosal lesions | Acantholytic blister formed in suprabasal layer of epidermis | Cell surface deposits of IgG on keratinocytes | Dsg3 (plus Dsg1 in patients with skin involvement) |
| **Paraneoplastic pemphigus** | Painful stomatitis with papulosquamous or lichenoid eruptions that progress to blisters | Acantholysis, keratinocyte necrosis and vacuolar interface dermatitis | Cell surface deposits of IgG and C3 on keratinocytes and (variably) similar immunoreactants in epidermal BMZ | Plakin protein family members and desmosomal cadherins (see text for details) |
| **Bullous pemphigoid** | Large tense blisters on flexor surfaces and trunk | Subepidermal blister with eosinophil-rich infiltrate | Linear band of IgG and/or C3 in epidermal MBZ | BPAG1, BPAG2 |
| **Pemphigoid gestationis** | Pruritic, urticarial plaques, rimmed by vesicles and bullae on the trunk and extremities | Teardrop-shaped, subepidermal blisters in dermal papillae; eosinophil-rich infiltrate | Linear band of C3 in epidermal BMZ | BPAG2 (plus BPAG1 in some patients) |

*Contd.*

**Table 13.1:** Immunologically mediated blistering diseases *Contd.*

| Disease | Clinical features | Histology | Immunopathology | Autoantigens |
|---|---|---|---|---|
| **Linear IgA disease** | Pruritic small papules on extensor surfaces; occasionally larger, arciform blisters | Subepidermal blister with neutrophil-rich infiltrate | Linear band of IgA in epidermal BMZ | BPAG2 (see text for specific details) |
| **Cicatricial pemphigoid** | Erosive and/or blistering lesions of mucous membranes and possibly the skin; scarring of some sites | Subepidermal blister that may or may not include a leukocytic infiltrate | Linear band of IgG, IgA, and/or C3 in epidermal BMZ | BPAG2, laminin 5, or others |
| **Epidermolysis bullosa acquisita** | Blisters, erosions, scars, and milia on sites exposed to trauma; widespread, inflammatory, tense blisters may be seen initially | Subepidermal blister that may or may not include a leukocytic infiltrate | Linear band of IgG and/or C3 in epidermal BMZ | Type VII collagen |
| **Dermatitis herpetiformis** | Extremely pruritic small papules and vesicles on elbows, knees, buttocks, and posterior neck | Subepidermal blister with neutrophils in dermal papillae | Granular deposits of IgA in dermal papillae | Epidermal transglutaminase |

- Blisters may be grouped in a herpetiform manner on erythematous plaque.
- Lesions are accompanied by intense itching or burning or stinging sensation and may precede a new lesion by 8–12 hrs.
- Lesions are symmetrically distributed over extensor surfaces of limbs.
- The areas of predilection are elbows, knees, buttocks, sacrum, shoulders, posterior hairline, and scalp.
- Face is occasionally affected but mucous membrane only rarely.
- Associated with gluten sensitive enteropathy and other autoimmune disorders like thyroid problems, SLE, RA, Sjögren's syndrome, and UC.
- Increased risk of lymphoma.
- **Gluten sensitive enteropathy**
- Less than 10% patients with DH have GIT symptoms suggestive of celiac disease, but virtually all patients suffer an enteropathy of varying severity.
- Usually asymptomatic but some have diarrhea, steatorrhea, abdominal distension, and weight loss.
- Abnormal absorption of D-xylose, iron, folate, glucose, water, and bicarbonate and low serum levels of iron and folate have been documented.
- Patchy involvement of small intestine, particularly the jejunum, biopsies from which show flattening of surfaces of epithelial cells, blunting of villi, elongation of intestinal crypts and an inflammatory infiltrate primarily of lymphocytes and plasma cells in the lamina propria.
- Enteropathy is due to non-allergic sensitivity to the gliadin fraction of gluten, the protein part that remains after removal of starch and water from defatted flour.
- **Histopathology**
  - Neutrophilic microabscesses at adjoining papillae intermingled with a few eosinophils, giving a multilocular appearance.
- **Immunopathology**
  - Perilesional noninvolved skin exhibits granular deposits of IgA in the dermal papillae.
  - No circulating anti-BM antibodies are found. Antiendomysial, antireticulin, and antigliadin antibodies have been identified in serum in 72%, 25%, and 45% of patients with DH, respectively.
  - Antiendomysial abs are of IgA class only and are diagnostic of DH.

- **Immunoelectron microscopy**
  - IgA deposits in the skin are in the form of amorphous grains 0.1 micrometer in size called DH bodies, mostly in sub-basal membrane region but also in the papillary dermis.
  - Recently tissue transglutaminase has been identified as the autoantigen of IgA antibodies in celiac disease.
  - Circulating IgA autoantibodies to tissue transglutaminase are detectable in DH as well and their levels reflect extent of changes of jejunal mucosa.
  - The ultrastructural site of blister formation in DH is the lamina lucida.
- **Treatment**
  - *Medications*
    - Drug therapy promptly suppresses the skin eruptions, but does not affect the IgA deposition in the skin, the enteropathy or its nutritional consequences.
    - *Dapsone* is the mainstay for Rx of DH.
      - o Dapsone inhibits proteolytic enzymes of neutrophils.
      - o Initial dose is 100 mg/day.
      - o Burning and itching usually cease within 24 hrs.
    - Sulfapyridine—poorly absorbed from GIT.
    - Colchicine—when dapsone and sulfapyridine are contraindicated.
  - *Gluten-free diet*
    - Though difficult to follow, treats the underlying precipitating cause of DH and results in a gradual resolution of the intestinal changes and in some patients of the IgA deposits in the skin and may protect against the risk of lymphoma.
    - The diet should be continued lifelong or the rash may return.
  - A gluten-free diet mandates strict avoidance of:

    - Barley
    - Rye     **BROW**
    - Oats
    - Wheat

## PEMPHIGUS

- **Pemphigus** refers to a group of autoantibody-mediated intraepidermal blistering diseases characterized by loss of cohesion between epidermal cells (a process termed acantholysis).

- Pemphigus is divided into 2 major subtypes:
  - ➢ Pemphigus vulgaris (includes pemphigus vegetans as variant)
  - ➢ Pemphigus foliaceus (includes pemphigus erythematosus and endemic pemphigus foliaceus)
- The most common subtype is **pemphigus vulgaris**, which presents with oral blisters and erosions in more than half of the patients. Skin lesions may appear after a period of several weeks.

## Pemphigus Vulgaris

- Presents with oral blisters and erosions in more than half of the patients.
- Skin lesions may appear after a period of several wks.
- The cutaneous lesions are vesicles and flaccid bullae on apparently normal skin (Fig. 13.2).
- Sites most commonly involved are: Scalp, face, axillae, and oral cavity.
- Bullae are initially **tense** and clear but become **flaccid and** turbid in 2–3 days.
- Nikolsky's sign is positive.
- Bulla spread sign is positive.

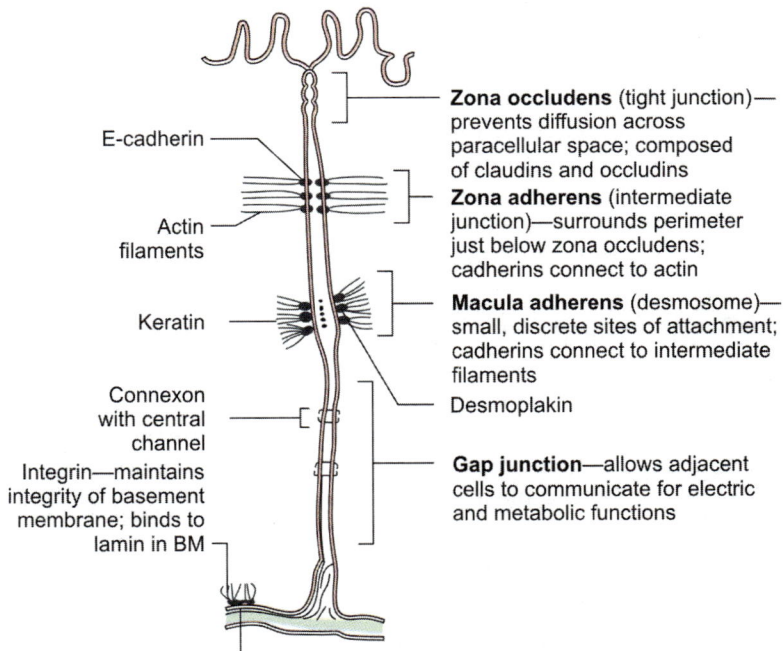

**Hemidesmosome**—connects cells to underlying extracellular matrix

**Fig. 13.2:** Cell junctions

- Almost all patients have oral involvement.
- Any stratified squamous mucosal surface (pharyngeal, laryngeal, esophageal, conjunctival, urethral, cervical, anal, may be affected particularly in severe disease).
- Itching may be present.
- Lesions usually heal without scarring, except at sites complicated by secondary infection or mechanically induced dermal wounds. Postinflammatory hyperpigmentation is usually present at sites of healed lesions for some time.
- Common causes of morbidity and mortality are infection and complications of treatment with glucocorticoids.
- **Bad prognostic factors include** advanced age, widespread involvement, and the requirement for high doses of glucocorticoids (with or without other immunosuppressive agents) for control of disease.
- Associated with thymoma and myasthenia gravis. Other autoimmune disorders like polymyositis, Sjögren's syndrome, RA, SLE, pernicious anemia (atrophic gastritis) may also be associated.
- Drugs containing a thiol group in their chemical structure (e.g. penicillamine, captopril, enalapril) are most commonly associated with drug-induced pemphigus. Nonthiol drugs linked to pemphigus include penicillins, cephalosporins, and piroxicam.
- **HPE**
  - ➤ The earliest changes are intercellular edema and disappearance of intercellular bridges in the lower most epidermis.
  - ➤ Intraepidermal vesicle formation secondary to loss of cohesion between epidermal cells (i.e. acantholytic blisters). Blister cavities contain acantholytic epidermal cells, which appear as round homogeneous cells containing hyperchromatic nuclei. Basal keratinocytes remain attached to the epidermal basement membrane.
  - ➤ *Tombstone appearance:* Basal cells remain attached to dermis.
  - ➤ Lesional skin may contain focal collections of intraepidermal eosinophils within blister cavities.
  - ➤ There is scanty perivascular inflammatory infiltrate composed of lymphocytes, histiocytes and occasional eosinophils, neutrophils, and plasma cells.
- **Immunopathology**
  - ➤ *Direct immunofluorescence*
    Deposition of IgG in the intercellular substance of epithelium.
  - ➤ *Indirect immunofluorescence*
    Circulating IgG abs directed against the cell surface of keratinocytes.

- **Autoantigens**
  - ➤ Desmoglein 3 mainly and desmoglein 1: All patients with PV have anti-Dsg3 abs.
  - ➤ Over 50% have anti-Dsg1 abs.
  - ➤ Desmoglein is a component of desmosome which binds the individual cells of epidermis.
  - ➤ Desmosome is a disc-like intercellular junction that is shared by two neighboring keratinocytes, each providing half of the structure.
  - ➤ In pemphigus, the desmosomes are disrupted and cell become round and separate.
- **Treatment**
  - ➤ *The mainstay of treatment is systemic glucocorticoids:* Patients with moderate to severe PV are usually started on prednisone, 1 mg/kg per day. If new lesions continue to appear after 1–2 weeks of treatment, the dose may need to be increased. Many regimens combine an immunosuppressive agent with systemic glucocorticoids for control of PV. The most frequently used are azathioprine (2–2.5 mg/kg per day), mycophenolate mofetil (20–35 mg/kg per day), or cyclophosphamide (1–2 mg/kg per day).
  - ➤ *Patients with severe, treatment-resistant disease may derive benefit from* plasmapheresis [six high-volume exchanges (i.e. 2–3 liters per exchange) over ~2 weeks], IV immunoglobulin (2 g/kg over 3–5 days every 6–8 weeks), or rituximab (375 mg/m$^2$ per week × 4).
  - ➤ *Dexamethasone: Cyclophosphamide pulse therapy*
- **DD of pemphigus vulgaris (Fig. 13.3)**
  - ➤ *Oral lesions*
    - – Aphthous ulcers
    - – Erythema multiforme
    - – Primary herpetic gingivostomatitis
    - – Candidiasis
    - – Erosive lichen planus
      Acantholytic cells on Tzanck smear = pemphigus vulgaris.
  - ➤ *Skin lesions*

| Subepidermal blisters | Bullous pemphigoid | Tense bullae |
| --- | --- | --- |
| | Cicatricial pemphigoid | Nikolsky's sign |
| | DH | negative |
| | Epidermolysis bullosa acquisita | |

- Pemphigus vegetans is a rare and more benign variant of pemphigus vulgaris.
  - It has 2 forms: Neumann and Hallopeau types.
  - It involves intertriginous areas and flexural surfaces.
  - Local moisture, heat, and friction are important factors in their development.

## Pemphigus Foliaceus

- Pemphigus foliaceus (PF) is distinguished from PV by several features. In PF, acantholytic blisters are located high within the epidermis, usually just beneath the stratum corneum (subcorneal). Hence, PF is a more superficial blistering disease than PV.
- The distribution of lesions in the two disorders is much the same, except that in PF mucous membranes are almost always spared.
- Patients with PF rarely demonstrate intact blisters but rather exhibit shallow erosions associated with erythema, scale, and crust formation. Mild cases of PF resemble severe seborrheic dermatitis; severe PF may cause extensive exfoliation.
- Seborrheic areas initially involved but latter disease may become generalized and patient presents as an erythroderma.
- Sun exposure (ultraviolet irradiation) may be an aggravating factor. Characteristic musty odor.
- **Fogo selvagem (FS)**, an endemic form of PF is thought to develop as a consequence of environmental stimuli (e.g. insect bites).
- **HPE**
  - The cleft is superficial usually in the granular layer.
  - It may develop into bulla with acantholysis at the floor as well as roof.

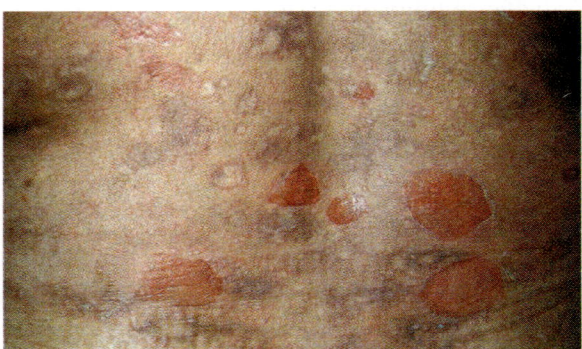

**Fig. 13.3:** Multiple erosions over back in a patient of pemphigus vulgaris

- Patients with PF have immunopathologic features in common with PV. Specifically, direct immunofluorescence microscopy of perilesional skin demonstrates IgG on the surface of keratinocytes.
- Similarly, patients with PF have circulating IgG autoantibodies directed against the surface of keratinocytes. Guinea pig esophagus is the optimal substrate for indirect immunofluorescence microscopy studies of sera from patients with PF.
- In PF, autoantibodies are directed against Dsg1, a 160-kDa desmosomal cadherin. As noted for PV, the autoantibody profile in patients with PF (i.e. anti-Dsg1 IgG) and the tissue distribution of this autoantigen (i.e. expression in oral mucosa that is compensated by coexpression of Dsg3) is thought to account for the distribution of lesions in this disease.
- PF is generally a less severe disease than PV and carries a better prognosis.
- Localized disease can sometimes be treated with topical or intralesional glucocorticoids; more active cases can usually be controlled with systemic glucocorticoids.
- Patients with severe, treatment-resistant disease may require more aggressive interventions as described above for patients with severe PV.

## Paraneoplastic Pemphigus

- Paraneoplastic pemphigus (PNP) is an autoimmune acantholytic mucocutaneous disease associated with an occult or confirmed neoplasm.
- Patients with PNP typically show painful mucosal erosive lesions in association with papulosquamous and/or lichenoid eruptions that often progress to blisters.
- Palm and sole involvement is common in these patients.
- The predominant neoplasms associated with PNP are:
  - ➤ Non-Hodgkin's lymphoma
  - ➤ Chronic lymphocytic leukemia
  - ➤ Thymoma
  - ➤ Spindle cell tumors
  - ➤ Waldenström's macroglobulinemia
  - ➤ Castleman's disease; the latter is particularly common among children with PNP
  - ➤ Biopsies of lesional skin from these patients show varying combinations of suprabasal acantholysis, dyskeratotic

keratinocytes, keratinocyte necrosis, and vacuolar-interface dermatitis.

- **Indirect immunofluorescence microscopy**: Circulating IgG autoantibodies.
- **Direct immunofluorescence microscopy of patient skin shows** deposits of IgG and complement 3 on the surface of keratinocytes and (variably) similar immunoreactants in the epidermal basement membrane zone.
- Patients with PNP have IgG autoantibodies against cytoplasmic proteins that are (autoantigens):
  - ➢ Members of the plakin family:
    - – Desmoplakins I and II
    - – Bullous pemphigoid antigen 1
    - – Envoplakin
    - – Periplakin
    - – Plectin
  - ➢ Cell surface proteins that are members of the cadherin family (e.g. Dsg3 and Dsg1).
- In addition to severe skin lesions, many patients with PNP develop life-threatening bronchiolitis obliterans.
- **Treatment**
  - ➢ No effective Rx exists.
  - ➢ PNP is generally resistant to conventional therapies (i.e. those used to treat PV); rare patients may improve (or even remit) following ablation or removal of underlying neoplasms.

## BULLOUS PEMPHIGOID

- Bullous pemphigoid (BP) is a polymorphic autoimmune subepidermal blistering disease.
- **Clinical features**
  - ➢ Usually seen in the elderly (**60–75 yrs**).
  - ➢ Initial lesions may consist of urticarial plaques
  - ➢ Most patients eventually display tense blisters on either normal-appearing or erythematous skin (Fig. 13.4).
  - ➢ The lesions are usually distributed over the lower abdomen, groins, and flexor surface of the extremities; oral mucosal lesions are found in some patients.
  - ➢ Pruritus may be nonexistent or severe.

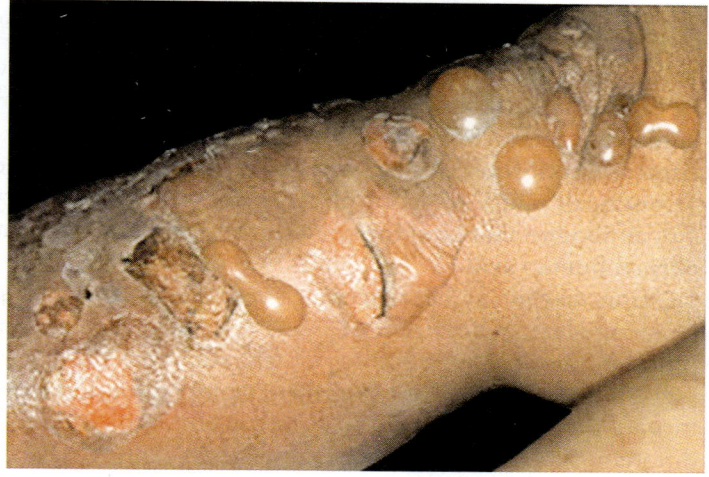

**Fig. 13.4:** Tense fluid-filled blisters in a case of bullous pemphigoid

- ➢ As lesions evolve, tense blisters tend to rupture and be replaced by erosions with or without surmounting crust.
- ➢ Nontraumatized blisters heal without scarring.
- ➢ Nikolsky's sign is negative.
- ➢ Bulla spread sign is negative
- ➢ Mucosal lesions are rare (10–40%); mild, transient, non-scarring.
- • **Genetics**
  - ➢ The major HLA II allele HLA-DQ7 is prevalent in patients with BP.
  - ➢ Patients with BP do not have an increased incidence of malignancy.
- • **Biopsies of early lesional skin demonstrate**
  - ➢ Subepidermal blisters with relatively intact epidermis.
  - ➢ Lesions on normal-appearing skin generally show a sparse perivascular leukocytic infiltrate with some eosinophils; conversely, biopsies of inflammatory lesions typically show an eosinophil-rich infiltrate at sites of vesicle formation and in perivascular areas.
  - ➢ In addition to eosinophils, cell-rich lesions also contain mononuclear cells and neutrophils.
  - ➢ It is not possible to distinguish BP from other subepidermal blistering diseases by routine histologic techniques alone.

- **Direct immunofluorescence microscopy**
  - ➤ In this, the normal-appearing perilesional skin from patients with BP shows linear deposits of IgG and/or C3 in the epidermal basement membrane.
- **Indirect immunofluorescence microscopy**
  - ➤ The sera of ~70% of these patients contain circulating IgG autoantibodies that bind the epidermal basement membrane of normal human skin.
  - ➤ IgG from an even higher percentage of patients shows reactivity to the epidermal side of 1 M NaCl split skin (an alternative immunofluorescence microscopy test substrate used to distinguish circulating IgG anti-basement membrane autoantibodies in patients with BP from those in patients with similar, yet different, subepidermal blistering diseases).
- **Autoantigen**
  - ➤ 230-kDa hemidesmosome-associated proteins/bullous pemphigoid antigen 1 (BPAG1).
  - ➤ 180-kDa hemidesmosome-associated proteins/BPAG2.
- **Autoantibodies**
  - ➤ Anti-basement membrane zone (BMZ) abs.
    Against BPAG2 are thought to deposit *in situ*, activate complement, produce dermal mast cell degranulation, and generate granulocyte-rich infiltrates that cause tissue damage and blister formation.
- **Treatment**
  - ➤ Systemic glucocorticoids (the **mainstay** of treatment).
    - Patients with local or minimal disease can sometimes be controlled with topical glucocorticoids alone; patients with more extensive lesions generally respond to systemic glucocorticoids either alone or in combination with immunosuppressive agents.
    - Patients will usually respond to prednisone, 0.75–1 mg/kg per day.
    - In some instances, azathioprine (2–2.5 mg/kg per day), mycophenolate mofetil (20–35 mg/kg per day), or cyclophosphamide (1–2 mg/kg per day) are necessary adjuncts.
    - Dapsone may be useful.
- **Prognosis**
  - ➤ BP may persist for months to years, with exacerbations or remissions.

Differences between pemphigus vulgaris and bullous pemphigoid are given in Table 13.2.

**Table 13.2:** Differences between pemphigus vulgaris and bullous pemphigoid

|  | PV | BP |
|---|---|---|
| Autoantibodies against | Desmosomal proteins (Desmoglein 3) | Hemidesmosomal proteins |
| Age | 40–60 yrs | 60–75 yrs |
| Initial site | Oral mucosa | Lower extremities |
| Bullae | Flaccid | Tense |
| Pruritus | Mild/– | Nonexistent or severe |
| Nikolsky's sign | + | – |
| Mucosal involvement | + (in almost all patients) | – (10–40% only) |
| HPE | Suprabasal acantholytic blisters (tombstone appearance) | Subepidermal blisters (eosinophil-rich dermal infiltrate) |
| DIF | IgG and C3 deposits at intercellular substance of epidermis ("Fishnet appearance") | IgG, C3, and IgA/IgM at BM zone |
| IIF | Circulating IgG antibodies to intercellular substance of epidermis. | Anti-BM zone antibodies IgG |
| Rx | Steroids + immunosuppressants Dapsone gold | Steroids Immunosuppressants Dapsone |
| Postinflammatory Hyperpigmentation | + | – |

## EPIDERMOLYSIS BULLOSA

- EB is of a group of similar disorders in which the skin and related epithelial tissues break and blister as the result of minor trauma. Mucous membranes and nails may be involved.
- Disease manifests at birth or thereafter.
- **Classification**
  - ➢ EB simplex for blistering in the epidermis
  - ➢ EB hemidesmosomal for fissures between keratinocytes and the basal lamina
  - ➢ EB junctional for blistering in the dermal–epidermal junction
  - ➢ EB dystrophica for blistering in the dermis.

- **Molecular defects**
  - ➤ Patients with EB simplex were found to have mutations in either keratin 14 or keratin 5, two of the major keratins in basal epithelial cells.
  - ➤ The new disease phenotype of hemidesmosomal EB has three clinical variants caused by mutations in one of four genes:
    - – A generalized atrophic and benign form of EB, caused by mutations in the COL17A1 gene for type XVII collagen.
    - – EB associated with pyloric atresia and other intestinal abnormalities, caused by mutations in either the gene for β6 integrin (ITGβ6) or the gene for the β4 integrin (ITGβ4).
    - – Relatively mild blistering at birth, but associated with late onset muscular dystrophy, caused by mutations in the gene for plectin (PLEC-1).
  - ➤ Junctional EB is caused by mutations in any one of three genes for laminin (LAMA-3, LAMB-3, LAMC-2), a major component of the dermal–epidermal junction.
  - ➤ The most severe dystrophic form of EB is caused by mutations in the gene for type VII collagen (COL7A1) that forms the anchoring fibers binding the epidermis to the dermis.
- **Diagnosis**
  - ➤ Histopatholgy
  - ➤ Electron microscopy
  - ➤ Antigen mapping using indirect immunohistochemical staining
  - ➤ Use of specific antibody probes
  - ➤ Molecular diagnosis
- **Treatment**
  - ➤ Avoid trauma
  - ➤ Prevent infection
  - ➤ Systemic drugs like phenytoin, vitamin E, minocycline, retinoids, and cyclosporine have been used
  - ➤ Skin grafts
  - ➤ Gene therapy

## EPIDERMOLYSIS BULLOSA ACQUISITA

- Epidermolysis bullosa acquisita (EBA) is a rare, noninherited, polymorphic, chronic, subepidermal blistering disease.
- Patients with classic or noninflammatory EBA have blisters on noninflamed skin, atrophic scars, milia, nail dystrophy, and oral lesions. Because lesions generally occur at sites exposed to minor trauma, classic EBA is considered to be a mechanobullous disease.

- Other patients with EBA have widespread inflammatory, scarring, and bullous lesions that resemble severe BP. Inflammatory EBA may evolve into the classic, noninflammatory form of this disease. Rare patients present with lesions that predominate on mucous membranes.
- The HLA-DR2 haplotype is found with increased frequency in EBA patients.
- Recent studies suggest that EBA is often associated with inflammatory bowel disease (especially Crohn's disease).
- Noninflammatory bullae show subepidermal blisters with a sparse leukocytic infiltrate. Inflammatory lesions consist of neutrophil-rich subepidermal blisters.
- EBA patients have continuous deposits of IgG (and frequently C3 as well as other complement components) in a linear pattern within the epidermal basement membrane zone. Ultrastructurally, these immunoreactants are found in the sublamina densa region in association with anchoring fibrils.
- Approximately 50% of EBA patients have demonstrable circulating IgG anti-basement membrane autoantibodies directed against type VII collagen—the collagen species that comprises anchoring fibrils. Such IgG autoantibodies bind the dermal side of 1 M NaCl split skin (in contrast to IgG autoantibodies in patients with BP).
- Treatment of EBA is generally unsatisfactory.
- Some patients with inflammatory EBA may respond to systemic glucocorticoids, either alone or in combination with immuno-suppressive agents.
- Other patients (especially those with neutrophil-rich inflammatory lesions) may respond to dapsone.
- The chronic, noninflammatory form of this disease is largely resistant to treatment, although some patients may respond to cyclosporine, azathioprine, or IV immunoglobulin (IVIg).
  Some skin diseases known to be associated with particular human leukocyte antigens (HLA) (Tables 13.3 to 13.5).

| Table 13.3: Diseases and target antigens | |
|---|---|
| *Disease* | *Antigen* |
| Dermatitis herpetiformis | B8; and Dw3/DRw3 |
| Pemphigus | DRw4 |
| Reiter's disease | B27 |
| Behçet's disease | B5 |
| Psoriasis | B13; B17; B37; Cw6; and Dw7 |
| Psoriatic arthropathy (central) | B27 |
| Psoriatic arthropathy (peripheral) | Bw38 |

**Table 13.4:** Autoantigens in different autoimmune diseases

| *Autoantigen* | *Autoimmune diseases* |
|---|---|
| Desmoglein 1 | Pemphigus foliaceus |
| Desmoglein 3 | Pemphigus vulgaris |
| Hemidesmosomal protein 180 | Bullous pemphigoid, herpes gestationis, cicatricial pemphigoid |
| Desmoplakin | Paraneoplastic pemphigus |
| SOX-10 | Vitiligo |
| Tissue transglutaminase | Celiac disease |
| Transcription coactivator p75 | Atopic dermatitis |
| Tyrosinase | Vitiligo, metastatic melanoma |
| Aminoacyl-tRNA histidyl synthetase | Myositis, dermatomyositis |
| Aminoacyl-tRNA synthetase (several) | Polymyositis, dermatomyositis |
| Carbonic anhydrase II | SLE, Sjögren syndrome, systemic sclerosis |
| DNA-dependent nucleosine-stimulated ATPase | Dermatomyositis |
| Fibrillarin | Scleroderma |
| Fibronectin | SLE, RA, morphea |
| Histone H2A-H2B-DNA | SLE |
| IgE receptor | Chronic idiopathic urticaria |

- **Direct immunofluorescence**

**Table 10.5:** Findings on direct immunofluorescence

| *Diagnosis* | *Deposits* | *Pattern* | *Site* |
|---|---|---|---|
| 1. Pemphigus | IgG | Reticulate | Intercellular |
| 2. Bullous pemphigoid | IgG | Linear | BMZ |
| 3. Cicatricial pemphigoid | IgG | Linear | BMZ |
| 4. EB acquisita | IgG | Linear | BMZ |
| 5. DH | IgA | Granular | Papillary dermis |
| 6. Linear IgA dermatosis | IgA | Linear | BMZ |
| 7. Lupus erythematosus | IgG | Granular | BMZ |
| 8. HSP | IgA | Granular | Vessel wall |

## QUESTIONS FROM PREVIOUS EXAMINATIONS

1. Pemphigus vulgaris
2. Dermatitis herpetiformis
3. Bullous pemphigoid
4. Cicatricial pemphigoid

5. Hailey-Hailey disease
6. Epidermolysis bullosa

## MULTIPLE CHOICE QUESTIONS

1. **What can patient with gluten sensitive hypersensitivity consume as food?** *(PGI 06)*
   - (a) Rice
   - (b) Barely
   - (c) Oat
   - (d) Corn
   - (e) Rye

2. **HLA associated with dermatitis herpetiformis:** *(PGI 06)*
   - (a) HLA A5
   - (b) HLA B8
   - (c) HLA B27
   - (d) HLA B28

3. **A 28-year-old patient has multiple grouped papulovesicular lesions on both elbows, knees, buttocks, and upper back associated with severe itching. The diagnosis is:** *(AIIMS 02)*
   - (a) Pemphigus vulgaris
   - (b) Bullous pemphigoid
   - (c) Dermatitis herpetiformis
   - (d) Herpes zoster

4. **A 30-year-old male had severely itchy papulovesicular lesions of the extremities, knees, elbows and buttocks for one year. Direct immunofluorescence staining of lesions showed IgA deposition at dermoepidermal junction. The most probable diagnosis is:** *(AI 04)*
   - (a) Pemphigus vulgaris
   - (b) Bullous pemphigoid
   - (c) Dermatitis herpetiformis
   - (d) Nummular eczema

5. **Extremely pruritic excoriation and papules on buttocks with autoantibodies against epidermal transglutaminase and IgA deposition in dermis on immunohistological examination of normal perilesional skin. Diagnosis is:** *(SGPGI 02)*
   - (a) Pemphigus vulgaris
   - (b) Pemphigoid
   - (c) Linear IgA disease
   - (d) Dermatitis herpetiformis

6. **The Rx of dermatitis herpetiformis:** *(AIIMS 02)*
   - (a) Gluten-free diet with minerals and vitamins
   - (b) Carbamazepine
   - (c) Acyclovir
   - (d) Steroids

7. **Drug of choice for dermatitis herpetiformis:** *(AI 91; AIIMS May 05)*
   - (a) Dapsone
   - (b) Methotrexate
   - (c) Clotrimazole
   - (d) Thiobendazole

8. **HLA DR4 is associated with:**                  *(Manipal 2008)*
   (a) Dermatitis herpetiformis
   (b) Erythema multiforme
   (c) Epidermolysis bullosa aquisita
   (d) Toxic epidermal necrolysis (TEN)

9. **Bullous skin lesions are seen in the following** *except:* *(MH 2005)*
   (a) Impetigo                (b) Diabetes mellitus
   (c) Porphyria              (d) Lupus vulgaris

10. **Subepidermal blistering is seen in all** *except:*        *(PGI 08)*
    (a) Pemphigus vulgaris
    (b) Dermatitis herpetiformis
    (c) Toxic epidermal necrolysis
    (d) Bullous pemphigoid
    (e) Hailey-Hailey disease

11. **Commonest variety of pemphigus:**                *(TN 99)*
    (a) Pemphigus vulgaris      (b) Pemphigus vegetans
    (c) Pemphigus foliaceus     (d) Pemphigus erythematosis

12. **Rarest variety of pemphigus:**                *(TN 99)*
    (a) Pemphigus vulgaris      (b) Pemphigus foliaceus
    (c) Pemphigus vegetans      (d) Pemphigus erythematosis

13. **A 24-year-old female has flaccid bullae in the skin and oral erosions. Histopathology shows intraepidermal acantholytic blister. Diagnosis is:**         *(AIIMS May 03)*
    (a) Pemphigoid            (b) Erythema multiforme
    (c) Pemphigus vulgaris    (d) Dermatitis herpetiformis

14. **A middle-aged female has flaccid bullae in skin and oral mucosa. HPE shows intraepidermal acantholytic blisters. The most likely diagnosis is:**        *(PGI 05)*
    (a) Pemphigus vulgaris
    (b) Paraneoplastic pemphigus
    (c) Bullous pemphigoid
    (d) Dermatitis herpetiformis

15. **A 40-year-old male developed persistent oral ulcers followed by multiple flaccid bullae on trunk and extremities. Direct examination of a skin biopsy immunofluorescence showed intercellular IgG deposits in the epidermis. The most probable diagnosis is:**        *(AI 93)*
    (a) Pemphigus vulgaris
    (b) Bullous pemphigoid
    (c) Bullous lupus erythematosus
    (d) Epidermolysis bullosa acquisita

16. **An autoimmune disease:** *(AI 2000)*
    (a) Pemphigus vulgaris      (b) Psoriasis
    (c) Lichen planus           (d) Acne vulagris

17. **Subepidermal splitting is not seen in:** *(PGI 99)*
    (a) Bullous pemphigoid      (b) Pemphigus foliaceus
    (c) Dermatitis herpetiformis (d) Burns

18. **Intradermal acantholytic blister is seen in:** *(PGI 06)*
    (a) Pemphigus vulgaris      (b) Bullous pemphigoid
    (c) Paraneoplastic pemphigus (d) Dermatitis herpetiformis

19. **Commonest site for herpes gestationis:** *(AIIMS 02)*
    (a) Periumbilical region    (b) Flanks of abdomen
    (c) Vulva                   (d) Infraorbital

20. **Acantholysis is seen in:** *(AI 95)*
    (a) Epidermis               (b) Dermis
    (c) Dermoepidermal junction (d) Subcutaneous tissue

21. **Acantholytic cells in pemphigus are:** *(PGI 96)*
    (a) Cells with hyperchromatic nuclei and perinuclear halo
    (b) Cells with hypochromatic nuclei and  perinuclear halo
    (c) Multinucleated cells
    (d) Non-nucleated cells

22. **Acantholysis is due to destruction of:**
    (a) Epidermis               (b) Subepidermis
    (c) Basement membrane       (d) Intercellular substance

23. **In Tzanck smear multinucleated cells are seen in:** *(PGI 097)*
    (a) Chickenpox              (b) Psoriasis
    (c) Molluscum contagiosum   (d) Pemphigus vulgaris

24. **Tzanck smear helps in diagnosis of:**
    (a) Herpes viral infection  (b) Bullous pemphigoid
    (c) Ca cervix               (d) All of the above

25. **Tzanck smear in a patient with bullous skin lesion will show:**
    *(AI 96)*
    (a) Langerhans' cells       (b) Acantholysis
    (c) Leukocytosis            (d) Absence of melanin pigment

26. **Acantholysis is seen in:** *(AIIMS 91; AI 03)*
    (a) Pemphigoid              (b) Pemphigus vulgaris
    (c) Erythema multiforme     (d) Dermatitis herpetiformis

27. **Intraepidermal bullae are seen in:** *(AIIMS 95)*
    (a) Pemphigoid              (b) Pemphigus vulgaris
    (c) Light reaction          (d) Dermatitis herpetiformis

28. Following are associated with pemphigus *except:*

    *(SGPGI 02; PGI 98)*

    (a) Thymoma          (b) MG
    (c) NHL              (d) CLL
    (e) Atrophic gastritis

29. A 50-year-old male known case of MG, presents with erythematous shallow erosions with blisters and scales. Oral mucosa is not involved. Immunopathology demonstrates IgG deposition on keratinocytes and autoantibodies against Dsg1. The diagnosis is:          *(PGI 98)*

    (a) Pemphigoid          (b) Pemphigus vulgaris
    (c) Pemphigus foliaceus (d) Dermatitis herpetiformis

30. In pemphigus vulgaris antibodies are present against:

    *(PGI 2000)*

    (a) Basement membrane   (b) Intercellular substance
    (c) Keratin             (d) Cell nucleus

31. Direct immunofluorescence is positive in:     *(PGI 02)*

    (a) Atopic dermatitis   (b) SLE
    (c) Pemphigus           (d) Secondary syphilis

32. A 23-year-old lady presents with vesicular lesions in the buccal mucosa and crusted lesions on the skin. The possible diagnosis is:

    (a) Pemphigus vulgaris  (b) Pemphigus foliaceus
    (c) Pemphigoid          (d) Dermatitis herpetiformis

33. A 40-year-old male reported with recurrent episodes of oral ulcers, large areas of denuded skin and flaccid vesiculobullous eruptions. Which of the following would be the bedside investigation helpful in establishing the diagnosis?

    (a) Gram staining of the blister fluid
    (b) Culture and sensitivity
    (c) Skin biopsy and immunofluorescence
    (d) Tzanck smear from the floor of bulla

34. A 40-year-old male has multiple blisters over the trunk and extremities. Direct immunofluorescence studies show linear IgG deposits along the BM. Diagnosis is:     *(AIIMS Nov 04)*

    (a) Pemphigus vulgaris  (b) Bullous pemphigoid
    (c) Pemphigus foliaceus (d) Dermatitis herpetiformis

35. A 56-year-old male presents with painful bullous lesion in lower extremity. Most likely diagnosis:

    (a) Pemphigus vulgaris  (b) Bullous pemphigoid
    (c) Necrotic pemphigus  (d) Contact eczema

36. Mucous membrane lesions are seen in:    *(AIIMS 90)*
    (a) Dermatitis herpetiformis  (b) Pemphigus
    (c) Impetigo                   (d) Pemphigoid

37. A 85-year-old female developed multiple blisters on trunk and thighs. Nikolsky's sign  negative. The lesions came on and off. The most probable diagnosis is:    *(PGI 2000)*
    (a) Pemphigus vulgaris    (b) Bullous pemphigoid
    (c) Lichen planus         (d) Lepra reaction

38. Etiology of epidermolysis bullosa is:    *(Rohtak 97)*
    (a) Genetic      (b) Infections
    (c) Senile       (d) Malignant
    (e) Metabolic

39. "Row of tombstones" appearance is seen in:    *(JIPMER 08)*
    (a) Irritant dermatitis    (b) Pemphigus
    (c) Pemphigoid             (d) Herpes zoster

40. A young boy presents with multiple flaccid bullous lesions over trunk with some oral mucosal lesions. Most likely finding on immunofluorescence study of the biopsy specimen would be:    *(AIIMS Nov 09)*
    (a) Fishnet IgG deposits in epidermis
    (b) Linear IgG in deposits
    (c) Linear IgA in dermal papillae
    (d) Granular IgA in reticular dermis

41. Granular IgA deposits in the dermal papillae are seen in:    *(AIIMS Nov 09)*
    (a) Dermatitis herpetiformis
    (b) Epidermolysis bullosa
    (c) Bullous pemphigoid
    (d) IgA papillomatosis of childhood

42. Intraepidermal IgG deposition is seen in:    *(AIIMS Nov 09)*
    (a) Pemphigus             (b) Herpes gestationis
    (c) Bullous pemphigoid    (d) Impetigo

43. Acantholytic cells are present in:    *(AMU 09)*
    (a) Stratum germinatum    (b) Stratum spinosum
    (c) Stratum granulosum    (d) Stratum corneum

44. Subepidermal bullae on trunk and flexural surface with linear C3/IgG basement membrane deposits are features of:    *(MH 08)*
    (a) Bullous pemphigoid    (b) Pemphigus vulgaris
    (c) Linear IgA disease    (d) Dermatitis herpetiformis

45. **A 50-year-old female presents with extensive flaccid bullous oral and skin lesions. The lesions are found to involve the supra-basal layer of epidermis. The likely diagnosis is:**    *(AI 08)*
    (a) Pemphigus vulgaris
    (b) Dermatitis herpetiformis
    (c) Epidermolysis bullosa
    (d) Bullous pemphigoid

46. **Which of the following is not true about pemphigus foliaceus?**
    *(JIPMER 09)*
    (a) Crusts and shallow erosions on scalp, face, chest, and back
    (b) Acantholytic blister formed in superficial layer of epidermis
    (c) Cell surface deposits of IgG on keratinocytes
    (d) Dsg3 is the main responsible pathogenic autoantigen

47. **Nikolsky's sign is positive in following conditions** *except:*
    *(DNB 2009)*
    (a) Pemphigus vulgaris
    (b) Toxic epidermal necrolysis
    (c) Epidermolysis bullosa
    (d) Pemphigoid

48. **Paraneoplastic pemphigus is seen in:**    *(SGPGI 09)*
    (a) Thymomas
    (b) Neuroma
    (c) Glioma
    (d) Hodgkin's lymphoma

49. **Acantholysis is characteristic of:**    *(AI 03)*
    (a) Pemphigus vulgaris
    (b) Pemphigoid
    (c) Erythema multiforme
    (d) Dermatitis hepetiformis

50. **A 40-year-old male developed persistent oral ulcers followed by multiple flaccid bullae on trunk and extremities. Direct examination of a skin biopsy immunofluorescence showed intercellular IgG deposits in the epidermis. The most probable diagnosis is:**    *(HP 07)*
    (a) Pemphigus vulgaris
    (b) Bullous pemphigoid
    (c) Bullous lupus erythematosus
    (d) Epidermolysis bullosa acquisita

51. **Characteristic of direct immunofluorescence findings in herpes gestationis:** *(PGI 09)*
    (a) Epidermal cell surface deposits of IgG and C3
    (b) Linear homogeneous deposits of IgG and C3 at the dermal–epidermal junction
    (c) Linear homogeneous deposits of C3 at the dermal–epidermal junction
    (d) Focal granular deposits of IgA at the papillary tips
    (e) Linear deposits of multiple immunoglobulins, C3 and fibrin at the dermal–epidermal junction

52. **Subepidermal bullae are seen in:** *(AIIMS 13)*
    (a) Pemphigoid                (b) Pemphigus
    (c) Pityriasis rosea          (d) Psoriasis

## Answers

1. **Ans. (a, d).**
2. **Ans. (b)** HLA B8 *(Ref. IADVL, 2nd edn/875; Rook'S Dermatology, 87th edn/ Table 12.2)*
3. **Ans. (c)** Dermatitis herpetiformis *(Ref. IADVL, 2nd edn/875–878)*
4. **Ans. (c)** Dermatitis herpetiformis
5. **Ans. (d)** Dermatitis herpetiformis *(Ref. IADVL, 2nd edn/875–878)*
6. **Ans. (a)** Gluten-free diet with minerals and vitamins *(Ref. IADVL, 2nd edn/877)*
7. **Ans. (a)** Dapsone *(Ref. IADVL, 2nd edn/877, 878)*
8. **Ans. (a)** Dermatitis herpetiformis
9. **Ans. (d)** Lupus vulgaris *(Ref. Harrison's Internal Medicine, 17th edn, 322)*
10. **Ans. (a, d)** *(Ref. IADVL, 2nd edn/857)*
11. **Ans. (a)** Pemphigus vulgaris *(Ref. IADVL, 2nd edn/858–861)*
12. **Ans. (c)** Pemphigus vegetans
13. **Ans. (c)** Pemphigus vulgaris *(Ref. IADVL, 2nd edn/859–866)*
14. **Ans. (a)** Pemphigus vulgaris *(Ref. IADVL, 2nd edn/859)*
15. **Ans. (a)** Pemphigus vulgaris *(Ref. Harrison's Medicine, 17th edn/328)*
16. **Ans. (a)** Pemphigus vulgaris *(Ref. IADVL, 2nd edn/857; Harrison's Medicine, 17th edn/ Table 55–1)*
17. **Ans. (b)** Pemphigus foliaceus *(Ref. IADVL, 2nd edn/859, 861; Harrison's Medicine, 17th edn/337)*
18. **Ans. (a, d)** *(Ref. IADVL, 2nd edn/859, 861; Harrison's Medicine 17th edn/337)*
19. **Ans. (a)** Periumbilical region *(Ref. IADVL, 2nd edn/874)*
20. **Ans. (a)** Epidermis *(Ref. IADVL 2nd edn/54, 68)*

21. **Ans. (a)** Cell with hyperchromatic nuclei and perinuclear halo. *(Ref. IADVL, 2nd edn/68)*
22. **Ans. (d)** Intercellular substance *(Ref. IADVL, 2nd edn/68)*
23. **Ans. (a)** Chickenpox *(Ref. IADVL, 2nd edn/81)*
24. **Ans. (a)** Herpes viral infection *(Ref. IADVL, 2nd edn/54)*
25. **Ans. (b)** Acantholysis *(Ref. IADVL, 2nd edn/54)*
26. **Ans. (b)** Pemphigus vulgaris *(Ref. IADVL, 2nd edn/54)*
27. **Ans. (b)** Pemphigus vulgaris *(Ref. IADVL, 2nd edn/859)*
28. **Ans. (c, d)** *(Ref. IADVL, 2nd edn/861, 866)*
29. **Ans. (c)** Pemphigus foliaceus *(Ref. IADVL, 2nd edn/860; Harrison's Medicine, 17th edn/ Table 308–12)*
30. **Ans. (b)** Intercellular substance *(Ref. IADVL, 2nd/861)*
31. **Ans. (c)** Pemphigus *(Ref. IADVL 2nd/52)*
32. **Ans. (a)** Pemphigus vulgaris *(Ref. IADVL, 2nd/859–866)*
33. **Ans. (d)** Tzank smear from the floor of bulla
34. **Ans. (b)** Bullous pemphigoid *(Ref. Harrison's Medicine, 17th edn/338; IADVL, 2nd edn/859–866)*
35. **Ans. (b)** Bullous pemphigoid *(Ref. IADVL, 2nd edn/867–872)*
36. **Ans. (a)** Dermatitis herpetiformis *(Ref. IADVL, 2nd edn/859)*
37. **Ans. (b)** Bullous pemphigoid *(Ref. IADVL, 2nd edn/867–872)*
38. **Ans. (a)** Genetic *(Ref. Harrison's Medicine, Chapter 357; IADVL, 2nd edn/883)*
39. **Ans. (b)** Pemphigus *(Ref. IADVL, 2nd edn/861)*
40. **Ans. (a)** 'Fishnet' IgG deposits in epidermis *(Ref. Harrison's Principles of Internal Medicine, 17th edn/ Table 55–1)*
41. **Ans. (a)** Dermatitis herpetiformis *(Ref. Robbin's Pathology, 7th/ 1259, 1260)*
42. **Ans. (a)** Pemphigus *(Ref. Robbin's Pathology, 7th edn/1259, 1260)*
43. **Ans. (a)** Stratum germinatum
44. **Ans. (a)** Bullous pemphigoid *(Ref. Harrison's Principles of Internal Medicine, 17th edn, Table 55–1)*
45. **Ans. (a)** Pemphigus vulgaris
46. **Ans. (d)** Dsg3 is the main responsible pathogenic autoantigen *(Ref. Harrison's Medicine, 17th edn/ Table 55–1)*
47. **Ans. (d)** Pemphigoid
48. **Ans. (a)** Thymomas
49. **Ans. (a)** Pemphigus vulgaris
50. **Ans. (a)** Pemphigus vulgaris
51. **Ans. (c)** Linear homogeneous deposits of C3 at the dermal–epidermal junction *(Ref. Rook's Dermatology, 7th edn/ Table 7.9)*
52. **Ans. (a)** Pemphigoid *(Ref. IADVL, 2nd edn/857).*

# 14 Scabies and Other Infestations

Scabies in humans and other animals is caused by mites (Acari) of the family Sarcoptidae which includes *Sarcoptes scabiei*, the scabies, mite and *Notoedres cati*, mange mite of cats.

## HUMAN SCABIES

- The human itch mite, *Sarcoptes scabiei* var *hominis*, is a common cause of itching dermatosis infesting ~300 million persons worldwide.
- Gravid female mites, measuring ~0.3 mm in length, burrow superficially beneath the stratum corneum, depositing three or fewer eggs per day.
- The female mite excavates a small burrow in which copulation takes place.
- After copulation, the fertilized female enlarges the burrow and begins laying eggs. About 40–50 eggs are laid by each female during a lifespan of 4–6 weeks, during which she does not leave the burrow. The eggs hatch into larvae in 3–4 days. These are transformed into nymphs. Nymphs mature in ~2 weeks and then emerge as adults to the surface of the skin, where they mate and (re)invade the skin of the same or another host.
- On an average, an adult has 10–11 mites and an infant 20 mites.
- **Transmission:** Transfer of newly fertilized female mites from person-to-person occurs mainly by intimate contact and is facilitated by overcrowding, poor hygiene, and multiple sexual partners.
- **Incubation period:** The onset of clinical features of scabies occurs 3–4 weeks after the infection is acquired. Subsequent episodes manifest in 2 weeks or so.
- **Clinical features:** Itching is usually the most obvious manifestation of scabies. It is generally worst at the night and when patient is

warm. Burrows are the characteristic lesions produced by female mites. They appear as tortuous S-shaped threads which are a few mm long.

- The **point of entry** of the mite, the most common superficial part of the burrow has slight scaly appearance and at the distal end there may be a tiny vesicle adjacent to which is the female mite.
- **Site of burrows:** Burrows occur on the wrists, the borders of the hands, the sides of the fingers, and the finger web spaces, nipples of women and in males the genitalia. They are often present on palms and soles of young children.
- Hypersensitivity reaction to mites and mite products result in a pruritic papular eruption which is more pronounced on abdomen, the lower portions of the buttocks, the axillary folds and the elbows. These main sites form a circle called the circle of hebra.
- Except in infants, the **face, scalp, neck, palms, and soles** are spared in scabies (Table 14.1).
- **Crusted scabies or Norwegian scabies**
  - ➤ Immunity and associated scratching limit most infestations to <15 mites per person.
  - ➤ Hyperinfestation with thousands of mites, a condition known as crusted scabies, or
  - ➤ Norwegian scabies may result from:
    - Glucocorticoid use
    - Immunodeficiency
    - Neurologic and psychiatric illnesses that limit itching and scratching.
- **Crusted scabies** resembles psoriasis in its typical widespread erythema, thick keratotic crusts, scaling, and dystrophic nails. In addition to classical sites, these lesions are seen on scalp, face, palms, soles, neck, and lumbosacral area.
  - ➤ Characteristic burrows are not seen in crusted scabies.
  - ➤ Patients usually do not itch.

| Table 14.1: Differences between scabies in adults and children | |
|---|---|
| *Scabies in adults* | *Scabies in infants and children* |
| 1. Widespread eruptions of inflammatory papules with itching | Florid excoriation, crusting, secondary pyoderma and eczematization |
| 2. Classical burrows noted | Vesicles and pustules are common |
| 3. Scalp, face, palms and soles are classically spared | Scalp, face, palms and soles are commonly involved |

➤ Highly contagious
➤ *Treatment:* Patients with crusted scabies may require two doses of ivermectin (200 µg/kg) separated by an interval of 1–2 weeks.

- **Scabies incognito**

Scabies wrongly treated with corticosteroids.

- **Nodular scabies**

Itchy nodules are seen. Most common over scrotum.

- **Animal scabies**

➤ Itchy papular eruption localized to the site of contact with the animals, usually dogs and cats.
➤ Animals need to be treated with anti-scabetic agents.

- **Complications**

➤ Secondary infection
➤ Eczematization
➤ Post-streptococcal glomerulonephritis

- **Diagnosis**

### The four cardinal features suggestive of scabies

1. Presence of burrow especially on the hand or penis
2. Characteristic distribution of pattern of lesions
   - Web of fingers
   - Flexor aspect of wrist
   - Elbow
   - Anterior axillary fold
   - Umbilicus
   - Periumbilical region
   - Genitalia and upper thighs
   - Knees and ankles
   - Nipple and areola (in females)
   - Lower part of buttocks and natal cleft
3. History of similar illness in other family members
4. Intense pruritus, which tends to worsen at night

- **Treatment**

➤ The anti-scabetic agent should be applied to entire body sparing scalp and face.
➤ It is preferably applied after a good scrub bath with soap and water.
➤ All the clothes worn should be washed, dried in hot sun, and ironed.

- ➤ All the members if personal household and other intimates should be treated even if they do not have obvious symptoms or signs.
- ➤ Systemic antibiotics seldom required for mild secondary pyoderma seen in early stages of scabies.
- ➤ For severe pyoderma especially in debilitated patients, a systemic antibiotic may be given.
- ➤ 5% permethrin cream is less toxic.
- ➤ 1% lindane
  - – Once commonly used
  - – Overuse has led to seizures and aplastic anemia.
  - – It should not be applied to pregnant women or infants.
- ➤ Crotamiton cream (10%) preferred in infants. Also has antipruritic effect
- ➤ Benzyl benzoate (25%)
- ➤ Sulfur ointment (10%) preferred in pregnant women
- ➤ 6% salicylic acid (for crusted scabies use keratolytic agent to improve the penetration of scabicides).
- ➤ **Ivermectin**
  A single oral dose of ivermectin (200 µg/kg) effectively treats scabies in otherwise healthy persons.

## Gammabenzene Hexachloride (Gammexane)

- It is used as 1% lotion or cream.
- One application of GBH for 2 hrs gives a cure rate of 82%.
- In infants and children there is risk of absorption and toxic effects.
- Adverse effects:
  - ➤ Skin rash
  - ➤ Conjunctivitis
  - ➤ Insomnia
  - ➤ Vertigo
  - ➤ Stupor
  - ➤ Ataxia
  - ➤ Tremors
  - ➤ Prostrations
  - ➤ Convulsions
  - ➤ Arrhythmias
  - ➤ Respiratory failure
- Diazepam is appropriate antagonist.

## Ivermectin

- It the only drug effective orally in scabies and pediculosis.
- Basically an antihelminthic drug used to Rx onchocerciasis.
- Inhibits glutamate and other ligand-gated chloride channels present in invertebrate nerve and muscle cells leading to increased permeability of the cell membrane to chloride ion with hyperpolarization of nerve/muscle cells resulting in paralysis and death of parasite.

## PEDICULOSIS CAPITIS

- Caused by *Pediculus humanus* var *capitis* (head louse)
  More common in 3–11 yrs age of group
- Girls are more frequently affected than boys
- Transmission is through close personal contact
- Scalp pruritus is the characteristic manifestation
- Secondary bacterial infection may occur as the result of scratching
- In severe neglected cases pus and exudates may produce matting of hair—Plica Polonica.
- The empty egg cases (nits) are seen in greater density on parietal and occipital regions.
- **Treatment:** Chemical pediculicides like 1% permethrin, lindane, crotamiton or malathion. Repeat treatment after 10 days because of limited ovicidal activity. Oral ivermectin has also been used.
- Oral therapy with cotrimoxazole has been reported to be effective in eradicating head lice. This is probably because the antibiotic is ingested by the louse and affects its symbiotic bacteria. These bacteria are essential for louse survival.
- Contacts and family members should also be treated.

## PEDICULOSIS CORPORIS

- Caused by *Pediculus humanus* var *corporis.*
- Common in unhygienic people.
- Overcrowding and poverty helps in the spread.
- Body louse is vector of epidemic typhus, louse borne relapsing fever and trench fever.
- Itching is the principal complaint. Pruritus is the result of sensitization to louse salivary antigens. Others, who have not become sensitized or have acquired tolerance to the bites, are asymptomatic.
- The body is often covered in excoriations, and there may be secondary bacterial infection.

- In those who have harboured clothing lice for long periods of time the skin is often hyperpigmented (so-called 'vagabonds' disease; morbus errorum).
- Lice and eggs should be sought in the clothing.
- **Treatment:** It is the clothing, not the patient, which requires treatment.
- Tumble-drying is a most effective means of killing both lice and eggs. High temperature laundering of undergarments and dry cleaning of outer clothing are also effective.

## PEDICULOSIS PUBIS

- Caused by *Phthirus pubis*.
- Transmitted by close physical contact, usually sexual.
- Occurs most frequently among sexually active young adults.
- Itching, mainly in the evening and at night, is the principal symptom.
- Later secondary infection and eczematization occurs.
- Close inspection of affected areas will reveal lice grasping hairs close to the skin surface, and louse eggs attached to the hair shafts.
- Mainly seen on pubic hair. May colonize eyebrows, eyelashes, beard, axillae, scalp margins and areolar hair.
- Blue–grey macules ("**Maculae ceruleae**") may be seen on skin of lower abdomen and upper thighs. These are probably produced by altered blood pigment or a reaction to louse's saliva.
- **Treatment:** Malathion and permethrin can be used. Sexual contacts should also be treated. Treatment should be repeated after an interval of 7–10 days.

## VAGABOND'S DISEASE

- **Vagabond's disease** occurs classically in person affected by triad of:
  - ➢ Inadequate food
  - ➢ Low personal hygiene
  - ➢ Heavy infestation of pediculi
- They usually show an addisonian pattern of pigmentation with frequent involvement of mucous membrane.
- The exact pathogenesis of hyperpigmentation is not known but considered to be post-inflammatory. The adrenal function is normal in most of the cases.

Biological and epidemiological characteristics of the six major EPSDs are given in Table 14.2.

**Table 14.2:** Biological and epidemiological characteristics of the six major EPSDs

| Characteristics | Scabies | Pediculosis capitis | Pediculosis corporis | Pediculosis pubis | Tunglasis | HrCLM |
|---|---|---|---|---|---|---|
| **Biological** | | | | | | |
| Infective agent | Sarcoptes scabies | Pediculus humanus var capitis | Pediculus humanus corporis | Phthirus pubis | Tunga penetrans | Animal hookworm sp. such as A. caninum, A. braziliense, Uncinaria stenocephala |
| Taxonomical classification | Acaridae (mite) | Phthiraptera (louse) | Phthiraptera (louse) | Phthiraptera (louse) | Siphonaptera (flea) | Helminths (nematode) |
| Life cycle | Completely on-host | Completely on-host | Completely on-host | Completely on-host | Partialy on-host[a] | Partially on-host (biological impasse) |
| **Epidemiological** | | | | | | |
| Transmission | | | | | | |
| Person-to-person[b] | +++ | +++ | +++ | (+) | | |
| Sexual | + | | +++ | +++ | | |
| Fomite | + | + | +++ | + | (+) | (+) |
| Soil-to-skin | + | + | +++ | + | +++ | +++ |
| Capacity to transfer pathogenic microorganisms | | | | | | |
| Actively | Not known | (+) | +++ | | + | Not known |
| Passively | + | ++ | ++ | ++ | +++ | ++ |

Contd.

**Table 14.1:** Biological and epidemiological characteristics of the six major EPSDs *Contd.*

| Characteristics | Scabies | Pediculosis capitis | Pediculosis corporis | Pediculosis pubis | Tunglasis | HrCLM |
|---|---|---|---|---|---|---|
| Occurrence | Worldwide | Worldwide | Restricted mainly to cold-climate regions | Worldwide | Caribbean, sub-Saharan Africa, South America | Predominantly in hot-climate countries |
| Seasonal variation | Peak during cold season[c] | Peak during cold season[c] | Inconsistent data | Peak during cold season | Peak in hot and dry season | Peak in rainy season |
| Animal reservoir | No[d] | No | No | No | Dogs, cats, pigs, rats[e] | Dogs, cats[e] |

EPSDs: epidermal parasitic skin diseases, HrCLM: hookworm-related cutaneous larva migrans.

+ : rare; ++: frequent; +++: very frequent.

[a] Female fleas penetrate into the epidermis, develop and produce eggs; eggs develop into larvae, adults off-host in soil.

[b] Other than sexual.

[c] Only than sexual.

[d] Sarcoptic mange may be transmitted to humans from pet dogs but causes self-limiting manifestations

[e] Other animals may serve as a reservoir.

# QUESTIONS FROM PREVIOUS EXAMINATIONS

1. Leishmaniasis
2. Scabies + morphology of mite
3. Papular urticaria
4. Pthriasis
5. Arachnoides
6. Nephritis in scabies
7. Papular dermatosis in pregnancy
8. Larva migrans
9. Cysticercosis
10. Oriental sore
11. PKDL
12. Malabar ulcer
13. Vagabond's disease
14. Onchocerciasis skin

# MULTIPLE CHOICE QUESTIONS

1. **Scabies is caused by:**                         *(AI 90; Kar 2002)*
   - (a) Tick
   - (b) Louse
   - (c) Mite
   - (d) Flea
2. *Acaros* **is causative agent of:**                *(Kar 92)*
   - (a) Pediculosis corporis
   - (b) Papular urticaria
   - (c) Scabies
   - (d) *Tinea corporis*
3. **Incubation period of scabies is:**               *(WB 2007)*
   - (a) 7 days
   - (b) 2 weeks
   - (c) 4 weeks
   - (d) 2–3 days
4. **Characteristic lesion of scabies is:**           *(AI 90, AP 2000)*
   - (a) Burrow
   - (b) Fissure
   - (c) Vesicle
   - (d) Papule
5. **The burrows in scabies are present in:**         *(Kar 98; AFMC 2000)*
   - (a) Stratum basale
   - (b) Stratum granulosum
   - (c) Stratum corneum
   - (d) Dermis
6. **Scabies in children differs from that in adults in that it affects:**
                                                        *(JIPMER 2000)*
   - (a) Web space
   - (b) Face
   - (c) Genitalia
   - (d) Axilla

7. **A 9-month-old infant has itchy papules on face and papulovesi-cular lesions on palms and soles and also on trunk. The most likely diagnosis would be:**    *(AIIMS 95)*
   (a) Atopic dermatitis       (b) Scabies
   (c) Seborrheic dermatitis    (d) Tinea

8. **Norwegian scabies is most commonly seen in:**    *(Manipal 2000)*
   (a) Immunocompromised individuals
   (b) Infants
   (c) Elderly
   (d) Males

9. **Gammexane is used in the Rx of:**    *(JIPMER 91)*
   (a) *Tinea versicolor*       (b) Scabies
   (c) Pediculosis corporis     (d) All of the above

10. **All the following are used for treatment of scabies *except*:**    *(AP 92)*
    (a) Benzyl benzoate         (b) Sodium thiosulfate
    (c) Tetmesol solution       (d) Sulfur ointment

11. **A child has multiple itchy papular lesions on genitalia and fingers. Similar lesions are also noted in his younger brother. What is the diagnosis?**    *(AI 2002)*
    (a) Papular urticaria        (b) Scabies
    (c) Atopic dermatitis        (d) Allergic contact dermatitis

12. **An 8-month-old child presented with itchy, exudative lesions on face, palms and soles. Siblings also have similar complaints. The treatment of choice in such a patient would be:**    *(AI 2003)*
    (a) Systemic ampicillin      (b) Topical betamethasone
    (c) Systemic prednisolone    (d) Topical permethrin

13. **In a child with itchy lesions over the groin and prepuce. Which of the following should not be advised?**    *(AI 2001)*
    (a) Bathe and apply scabicidal  (b) Treat family
    (c) Boil the clothes         (d) IV antibiotics

14. **All the following are used in scabies *except*:**    *(AIIMS May 2008)*
    (a) BHC                      (b) Permethrin
    (c) Crotamiton               (d) Cyclopirox oleamine

15. **Ivermectin is indicated in Rx of:**    *(AIIMS 06)*
    (a) Scabies                  (b) Syphilis
    (c) TB                       (d) Dermatophytosis

16. **Nodular scabies is found in:**    *(AIIMS 97)*
    (a) Web space of fingers     (b) Axilla
    (c) Abdomen                  (d) Scrotum

17. **An 8-month-old child presented with itchy, exudative lesions on the face, palms and soles. The siblings also have similar complaints. The treatment of choice in such a patient is:** *(AI 03)*
    (a) Topical betamethasone    (b) Systemic prednisolone
    (c) Sytemic ampicillin    (d) Topical permethrin

## Answers

1. **Ans. (c)** Mite *(Ref. Rook's Textbook of Dermatology, 7th edn/33.41; 33.37)*
2. **Ans. (c)** Scabies *(Ref. Rook's Textbook of Dermatology, 7th edn/33.37)*
3. **Ans. (c)** Four weeks *(Ref. Rook's Textbook of Dermatology, 7th edn/ 33.39)*
4. **Ans. (a)** Burrow *(Ref. Rook's Textbook of Dermatology, 7th edn/33.39)*
5. **Ans. (c)** Stratum corneum *(Ref. Rook's Textbook of Dermatology, 7th edn/33.37)*
6. **Ans. (b)** Face *(Ref. Rook's Textbook of Dermatology, 7th edn/33.40)*
7. **Ans. (b)** Scabies *(Ref. IDVL Textbook of Dermatology, 2nd/348)*
8. **Ans. (a)** Immunocompromised individuals *(Ref. IDVL Textbook of Dermatology, 2nd edn/349)*
9. **Ans. (b)** Scabies *(Ref. IDVL Textbook of Dermatology, 2nd edn/350)*
10. **Ans. (b)** Sodium thiosulfate *(Ref. IDVL Textbook of Dermatology, 2nd edn/350, 351)*
11. **Ans. (b)** Scabies *(Ref. IDVL Textbook of Dermatology, 2nd edn/350)*
12. **Ans. (d)** Topical permethrin *(Ref. IDVL Textbook of Dermatology, 2nd edn/350, 351)*
13. **Ans. (d)** IV antibiotics *(Ref. IDVL Textbook of Dermatology, 2nd edn/ 350, 351)*
14. **Ans. (d)** Cyclopirox oleamine *(Ref. Ref. KDT, 6th edn, 706)*
15. **Ans. (a)** Scabies *(Ref. Fitzpatrick's Dermatology, 6th edn/2283)*
16. **Ans. (d)** Scrotum *(Ref. Nelson's Paediatrics, 18th edn/ 95)*
17. **Ans. (d)** Topical permethrin

# 15 Fungal Infections

## Cutaneous Fungal Infections

- Superficial: Confined to stratum corneum—dermatophytosis, *tinea versicolor*, candidiasis.
- Deep forms: Invade deeper tissues—mycetoma, sporotrichosis.

| Organism | Disease | Notes |
|---|---|---|
| *Malassezia furfur* | Pityriasis of *tinea versicolor* | • Superficial infection of keratinized cells<br>• Hypopigmented spots on the chest/back (blotchy suntan)<br>• KOH mount of skin scales "spaghetti and meatballs," yeast clusters and short, curved septate hyphae<br>• Treatment is topical selenium sulfide; recurs |
| | Fungemia | • In premature infants |
| *Candida albicans*, *Candida* spp. | Cutaneous or mucocutaneous candidiasis | • Causes oral thrush and vulvovaginitis in immunocompetent individuals<br>• Source of opportunistic infections in hospitalized and immunocompromised (see opportunistic mycoses)<br><br>Pseudohyphae  Budding yeasts  Germ tubes  True hyphae |
| Trichophyton, Microsporum, Epidermophyton | *Tinea* (*capitis, barbae, corporis, cruris, pedis*) | • Infects skin, hair, and nails<br>• Monomorphic filamentous fungi<br>• KOH mount shows arthroconidia, hyphae<br>• Pruritic lesions with serpiginous borders and central clearing |
| *Sporothrix schenckii*<br><br>Hyphae<br><br>Conidia | • Sporotrichosis (Rose Gardener's disease)<br>• Pulmonary sporotrichosis (in alcoholics/ homeless) | Dimorphic fungus:<br>• Environmental form: Hyphae with rosettes and sleeves of conidia<br>• Tissue form: Cigar-shaped yeast |

## DERMATOPHYTOSIS

- Dermatophytosis is a superficial fungal infection of keratinized tissue.
- The infection is commonly designated as ringworm or tinea, caused by dermatophytes (Microsporum, Trichophyton, Epidermophyton).
- The three asexual dermatophyte genera are distinguished by the morphology of the large, multicellular macroconidia that are produced.
- In the genus Microsporum, the macroconidia are rough, usually thick-walled and range from fusiform to obovate in shape with 1–12 or more septa.
- Those of Trichophyton species are thin walled, smooth and may be cylindrical, fusiform or clavate in shape with up to 12 transverse septa.
- In Epidermophyton, the macroconidium is clavate, broadened and rounded at its distal pole, thin walled and has up to five septa; the conidia are smooth when first formed, but as the colony ages discrete wall thickenings may be observed (Fig. 15.1).
- The fungi may be of:
  - ➢ Geophilic species originating in the soil
  - ➢ Zoophilic species having animal origins
  - ➢ Anthropophilic species, which are largely restricted to human skin

    Table 15.1 shows the type of tinea.

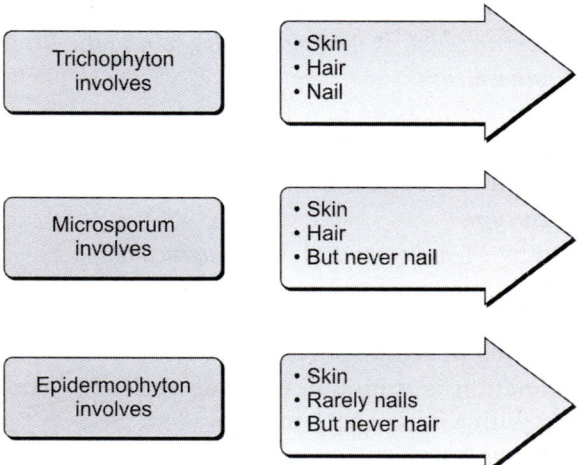

**Fig. 15.1:** Involvement of different genus of fungi

| Dermatophytes | T. capitis | T. pedis | T. cruris | T. corporis |
|---|---|---|---|---|
| Epidermophyton flocculosum | – | – | + | – |
| Microsporum canis | + | – | + | + |
| M. gypseum | + | – | + | – |
| Trichophyton mentagrophytes | + | + | + | + |
| T. rubrum | + | + | + | + |
| T. schoenleinii | + | – | + | |
| T. soudanense | + | – | + | + |
| T. violaceum | – | – | + | + |
| T. verrucosum | – | – | + | + |

**Table 15.1: Type of tinea**

## Tinea Capitis

- *Tinea capitis* signifies infection of scalp and hair with a dermatophyte (Table 15.2).
- Most common in children.
- Uncommon after puberty—could be due to inhibitory affect of sebaceous secretions
- Most common organisms:
  - ➤ **T. tonsurans**—most common
  - ➤ **M. canis**—seen in children with infected animals.
  - ➤ **M. audouini**

  Presentations of tinea capitis: There are 4 clinical patterns
- *Grey patch type:* Caused by ectothrix organisms
- *Black dot pattern:* Caused by endothrix organisms
- *Kerion: T. verrucosum, T. mentagrophytes* (zoophilic fungi)
- *Favus: T. schoenleinii*
- The type of hair invasion may be:
  - ➤ *Endothrix:* Invasion inside the hairshaft
  - ➤ *Ectothrix*: Invasion outside the hairshaft
- *Grey patch type*
  - ➤ Caused by *M. audouini* and *M. ferrugineum*
  - ➤ The basic lesions are patches of partial alopecia, often circular in shape, but showing numerous broken-off hairs, dull grey from their coating of arthrospores (Table 15.2).
  - ➤ Inflammation is minimal, but fine scaling is characteristic, usually with a fairly sharp margin.
- *Black dot type*
  - ➤ In *T. tonsurans* and *T. violaceum* infections, a relatively non-inflammatory type of patchy baldness occurs.

➢ Formation of black dots (swollen hair shafts) as the affected hair breaks at the surface of the scalp is classical in this condition.

- **Favus**
  - ➢ The classical picture of *tinea capitis* caused by this organism is characterized by the presence of yellowish cup-shaped crusts known as scutula.
  - ➢ Each scutulum develops round a hair, which pierces it centrally.
  - ➢ Adjacent crusts enlarge to become confluent and form a mass of yellow crusting.
  - ➢ Seen in families in Kashmir.
  - ➢ A characteristic mousy odor may be there.
- **Kerion**
  - ➢ It is mostly due to infection with zoophilic *(M. canis)* or geophilic species *(M. gypseum)*.
  - ➢ Clinically, a spectrum of inflammatory changes may be seen, ranging from a pustular folliculitis to kerion formation.
  - ➢ Kerion is a boggy and indurated swelling studded with broken or unbroken hair, vesicles, and pustules.
  - ➢ There may be sinus formation.
  - ➢ Thick crusting with matting of adjacent hair.
  - ➢ Occipital lymphadenopathy is frequent.
  - ➢ Secondary bacterial infection often occurs.
  - ➢ This type of *tinea capitis* heals with scarring.
  - ➢ Agminate folliculitis, a somewhat less severe inflammatory ringworm of the scalp consisting of sharply defined, dull red plaques studded with follicular pustules, is also seen in zoophilic infections.
- **Diagnosis**
  - ➢ Morphology of lesion
    - – Broken hairs, black dots, localized.
  - ➢ Wood's lamp
    - – Blue green fluorescence
  - ➢ Hair shaft examination (KOH)
    - – Endo-/Exothrix
  - ➢ Culture
- **Treatment**
  - ➢ Topicals not effective
  - ➢ Systemic agents should be used.
  - ➢ Griseofulvin for children—liquid with good taste.
  - ➢ Imidazoles, terbinafine.

**Table 15.2:** Differences between tinea capitis and alopecia areata

|  | Tinea capitis | Alopecia areata |
|---|---|---|
| Age | Children | Adults |
| Itching and scales | + | – |
| Exclamation mark | Not seen | Stumps are exclamation mark shaped |
| Density of hair | Numerous broken hair | Scanty hair |

- ➤ Steroids for inflamed lesions like kerion.
- ➤ Treat until no visual evidence, culture (–)... plus 2 weeks
- ➤ Average of 6–12 weeks of treatment.
- ➤ Examine/treat family in recurrent cases.
- ➤ The usual adult dose of griseofulvin for *tinea capitis* is 1 g microsized or 0.5 g ultramicrosized given daily.
- ➤ Children should be treated with 15 to 20 mg/kg as a single daily dose given with a fatty meal.
- ➤ Recent studies in children have also suggested that both itraconazole (3 to 5 mg/kg for 6 to 10 weeks) and terbinafine (125 mg/d for 6 weeks) may be effective treatments for *tinea capitis.*
  - – *Oral antifungal agents must be used in the management of tinea capitis.*
  - – *Griseofulvin currently remains the Rx of choice because of its affordability and safety.*

## Tinea Corporis

- Ringworm infection of the non-hair bearing skin of the body. Classically presents with slightly itchy, asymmetrical, scaly, annular erythematous patches which show central clearing and an advancing, scaly, raised edge (Fig. 15.2).

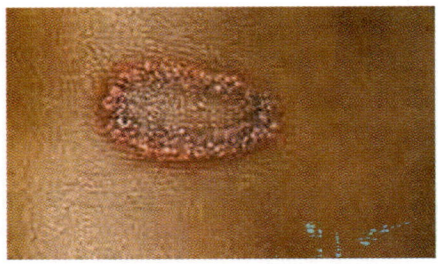

**Fig. 15.2:** Scaly annular plaque with central clearing and raised border

- The active border consists of papulovesicular lesions.
- *Tinea imbricata* is caused by *T. concentricum.* It is characterized by ring-like lesions inside another ring.
- *T. rubrum* is the most common dermatophyte causing *tinea corporis.*

## Tinea Faciei

- Infection of the glabrous skin of the face with a dermatophyte fungus (the moustache and beard areas of the adult male are excluded).
- *T. mentagrophytes* var *mentagrophytes* and *T. rubrum* predominate.
- Facial lesions are annular, infiltrated and erythematous.
- Lack of scaling.
- Burning, stinging and exacerbation after sun exposure are common.

## Tinea Barbae

- Ringworm of the beard and moustache areas of the face with invasion of coarse hairs. It is thus a disease of the adult male.
- The animal species *T. verrucosum* and *T. mentagrophytes* var. *mentagrophytes* are responsible for the great majority of cases.
- The clinical picture in these is that of a highly inflammatory pustular folliculitis, often showing all the features of a kerion. Hairs of the beard or moustache regions are surrounded by red inflammatory papules or pustules, usually with exudation or crusting. Many hairs within the affected areas are loose and easily removed with the forceps without causing pain.
- Some infections are less severe and consist of dry, circular, reddish, scaly lesions enclosing lustreless hair stumps, which are either broken off close to the surface of the skin or plug the follicles.

## Tinea Pedis

- *Tinea pedis* is a dermatophyte infection of feet and is also referred as athlete's foot.
- Commonly affects shoe bearing population.
- It is caused by *T. rubrum* (commonest), *T. mentagrophytes,* and *E. flocculosum.*
- The most common form of *tinea pedis* is an intertriginous dermatitis characterized by peeling, maceration and fissuring affecting the lateral toe clefts, and sometimes spreading to involve the undersurface of the toes. Itching is a common in warm weather.

- In *T. rubrum* infections, a scaling hyperkeratotic variety, which is particularly chronic and resistant to treatment and which affects the soles, heels and sides of the feet, is often found. The affected areas are pink and covered with fine silvery white scales. If the foot is extensively involved, the term 'moccasin foot' or dry type infection are sometimes applied. Different types of tinea lesions are given in Table 15.3
- The changes produced by *T. mentagrophytes* var *interdigitale* vary from mild insignificant scaling in the toe clefts to severe acute inflammatory reactions affecting all parts of the feet. A vesiculobullous reaction is more likely to be caused by this species than by any other fungus. Vesicles may become pustules, and when they rupture they tend to leave collarettes of scaling with the intervening skin normal.
- When the lesions on the feet are acutely vesicular, a vesicular allergic reaction (id) may develop on the uninfected hands.
- **Treatment** (Table 15.4)
  - ➤ *Dry feet*
    - – Alternate shoes, absorbent powders, change socks
    - – Scale my be reduced with keratolytics.
  - ➤ *Topicals and/or systemics*
    - – Topical: Naftine, lamisil, mentax may be more effective than azoles. Steroids, if inflamed.
    - – Systemic allylamines or azoles
    - – Treat secondary bacterial infections.
    - – Steroids for severe inflammation and id.

## Tinea Cruris

- Dermatophyte infection of groin is referred as *tinea cruris* (Fig. 15.3).
- It predominantly occurs in adult males predisposed to warm and humid environment and is also known as Dhobi's itch.
  It is caused by:
  - ➤ *Trichophyton rubrum* (common in India)
  - ➤ *T. mentagrophytes*
  - ➤ *Epidermophyton flocculosum* (common in Western world)
- Lesions are seen in the genitocrural area and on medial aspect of upper thigh.
- Lesions are usually bilateral but asymmetrical.
- Typical lesions have annular (ring-like) appearance of 'ringworm'. Start off as macules but clear in the center making ring-like annular lesions.
- Presents as large, scaling, well demarcated dull red tan brown plaques.

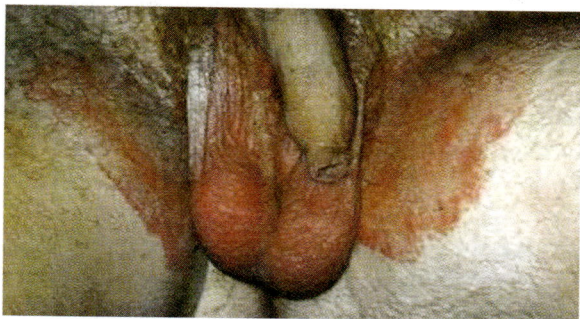

**Fig. 15.3:** Erythematous plaques involving groin area

- Show central clearing and advance centrifugally (at the periphery)
- Papules and pustules may be present at periphery.
- Itching is the predominant feature.
- Treatment involves topical antifungal agents.

## Tinea Incognito

It is extensive ringworm infection with atypical appearance due to inappropriate use of steroids.

## Tinea Unguium

- *Tinea unguium* is clinically defined as dermatophytic infection of the nail plate.
- The term onychomychosis includes all infections of nail plate caused by any fungus including non-dermatophytes and yeasts.
- The principal dermatophytes concerned are:
  - ➤ With associated foot and hand infections—*T. rubrum, T. mentagrophytes* var *interdigitale* and *E. flocculosum*
  - ➤ With associated scalp infections—*T. tonsurans, T. violaceum* and *T. soudanense*
- Five patterns have been described.
  - ➤ ***Distal and lateral subungual onychomycosis:*** Most common pattern of infection, and usually presents as a streak or a patch of discoloration, white or yellow at the free edge of the nail plate, often near the lateral nail fold. The initial invasion of the hyponychium shows through a relatively normal dorsal nail plate. It commonly spreads towards the base of the nail and may occasionally become darker brown or black. A later phase of invasion may lead to massive destruction of the nail plate (total dystrophic onychomycosis—TDO).

**Table 15.3:** Different types of tinea lesions

| Dermatophytic skin disease | Location of lesions | Clinical features | Fungi responsible |
|---|---|---|---|
| **Tinea corporis** (ringworm) | Nonhairy, smooth skin | Circular patches with advancing red, vesiculated border and central scaling Pruritic | T. rubrum, E. flocculosum |
| **Tinea pedis** (athlete's foot) | Interdigital spaces on feet of persons wearing shoes | Acute: Itching, red vesicular Chronic: Itching, scaling, fissures | T. rubrum, T. mentagrophytes, E. flocculosum |
| **Tinea cruris** (jock itch) | Groin | Erythematous scaling lesion in intertriginous area | T. rubrum, T. mentagrophytes, E. flocculosum |
| | Scalp hair. Endothrix: Fungus inside hair shaft | Pruritic: Circular bald patches with short hair stubs or broken hair within hair follicles | T. mentagrophytes, M. canis |
| **Tinea capitis** | Ectothrix: Fungus on surface of hair | **Kerion** rare: Microsporum-infected hairs fluoresce | – |
| **Tinea barbae** | Beard hair | Edematous, erythematous lesion | T. mentagrophytes |
| **Tinea unguium** (onychomycosis) | Nail | Nails thickened or crumbling distally; discolored; lusterless. Usually associated with tinea pedis. | T. rubrum, T. mentagrophytes, E. flocculosum |
| **Dermatophytid** (id reaction) | Usually sides and flexor aspects of fingers Palm: Any site on body | Pruritic vesicular to bullous lesions. Most commonly associated with tinea pedis | No fungi present in lesion May become secondarily infected with bacteria |

**Table 15.4:** Treatment of tinea

| Infection | Recommended | Alternative |
|---|---|---|
| Tinea unguium (Onychomycosis) | Terbinafine 250 mg/day, 6 weeks for fingernails, 12 weeks for toenails. | Itraconazole 200 mg/day for 3–5 months or 400 mg/day for one week per month for 3–4 consecutive months<br>Fluconazole 150–300 mg/wk until cure (6–12 months)<br>Griseofulvin 500–1000 mg/day until cure (12–18 months) |
| Tinea capitis | Griseofulvin 500 mg/day (not less than 10 mg/kg/day) until cure (6–8 weeks). | Terbinafine 250 mg/day for 4 wks<br>Itraconazole 100 mg/day for 4 wks<br>Fluconazole 100 mg/day for 4 wks |
| Tinea corporis | Griseofulvin 500 mg/day until cure (4–6 weeks), often combined with a topical imidazole agent | Terbinafine 250 mg/day for 2–4 weeks<br>Itraconazole 100 mg/day for 15 days or 200 mg/day for 1 week<br>Fluconazole 150–300 mg/week for 4 weeks |
| Tinea cruris | Griseofulvin 500 mg/day until cure (4–6 weeks) | Terbinafine 250 mg/day for 2–4 weeks<br>Itraconazole 100 mg/day for 15 days or 200 mg/day for 1 week<br>Fluconazole 150–300 mg/week for 4 weeks |
| Tinea pedis | Griseofulvin 500 mg/day until cure (4–6 weeks) | Terbinafine 250 mg/day for 2–4 weeks<br>Itraconazole 100 mg/day for 15 days or 200 mg/day for 1 week<br>Fluconazole 150–300 mg/week for 4 weeks |
| Chronic and/or widespread non-responsive tinea | Terbinafine 250 mg/day for 4–6 weeks | Itraconazole 200 mg/day for 4–6 weeks<br>Griseofulvin 500–1000 mg/day until cure (3–6 months) |

➤ **Superficial white onychomycosis (SWO):** It is a less common presentation and can produce a distinct form of nail invasion in which the dorsal surface of the nail plate is eroded in well-circumscribed powdery white patches, often away from the free edge.

➤ **Proximal subungual onychomycosis:** Particularly associated with AIDS patients. Rapid invasion of the nail plate from the posterior nail fold may develop to produce a white nail with only marginal increase in thickness. The most commonn cause is currently *T. rubrum.*

➤ **Endonyx onychomycosis:** This is seen with infection caused by dermatophytes that cause endothrix scalp infections, notably *T. soudanense.* The nail plate is scarred with pits and lamellar splits. The invasion occurs from the top surface, but penetrates deeply into the nail plate.

➤ **Totally dystrophic onychomycosis:** This is the final common pathway for severe infection where the nail plate is completely destroyed.

## Tinea Mannum

- Ringworm of the  palmar skin.
- *T. rubrum* is the most common cause. *E. flocculosum* and *T. mentagrophytes* var. *interdigitale* are involved in a small minority of cases.
- Hyperkeratosis of the palms and fingers affecting the skin diffusely is the most common variety, and is unilateral in about half of cases. The accentuation of the flexural creases is a characteristic feature.
- Other clinical variants include crescentic exfoliating scales, circumscribed vesicular patches, discrete red papular and follicular scaly patches, and erythematous scaly sheets on the dorsal surface of the hand.

## Dermatophytid Reactions

- A non-infective cutaneous eruption representing an allergic response to a distant focus of dermatophyte infection.
- Essential criteria required for the diagnosis of an id reaction to a dermatophyte infection are:
  ➤ Proven dermatophyte infection, which usually becomes highly inflamed before the appearance of the secondary rash.
  ➤ A distant eruption, which is demonstrably free of ringworm fungus.
  ➤ Spontaneous disappearance of the rash when the ringworm infection settles, with or  without treatment.

## Dermatophytosis Diagnosis

- *Wood's lamp examination:* Evaluation of *tinea capitis*
- *KOH preparation:* Skin scrapings, nail clippings and hair can be mixed with KOH and examined for septate and branching hyphae
- *Culture on Sabouraud's medium*
- Histopathological examination with special stains.

## Dermatophytosis Treatment

- Topical therapy is generally effective for uncomplicated *tinea corporis, tinea cruris,* and limited *tinea pedis.*
- It is not effective as a monotherapy for *tinea capitis* or onychomycosis.
- Topical imidazoles, triazoles, and allylamines may be effective therapies for dermatophyte infections, but nystatin is not active against dermatophytes.
- Topicals are generally applied twice daily, and treatment should continue 1 week beyond clinical resolution of the infection.
- *Tinea pedis* often requires longer treatment courses and frequently relapses.
- Oral antifungal agents may be required for recalcitrant *tinea pedis* or *tinea corporis.*
- Oral antifungal agents are required for dermatophyte infections involving the hair and nails and for other infections unresponsive to topical therapy. A fungal etiology should be confirmed by direct microscopic examination or by culture prior to prescribing oral antifungal agents.
- All of the oral agents may cause hepatotoxicity and should not be used in women who are pregnant or breastfeeding.

The 3 anti-fungals being increasingly used for Rx of onychomycosis are given in Table 15.5.

| Table 15.5: Antifungals used for onychomycosis | |
|---|---|
| *Drug for Rx onychomycosis* | *Dose* |
| 1. Terbinafine | 250 mg/day for 6 and 12 wks in fingernail and toenail onychomycosis respectively |
| 2. Itraconazole | **Pulse therapy:** 200 mg twice daily for 1 wk/month for 2 and 3 consecutive months for finger and toenail onychomychosis respectively<br>**Continuous regimen:** 200 mg/day for 6 wks |
| 3. Fluconazole | 150 mg weekly for maximum period of 12 months |

## TINEA (PITYRIASIS) VERSICOLOR

- It is common superficial skin infection in warm and humid climate. Caused by lipophilic yeasts of the genus Malassezia (*M. furfur*, *M. sympodialis*, *M. obtusa*, *M. globosa*, *M. restricta*, *M. slooffiae*, and *M. pachydermatis*.)
- Scaly hypo- or hyperpigmented well-defined multiple asymptomatic or mildly itchy macular lesions on the chest, back, neck, and arms (Fig. 15.4).
- Scraping the surface of the lesions accentuates the scalling (*Coup d'ongle sign*).
- Other cutaneous manifestations associated with Malassezia species include seborrheic dermatitis, folliculitis, atopic dermatitis, and dandruff.
- **Pathogenesis**
  - ➤ The pathogenesis of *tinea versicolor* is unclear but may involve the conversion of colonizing yeasts into the mycelial form, which then invades the stratum corneum.
  - ➤ Hyperpigmentation is believed to be due to the normal inflammatory stimulation of melanogenesis.
  - ➤ Hypopigmentation is believed to be a result of azelaic acid produced by the organism. It reduces the production of melanin and inhibits its transfer to keratinocytes.
- **Diagnosis**
  - ➤ Scrape lightly—fine white scales (branny scales)
  - ➤ KOH positive for short hyphae and spores ("Spaghetti and meatballs")
  - ➤ Wood's light—pale yellow fluorescence.
  - ➤ Culture rarely done (Sabouraud's medium).

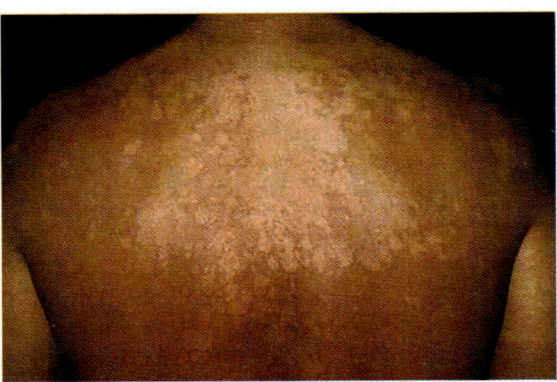

**Fig. 15.4:** Scaly hypo- and hyperpigmented macules over back and neck area

- **Treatment**
  - ➤ Topicals  for limited involvement.
    - – 2.5% selenium sulfide shampoos: Leather 10 minutes wash off × 7 days.
    - – Ketoconazole 2% shampoo
    - – 20% sodium hyposulphite
    - – Imidazoles topically  for  2–4 wks
    - – Terbinafine spray
  - ➤ Oral  for extensive
    - – Griseofulvin is not effective
    - – Oral ketoconazole (a single 400 mg dose or 200 mg daily orally for 5–10 days), fluconazole (a single 400 mg dose or 150 mg every week for 4 weeks), or itraconazole (200 mg daily  for 7 days) has proved effective.
- **Complications**
  - ➤ *M. furfur* is lipophilic and causes catheter-related fungemia in premature neonates and immunocompromised adults receiving IV lipids by central venous catheter.
  - ➤ Infection of the lungs is pronounced and frequently results in respiratory failure. *M. pachydermatis,* although not lipophilic, is an increasingly important pathogen in neonatal intensive care units.
  - ➤ Catheter-related Malassezia infections should be managed with prompt catheter removal and systemic antifungal therapy with amphotericin B or an azole.

## CANDIDIASIS

- **Most commonly caused by *Candida albicans***
- **Candida species** are normal commensals of the mouth affecting about 20–25% of adult population, GI tract, vaginal mucosa and in the patients with an indwelling catheter.
- Infants are particularly susceptible to superficial candidiasis that may reflect the immature immune response.
- Vaginal candidiasis is more common in pregnancy and its development may follow hormone related changes in the mucosa.
- Oral candidiasis is commonly associated with AIDS.
  Diabetes is particularly associated with increased susceptibility to vaginal infections.
- **Predisposing factors for candidiasis**
  - ➤ Obesity
  - ➤ Diabetes mellitus

- ➤ Pregnancy
- ➤ Broad spectrum antibiotics
- ➤ Immunosuppression
- ➤ HIV infection
- • **Oral candidosis**
  - ➤ *Acute pseudomembranous candidosis* (oral thrush; acute pseudomembranous candidiasis): A sharply defined patch of creamy, crumbly, curd-like white pseudomembrane, which, when removed, leaves an underlying erythematous base. This membrane consists of desquamated epithelial cells, fibrin, leukocytes and fungal mycelium that attaches it to the inflamed epithelium. The buccal epithelium on the cheeks, the gums or the palate may be affected. In immunocompromised patients, the tongue may be affected as well. In severe cases, extension to the pharynx or the esophagus may occur, and erosion and ulceration are occasional complications. The condition occurs most commonly in the first weeks of life, and the preterm infant may be especially susceptible. Apart from in neonatal oral candidosis (as distinct from Candida carriage), acute pseudomembranous candidosis is usually secondary to local or general predisposing factors.
  - ➤ *Acute erythematous candidosis* (acute atrophic oral candidiasis; 'antibiotic sore tongue'): There is marked soreness and denuded atrophic erythematous mucous membranes, particularly on the dorsum of the tongue. It is especially associated with antibacterial antibiotic therapy.
  - ➤ *Chronic pseudomembranous candidosis*: Lesions are very persistent. It occurs principally in immunocompromised patients.
  - ➤ *Chronic erythematous candidosis* (chronic atrophic candidiasis; denture sore mouth; denture stomatitis): Some soreness in the epithelium in the denture-bearing area is said to affect nearly one-quarter of all denture wearers and most, if not all cases appear to be caused by candidosis.
  - ➤ *Chronic plaque-like candidosis* (chronic hyperplastic candidiasis; Candida leukoplakia): Very persistent, firm, irregular white plaques occur in the mouth, commonly on the cheek or the tongue. Unlike the pseudomembrane of oral thrush, this plaque cannot be easily removed.  Smokers appear to be particularly prone to develop this form of oral candidosis.
  - ➤ *Chronic nodular candidosis*. This is a rare form, where the clinical appearance that usually affects the tongue is cobbled.

- ➤ *Angular cheilitis* (angular stomatitis; perleche): Soreness at the angles of the mouth extending outwards in the folds of the facial skin. Nutritional status and mechanical factors (e.g. the depth of the fold), the presence of moisture from persistent salivation or licking the lips may also be important.
- ➤ *Median rhomboid glossitis:* This condition, characterized by a more-or-less diamond-shaped area on the dorsum of the tongue with loss of papillae, occurs as an acquired condition. It is simply a variant of chronic plaque-like candidosis.

- **Candida intertrigo (flexural candidosis)**
  - ➤ Any skin fold may be affected, especially in the obese subject.
  - ➤ Signs are typically erythema and a little moist exudation starting deep in the fold. As the condition develops, it spreads beyond the area of contact, usually developing the typical features of candidosis with a fringed, irregular edge and subcorneal pustules rupturing to give tiny erosions, and then further peeling of the stratum corneum.
  - ➤ Satellite lesions, pustular or papular, are classical.
  - ➤ The differential diagnosis of intertriginous candidosis includes tinea, seborrheic dermatitis, bacterial intertrigo, flexural psoriasis, Hailey-Hailey disease and flexural Darier's disease.

- **Vulvovaginitis (vulvovaginal thrush)**
  - ➤ This condition affects around 75% of women of childbearing age and presents with itching and soreness, and with a thick, creamy white discharge.
  - ➤ It is more common in pregnancy. Typically, there is dusky red erythema of the vaginal mucosa and the vulval skin, with curdy white flecks of discharge, but on occasions the only sign is erythema.

- **Candida balanitis:** In the mildest cases, transient tiny papules or pustules develop on the glans penis a few hours after intercourse, and rupture, leaving a peeling edge. Some may settle spontaneously without going through the full evolution. This mild form is usually associated with a little soreness and irritation. In more severe and chronic cases, the inflammatory changes become persistent over the glans and the prepuce.

- **Napkin candidosis** (diaper candidiasis): *C. albicans* is commonly isolated from the moist skin of the buttocks and genitalia of the infant but is more prevalent where the skin is affected by napkin rash.

- **Nodular or granulomatous candidosis of the napkin area** (granuloma gluteale infantum): This rare condition presents with an eruption over the buttocks, genitalia, upper thighs and pubis, within which develop nodules, sometimes as large as 2 cm across, bluish or brownish in color, reminiscent of Kaposi's sarcoma. The primary napkin dermatitis may clear leaving only the nodules. Successful management involves removal of microorganisms, avoidance of topical steroids and general measures to ensure adequate dryness in the region.

- **Candida paronychia**
  - ➤ This condition is chiefly found among those whose hands are frequently immersed in water.
  - ➤ *Clinical features:* Typically, several fingers are chronically infected, but one or all may be involved. The nail fold is red and swollen, and there is loss of the cuticle, and detachment of the nail fold from the dorsal surface of the nail plate, leading to pocketing.
  - ➤ Occasionally, thick white pus may discharge; often force is needed to express it.
  - ➤ The patient usually has marked tenderness, and spontaneous pain is an occasional feature.
  - ➤ Nail dystrophy with buckling of the nail plate and some discoloration and onycholysis around the lateral nail fold frequently occur, but massive destruction of the nail plate is rare.
  - ➤ Onychomycosis resulting from Candida: The most common is distal and lateral subungual onychomycosis (DLSO) associated with paronychia.
  - ➤ Complete destruction of the nail plate is also seen in some patients with chronic mucocutaneous candidosis. Two important predisposing conditions are Raynaud's phenomenon or disease and Cushing's syndrome.
- **Congenital candidosis**
  - ➤ This, as the name implies, represents established candidosis, usually of the skin and birth membranes present at the time of birth, and following intrauterine infection.
  - ➤ It is quite distinct from oral thrush of the neonate in which the organism is acquired, at the very earliest, from the birth canal during delivery. The skin is the most common site for lesions, which are usually present at birth.
  - ➤ The lesions are typically discrete vesicles or pustules on an erythematous base.
  - ➤ The face and chest are first affected by the rash, which generally spreads over the next few days after delivery.

- **Chronic mucocutaneous candidiasis:** Recurrent and persistent candidal infection of the skin, nails and mucous membranes.
- **Diagnosis**
  - *KOH preparation:* Pseudohyphae, hyphae and budding yeast cells may be seen.
  - *Grams stain:* Gram-positive pseudohyphae, hyphae and budding yeast cells.
  - *Culture:* Sabouraud's medium, cornmeal agar, rice extract agar supplemented with Tween-80.
  - Reynolds-Braude phenomenon
  - Germ tubes of Candida species can be demonstrated by Reynolds-Braude phenonmenon. Incubation of the culture of Candida species with human or sheep serum at 37°C produces germ tubes within 2–4 hrs.
  - Tube-like projections without a constriction at the point of attachment to yeast cells (pseudohyphae) are seen extending from the cell wall.
- **Treatment of candidiasis** (Table 15.6)

**Table 15.6:** Treatment of candidiasis

| Type of disease | Preferred treatment | Alternatives |
|---|---|---|
| **Mucocutaneous** | | |
| Cutaneous | Topical azole | Topical nystatin |
| Vulvovaginal | Azole cream or suppository or oral fluconazole (150 mg) | Nystatin suppository |
| Oropharyngeal | Clotrimazole troche or fluconazole tablet (100 mg/d) or itraconazole | Nystatin suspension; for azole unresponsive disease: Caspofungin (50 mg/d) or amphotericin B (0.3–0.5 mg/kg daily) |
| Esophageal | Fluconazole tablet (100–200 mg/d) or itraconazole solution (200 mg/d) | For azole unresponsive disease: Caspofungin (70 mg once, then 50 mg/d) or amphotericin B (0.3–0.5 mg/kg daily) |
| **Deeply invasive** | | |
| Non-neutropenic | Fluconazole (400 mg/d) or amphotericin B or caspofungin (70 mg once, then 50 mg/d) | |
| Neutropenic | Amphotericin B | |

## TINEA NIGRA

- *Tinea nigra* is an asymptomatic, superficial fungal infection generally affecting the skin of the palms and characterized by deeply pigmented, macular, non-scaly patches.
- *Tinea nigra* is caused by *Hortaea werneckii*
- One or several, sharply defined brown to black macules that resemble silver nitrate stain.
- Soles may be affected rarely.
- Diagnosis is by KOH examination or culture
- Topical imidazoles are effective.

## PIEDRA

- Two types of piedra characterized by nodules of fungal elements on the hair shaft have been reported: **Black piedra** caused by *Piedraia hortae* and **white piedra** caused by Trichosporon species (which may also be associated with other superficial infections as well as with invasive trichosporosis). *T. beigelii* has historically been the most significant pathogen in the genus Trichosporon.
- Black piedra is characterized by the presence of firmly adherent, black, gritty, hard nodules on the hairs of the scalp, or less frequently of the beard, moustache or pubic area.
- White piedra is characterized by the presence of soft, white or light brown nodules. The infection is more common on the hairs of the beard, moustache and genital areas than the scalp.
- Diagnosis is by KOH preparation and culture.
- Treatment: Shaving or cutting the affected hair.

## SPOROTRICHOSIS

- Sporotrichosis most commonly presents as chronic cutaneous, lymphocutaneous, and/or subcutaneous disease.
- This infection may also be extracutaneous, occurring at pulmonary, osteoarticular, or disseminated sites.
- It is caused by the dimorphic fungus *Sporothrix schenckii*.
  It is usually an occupational disease of gardeners, farmers, forestry workers, florists, and horticulturists.
- It most often follows inoculation of the organism into the skin.

- **Clinical manifestations**
  - ➢ The majority of infections with *S. schenckii* present either as fixed cutaneous **sporotrichosis** or as lymphangitic or lymphocutaneous disease.
  - ➢ Fixed cutaneous disease (plaque **sporotrichosis**) is limited to the site of inoculation. The primary lesion enlarges and may ulcerate and become verrucous.
  - ➢ In lymphocutaneous disease, which accounts for ~80% of cases, secondary lesions ascend along the lymphatics that drain the area, producing small painless nodules that erupt, drain, and ulcerate.
  - ➢ Osteoarticular **sporotrichosis** is an uncommon complication but may cause granulomatous tenosynovitis and bursitis, particularly in alcoholic patients.
  - ➢ Pulmonary **sporotrichosis** following inhalation of *S. schenckii* conidia has been reported in alcoholic patients with chronic obstructive pulmonary disease.
  - ➢ Disseminated disease, including that involving the central nervous system, is most likely to occur in patients who have AIDS or are otherwise immunocompromised.
- **Diagnosis**
  - ➢ A definitive diagnosis is made by culture of *S. schenckii.*
  - ➢ Histopathologic examination of biopsy material may also contribute to the diagnosis, with detection of the characteristic ovoid or cigar-shaped yeast forms.
- **Sporotrichosis: Treatment** (Table 15.7)
  - ➢ Oral therapy with a saturated solution of potassium iodide (SSKI; 5 drops 3 times daily, increasing to 40–50 drops 3 times daily as tolerated) has been successful.
  - ➢ Oral itraconazole has replaced SSKI as the treatment of choice for cutaneous and lymphocutaneous **sporotrichosis**.
  - ➢ Patients with non-life-threatening pulmonary disease and those with osteoarticular disease should be treated with itraconazole for at least 12 months.
  - ➢ Amphotericin B is the preferred agent for patients with life-threatening pulmonary disease or disseminated infection, for patients who cannot tolerate itraconazole, and for patients in whom itraconazole treatment has failed.

| Table 15.7: Treatment of sporotrichosis | | |
|---|---|---|
| *Sporotrichosis* | *First-line therapy* | *Alternative therapy* |
| Cutaneous/ lymphocutaneous | Itraconazole (100–200 mg/d for 3–6 months) | Terbinafine, 500–1000 mg/d |
| Non-life-threatening pulmonary, osteoarticular, or disseminated disease | Itraconazole (200 mg bid for 12 months) | AmB (lipid formulation) or fluconazole (800 mg/d for 12 months) in patients who cannot tolerate AmB or itraconazole |
| Life-threatening pulmonary or disseminated disease | AmB | Selected patients may be switched to oral itraconazole (200 mg bid for 12 months) |

AmB: Amphotericin B

Sporotrichoid pattern, i.e. in a **linear arrangement** along the lymphatic channels are:
- *Sporothrix schenckii* (**sporotrichosis**)
- Leishmania
- *M. marinum* (atypical mycobacteria)
- Nocardia
- Other dimorphic fungi.

The organisms are introduced as a result of trauma, and a primary inoculation site is often seen in addition to the lymphatic nodules.

## QUESTIONS FROM PREVIOUS EXAMINATIONS

1. *Tinea capitis*
2. Opportunistic infections
3. Chromomycosis
4. *Tinea pedis*
5. Spore-bearing fungal dermatitis
6. Classify *tinea barbae;* how will you treat
7. Candidiasis
8. Lab diagnosis of superficial mycoses
9. Dermatophytids
10. Corn meal appearance recurrent vaginal candidiasis
11. Trichophyton test
12. Gentian violet
13. Favus

14. Majocci's granuloma
15. *Tinea nigra*
16. Deep fungal infections
17. Madura foot
18. Phycomycosis
19. Opportunistic fungus in dermatology, clinical features and management.
20. Rhinosporidiosis
21. Actinomycosis
22. Madura bodies
23. *Phialophora verrucosa*
24. Sporotrichosis
25. *Tinea circinata*
26. *Tinea amiantacea*
27. *Conidiobolus coronatus*
28. Endothrix
29. Recurrent vaginal candidiasis

## MULTIPLE CHOICE QUESTIONS

1. **Tinea corporis is common in:**    *(AIIMS 91)*
   (a) Adult male              (b) Adult female
   (c) Female child            (d) Male child
2. **Dhobi's itch is:**    *(DNB 91)*
   (a) *Tinea corporis*        (b) *Tinea cruris*
   (c) *Tinea barbae*          (d) *Tinea capitis*
3. **All are dermatophytes *except*:**    *(AI 97)*
   (a) *Malassezia furfur*     (b) Trichophyton
   (c) Epidermophyton          (d) Microsporum
4. **Ringworm group of fungi include:**    *(Kar 90)*
   (a) Trichophyton            (b) Epidermophyton
   (c) Microsporum             (d) All of the above
5. **Tinea ungium affects:**    *(AI 95)*
   (a) Nail fold               (b) Nail plate
   (c) Joints                  (d) Interdigital space
6. **Nail infection is caused by the following *except*:**
   *(Manipal 09, NEET 13)*
   (a) Trichophyton            (b) Epidermophyton
   (c) Microsporum             (d) Candida

7. **Trichophyton affects:**
   - (a) Skin only
   - (b) Hair only
   - (c) Skin, hair, and nails
   - (d) Skin and nails only

8. ***Tinea capitis* is not caused by:**
   - (a) *Microsporum canis*
   - (b) *Trichophyton mentagrophytes*
   - (c) *Epidermophyton*
   - (d) *Trichophyton rubrum*

9. **Boggy swelling on the head with easily plukable hair in a young child suggests the diagnosis of:** *(AIIMS 98)*
   - (a) Pyoderma capitis
   - (b) *Tinea capitis*
   - (c) Alopecia areata
   - (d) Favus

10 **In a child with cystic boggy swelling over the scalp with easily plukable hair, what should be the investigation of choice?** *(AIIMS 96)*
   - (a) Gram staining
   - (b) Bacterial culture
   - (c) KOH staining
   - (d) Tissue culture

11. **Kerion is caused by:** *(AIIMS 98)*
   - (a) Dermatophytes
   - (b) Pityrosporum
   - (c) Candida
   - (d) Piedra

12. ***Tinea versicolor* is caused by:** *(UP 2006)*
   - (a) *Malassezia furfur*
   - (b) *Candida tropicalis*
   - (c) *Trichophyton rubrum*
   - (d) *Trichophyton mentagrophytes*

13. **Ciclopirox olamine is used in treatment of infection with:** *(AP 96)*
   - (a) Epidermophyton
   - (b) Crusted scabies
   - (c) Dermatophytes
   - (d) Microsporum

14. **Rx of choice for *tinea unguium*:** *(AI 93)*
   - (a) Amphotericin B
   - (b) Benzyl benzoate
   - (c) Griseofulvin
   - (d) Whitefield's ointment

15. **Which of the following is the drug of choice for routine oral Rx of ringworm infestation of skin?** *(Kar 90)*
   - (a) Nystatin only
   - (b) Amphotericin B only
   - (c) Ketokonazole orally
   - (d) Griseofulvin orally

16. **Rx of choice for *tinea unguium*:** *(Manipal 2000)*
   - (a) Miconazole
   - (b) Systemic griseofulvin
   - (c) Topical griseofulvin
   - (d) Amphotericin B

17. **Griseofulvin in not useful in Rx of:** *(WB 2007)*
   - (a) *T. capitis*
   - (b) *T. cruris*
   - (c) *T. versicolor*
   - (d) *T. pedis*

18. **Direct examination of lesions of** *tinea versicolor* **with Wood's lamp shows:**
    - (a) No fluorescence
    - (b) Pale yellow fluorescence
    - (c) Coral-red fluoroscence
    - (d) Green fluorescence

19. **Commonest fungal infection of female genitalia in diabetes is:**
    *(Kar 98)*
    - (a) Cryptococcal
    - (b) Maduromycosis
    - (c) Candida
    - (d) Aspergillosis

20. **'Black dot' ringworm is caused by:**   *(DNB 99)*
    - (a) Microsporum
    - (b) Trichophyton
    - (c) Epidermophyton
    - (d) Candida

21. **'Favus' is caused by:**   *(DNB 2008)*
    - (a) *T. schoenleinii*
    - (b) *T. microsporum*
    - (c) Epidermophyton
    - (d) *Candida tropicalis*

22. **Ringworm infection affects:**   *(AIIMS 92)*
    - (a) Dermis
    - (b) Papillary layer
    - (c) Stratum corneum
    - (d) Prickle cell layer

23. **Which of the following is most effective against Candida and dermatophytes?**   *(AIIMS May 2008)*
    - (a) Nystatin
    - (b) Tolnaftate
    - (c) Ketoconazole
    - (d) Griseofulvin

24. **Voriconazole is used in the following** *except*:   *(AIIMS Nov 2009)*
    - (a) Aspergillosis
    - (b) *Candida albicans*
    - (c) *Candida tropicalis*
    - (d) Mucormycosis

25. **A 10-year-old boy presented with painful boggy swelling of scalp, multiple sinuses with purulent discharge, easily pluckable hair, and lymph nodes enlarged in occipital region. Which one of the following would be most helpful for diagnostic evaluation?**   *(AIIMS Nov 2009)*
    - (a) Biopsy
    - (b) Bacterial culture
    - (c) KOH mount
    - (d) Patch test

26. **Fungi with no sexual stage:**   *(PGI 96)*
    - (a) Imperfect fungi
    - (b) Phycomycetes
    - (c) Basidiomycetes
    - (d) Ascomycetes

27. **Athlete's foot is caused by:**
    - (a) Dermatophytes
    - (b) Madurella
    - (c) Actinomycosis
    - (d) Candida

28. **Wavelength of light produced in Wood's lamp is:**   *(DNB 2006)*
    - (a) 320 nm
    - (b) 360 nm
    - (c) 400 nm
    - (d) 480 nm

29. **Reynolds-Braude phenonmenon is seen with:**   *(MH 2001)*
    - (a) Candida
    - (b) Malasezzia
    - (c) Trichophyton
    - (d) Epidermophyton

30. **Whitfield's ointment consists of:**   *(AIIMS 90)*
    - (a) Benzoic acid and salicylic acid
    - (b) Salicylic acid and HCl
    - (c) HCl and nitric acid
    - (d) Nitric acid and benzoic acid

31. **Linear lesion is seen in:**   *(DNB 99)*
    - (a) Sporotrichosis
    - (b) Lichen planus
    - (c) Psoriasis
    - (d) Pemphigus

32. **Which of the following are fungal infections of skin?**   *(PGI 2005)*
    - (a) Sporotrichosis
    - (b) Piedra
    - (c) Madura foot
    - (d) Tinea
    - (e) Erysipelas

33. *Tinea incognito* **is seen with:**
    - (a) Steroid therapy
    - (b) 1% permethrin
    - (c) 5% permethrin
    - (d) Antibiotics

34. **Griseofulvin is given for Rx of fungal infection of fingernail for duration of:**   *(AI 02)*
    - (a) 4 weeks
    - (b) 6 weeks
    - (c) 2 months
    - (d) 3 months

35. **An 8-year-old child has localized noncicatricial alopecia over scalp with itching and scales. The diagnosis is:**   *(JK 2004)*
    - (a) *Tinea barbae*
    - (b) Alopecia areata
    - (c) *Tinea capitis*
    - (d) Lichen planus

36. **A 36-year-old male worker in a factory by occupation, presented with itchy, annular, scaly diffuse plaques in both the groins. Application of corticosteroid ointment relieved the symptoms temporarily but the plaques continued to spread at the periphery. The most likely diagnosis would be:**   *(AI 2007)*
    - (a) Erythema annulare centrifugum
    - (b) Granuloma annulare
    - (c) Annular lichen planus
    - (d) *Tinea cruris*

37. **The most common pattern of onychomycosis is:**   *(CMC 08)*
    - (a) Endonyx onychomycosis
    - (b) Superficial white onychomycosis
    - (c) Proximal subungual onychomycosis
    - (d) Distal and lateral subungual onychomycosis

38. An 11-year-old boy is having *tinea capitis* on his scalp. The most appropriate line of treatment is:    *(TN 09)*
    (a) Oral griseofulvin therapy
    (b) Topical griseofulvin therapy
    (c) Shaving of the scalp
    (d) Selenium sulphide shampoo

39. Coral-red fluorescence with Wood's light strongly suggests the diagnosis of:    *(Rajasthan 09)*
    (a) Ash leaf macules        (b) Acanthosis nigricans
    (c) Erysepeloid             (d) Erythrasma

## Answers

1. **Ans. (a)** Adult male *(Ref. IDVL Textbook of Dermatology, 2nd edn, 225)*
2. **Ans. (b)** *Tinea cruris (Ref. IDVL Textbook of Dermatology, 2nd edn, 225)*
3. **Ans. (a)** *Malassezia furfur (Ref. IDVL Textbook of Dermatology, 2nd edn/ 215)*
4. **Ans. (d)** All of the above *(Ref. IDVL Textbook of Dermatology, 2nd edn/215)*
5. **Ans. (b)** Nail plate *(Ref. IDVL Textbook of Dermatology, 2nd edn/228)*
6. **Ans. (c)** Microsporum *(Ref. Ananthanarayan Microbiology, 6th edn, 567)*
7. **Ans. (c)** Skin, hair, and nails
8. **Ans. (c)** Epidermophyton *(Ref. IDVL Textbook of Dermatology, 2nd/217)*
9. **Ans. (b)** *Tinea capitis (Ref. IDVL Textbook of Dermatology, 2nd edn/ 223)*
10. **Ans. (c)** KOH staining *(Ref. IDVL Textbook of Dermatology, 2nd edn/ 223, 231)*
11. **Ans. (a)** Dermatophytes *(Ref. IDVL Textbook of Dermatology, 2nd edn/ 223, 231)*
12. **Ans. (a)** *Malassezia furfur (Ref. IDVL Textbook of Dermatology, 2nd edn/242)*
13. **Ans. (c)** Dermatophytes *(Ref. IDVL Textbook of Dermatology, 2nd edn/249)*
14. **Ans. (c)** Griseofulvin *(Ref. IDVL Textbook of Dermatology, 2nd edn/ 245; KDT, 6th edn/760)*
15. **Ans. (d)** Griseofulvin orally *(Ref. IDVL Textbook of Dermatology, 2nd edn/245)*
16. **Ans. (b)** Systemic griseofulvin *(Ref. IDVL Textbook of Dermatology, 2nd edn/245)*
17. **Ans. (c)** *Tinea versicolor (Ref. IDVL Textbook of Dermatology, 2nd edn/245)*

18. **Ans. (b)** Pale yellow fluorescence *(Ref. IDVL Textbook of Dermatology, 2nd edn/243)*

19. **Ans. (c)** Candida *(Ref. IDVL Textbook of Dermatology, 2nd edn/235)*

20. **Ans. (b)** Trichophyton *(Ref. IDVL Textbook of Dermatology, 2nd edn, 223)*

21. **Ans. (a)** *Tinea schoenleinii (Ref. IDVL Textbook of Dermatology, 2nd edn/223)*

22. **Ans. (c)** Stratum corneum *(Ref. Ananthanarayan Microbiology, 6th edn/ 567)*

23. **Ans. (c)** Ketoconazole

24. **Ans. (d)** Mucormycosis *(Ref. Harrison's Internal Medicine, 17th edn/ Chapter 191)*

25. **Ans. (c)** KOH mount *(Ref. Harrison's Medicine, 17th edn, Table 54–5; Chapter 53, 54, 199)*

26. **Ans. (a)** Imperfect fungi *(Ref.Ananthanarayan Microbiology, 6th edn, 565)*

27. **Ans. (a)** Dermatophytes *(Ref. IDVL Textbook of Dermatology, 2nd edn/ 226)*

28. **Ans. (b)** 360 nm *(Ref. IDVL Textbook of Dermatology, 2nd edn/232)*

29. **Ans. (a)** Candida *(Ref. IDVL Textbook of Dermatology, 2nd edn, 242)*

30. **Ans. (a)** Benzoic acid and salicylic acid *(Ref. IDVL Textbook of Dermatology, 2nd edn/249)*

31. **Ans. (a)** Sporotrichosis *(Ref. Roxburgh's Common Skin Diseases, 17th edn/43)*

32. **Ans. (a)** Sporotrichosis, **(c)** madura foot, **(d)** tinea *(Ref. Harrison's Internal Medicine, 17th edn/ Chapter 199)*

33. **Ans. (a)** Steroid therapy *(Ref. Roxburgh's Common Skin Diseases, 17th edn/42)*

34. **Ans. (d)** 3 months *(Ref. KDT, 6th/761; 5th/719)*

35. **Ans. (c)** *Tinea capitis (Ref. Harrison's Internal Medicine, 17th edn/ 312, 1264)*

36. **Ans. (d)** *Tinea cruris (Ref. IADLV, 2nd/225; Roxbergh, 17th edn/16,40; Fitzpatrick's Colour Atlas and Synopsis of Dermatology, 5th edn/699, 700)*

37. **Ans.** (d) Distal and lateral subungual onychomycosis *(Ref. Rook's Dermatology, 7th edn/31.37)*

38. **Ans. (a)** Oral griseofulvin therapy *(Ref. KD Tripathi 6th, edn/774)*

39. **Ans. (d)** Erythrasma *(Ref. Rook, 7th edn/ 27.38).*

# Bacterial Skin Infections

## IMPETIGO

- The word *impetigo* is derived from latin meaning 'to attack'.
- Impetigo is a contagious superficial bacterial infection of skin caused most often by *S. aureus,* and in some cases by group A beta hemolytic streptococci
- The most common skin infection in children.
- Overcrowding, poor hygiene and pre-existing skin diseases predispose to infection
- Face and extremities are commonly affected.

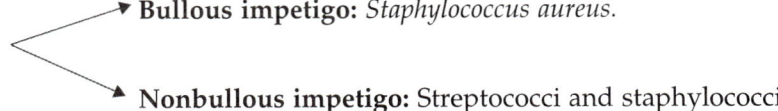

**Bullous impetigo:** *Staphylococcus aureus.*

**Nonbullous impetigo:** Streptococci and staphylococci

## Nonbullous Impetigo

- Usually presents as an erythematous macule over which a thin roofed vesicopustule appears.
- The vesicle fluid, clear in the beginning becomes turbid in less than a day.
- The roof of the vesicopustule soon ruptures and discharge dries up forming a loosely adherent, honey, or straw-colored or golden yellow, granular crust which appears stuck on (Fig. 16.1).
- Nonbullous impetigo is caused by *Streptococcus pyogenes or Staph. aureus*
- Streptococcal impetigo is responsible for majority of poststreptococcal acute GN.
- Rheumatic fever is not a complication of streptococcal impetigo.

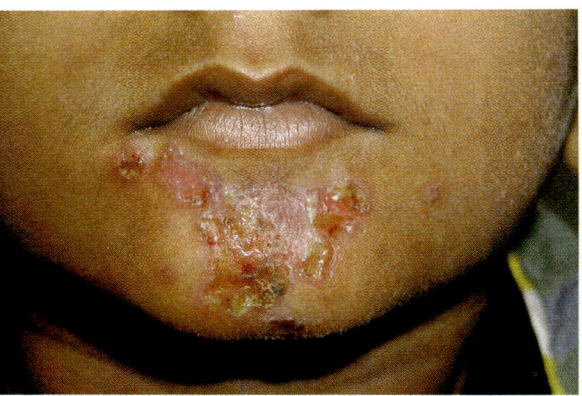

**Fig. 16.1:** Erythematous oozing and crusted lesion over chin in a child

## Bullous Impetigo

- Thin-walled flaccid bullae with a little or no surrounding erythema bullae persist for 2–3 days and then rupture.
- A thin, flat, honey-colored crust may appear in the center overlying superficial erosion.
- Central healing and peripheral extension may give rise to circinate lesions.
- The epidermis splits just below the stratum granulosum
- Blisters are caused by the production of exfoliative toxin by *S. aureus* phage type II.
- This is the same toxin responsible for staphylococcal scalded skin syndrome (SSSS), often resulting in dramatic loss of the superficial epidermis due to blistering.

## ECTHYMA

- Ecthyma is a pyogenic infection of the skin characterized by the formation of adherent crusts, beneath which ulceration occurs.
- It may result from neglected or inadequately treated impetigo.
- Small bullae or pustules on an erythematous base are soon surmounted by a hard crust of dried exudates. The base may become indurated and a red edematous areola is often present. The crust is removed with difficulty, to reveal a purulent ulcer. Healing occurs with scarring.
- Buttocks, thighs and legs are most commonly affected.
- Treatment of both ecthyma and impetigo involves gentle debridement of adherent crusts, which is facilitated by the use of

soaks and topical antibiotics, in conjunction with appropriate oral antibiotics. Topical mupirocin or fucidic acid may be used.

## STAPHYLOCOCCAL SCALDED SKIN SYNDROME (REITER'S DISEASE)

- Exfoliative toxin elaborated by *Staphylococcus aureus* phage group II.
- The syndrome was first described in children, but adults may be affected. Factors such as renal failure, malignancy, immuno-suppression or alcohol abuse predispose adults to the disease.
- Mucosae not involved.
- Staphylococcal organisms are not found in the skin lesions
- Focus of infection is extracutaneous (pharyngitis, otitis, tonsillitis, conjunctivitis, rhinorrhea).
- Redness and tenderness of central face, neck, trunk, and intertri-ginous zone followed by short-lived flaccid bulllae and slough or exfoliation or peeling of superficial epidermis.
- Nikolsky sign is positive.
- Children are not severely ill.
- Slight fever and systemic disturbances seen.
- Prognosis is good. Usually heals within 7–14 days.
- **Treatment: IV** antibiotics. Parenteral antibiotics such as methicillin, flucloxacillin, a cephalosporin or erythromycin are required.

## PYODERMA

- In India, particularly in poorer areas, children who are partially clad are exposed to various types of trauma which get secondarily infected. They have various lesions including impetiginized lesions, ecthyma, boils, etc. scattered over body. The diagnosis of pyoderma is made in such cases.

## TOXIC SHOCK SYNDROME

- Acute febrile multisystem illness caused by toxin producing strains of *S. aureus* most of which were initially isolated from the cervical mucosa in menstruating young women (Table 16.1).
- Recent cases are most often due to infections in wounds, catheters, contraceptive diaphragms or nasal packing.
- A very similar syndrome in which the cause is group A or rarely group B streptococci has been defined.

**Table 16.1:** Comparison of streptococcal and staphylococcal toxic shock

| Disease | Etiology | Description | Group affected | Clinical |
|---|---|---|---|---|
| **Streptococcal toxic shock syndrome** | Group A Streptococcus (associated with pyrogenic exotoxin A and/or B or certain M types) | When present, rash often scarlatiniform | May occur in setting of severe group A streptococcal infections, such as necrotizing fasciitis, bacteremia, pneumonia | Multiorgan failure, hypotension; 30% mortality rate |
| Staphylococcal toxic shock syndrome | S. aureus (toxic shock syndrome toxin 1, enterotoxin B or C) | Diffuse erythema involving palms; pronounced erythema of mucosal surfaces; conjunctivitis; desquamation 7–10 days into illness | Colonization with toxin-producing S. aureus | Fever >39°C (102°F), hypotension, multiorgan dysfunction |

## CELLULITIS

- Cellulitis is strictly an acute, subacute or chronic inflammation of loose connective tissue, but the term has been applied mainly to inflammation of subcutaneous tissue in which infective, generally bacterial, cause is proven or assumed.
- Most commonly caused by Group A beta hemolytic streptococci
- Diffuse erythema, edema, and tenderness.
  Edge is diffuse and in severe cases there may be bullae and dermal necrosis
- Constitutional symptoms are seen. Lymphangitis and lymphadenopathy may be seen.
- Leg is the commonest site.
- If untreated may lead to septicemia
- **Treatment:** IV or IM antibiotics.

## ERYSIPELAS

- Acute inflammation of lymphatics of skin caused by α-hemolytic streptococci.

- There is sudden onset of well marginated painful and swollen erythematous area usually on face and lower limb.
- There may be hemorrhage and blistering.
- Systemic symptoms may be acute and severe
- Milian's ear sign is positive. (Erysipelas extends to pinna whereas cellulitis does not.)
- **Treatment:** IV/IM antibiotics.

## FOLLICULITIS

### Superficial Folliculitis

- *Staphylococcus aureus* superficial folliculitis (follicular impetigo of Bockhart) is an infection of the follicular ostium with *S. aureus.*
- It is commonest in childhood, and occurs mainly in the scalp or scalp margins or on the limbs.
- The individual lesion is a domed, yellow pustule, sometimes with a narrow, red areola.
- The pustules develop in crops and may heal within 7–10 days, but sometimes become chronic.
- Chronic folliculitis of the legs has been described mainly in young adult males in India. The profuse eruption of superficial and deep follicular pustules on the thighs and lower legs persists for many years and is resistant to treatment.
- **Treatment:** Topical and systemic antibiotics.

### Deep Folliculitis

- **Sycosis barbae and nuchae**
  - ➢ Deep *Staphylococcus aureus* infection of hair follicle. Asymptomatic or painful and tender erythematous papules and pustules situated around coarse terminal hair in beard (barbae) and back of neck (nuchae).

- **Folliculitis keloidalis**
  - ➢ Folliculitis keloidalis is a chronic, inflmmatory process involving the hair follicles of the nape of the neck and leading to hypertrophic scarring in papules and plaques. It occurs in males after puberty and is most frequent between the ages of 14 and 25 years, especially in black males.

## FURUNCLE

- A furuncle is an acute, usually necrotic, infection of a hair follicle with *S. aureus.*
- Common in adolescence and early adult life

- Common in males than females
- Malnutrition, diabetes and HIV are predisposing factors.
- A furuncle first presents as a small, follicular, inflammatory nodule, soon becoming pustular and then necrotic and healing after discharge of a necrotic core to leave a violaceous macule, and ultimately, a permanent scar (Fig. 16.2).
- Tenderness is common
- Occasionally, there may be fever and mild constitutional symptoms.
- Pyemia and septicemia are favored by malnutrition.
- On the upper lip and cheek, cavernous sinus thrombosis is a rare and dangerous complication.
- The sites commonly involved are the face and neck, the arms, wrists and fingers, the buttocks and the anogenital region.
- Systemic antibiotics are needed.

### CARBUNCLE

- A carbuncle is a deep infection of a group of contiguous follicles with *S. aureus*, accompanied by intense inflammatory changes in the surrounding and underlying connective tissues, including the subcutaneous fat.
- Carbuncles occur predominantly in men, and usually in middle or old age.

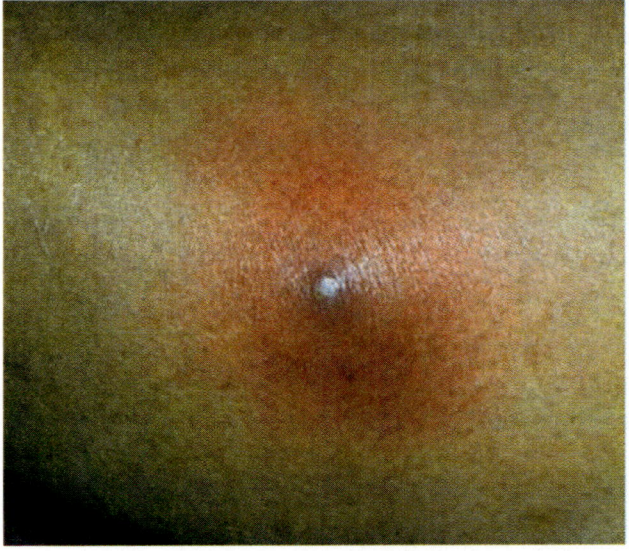

**Fig. 16.2:** Erythematous follicular nodule

- More common in the presence of diabetes, malnutrition, cardiac failure, drug addiction or severe generalized dermatoses and during prolonged steroid therapy.
- Most lesions are on the back of the neck, the shoulders or the hips and thighs.
- Constitutional symptoms are seen.
- Healing occurs with scarring.
- Systemic antibiotics are needed.

## ERYTHEMA MARGINATUM (RHEUMATIC FEVER)

- Caused by group A Streptococcus
- Seen in patients with rheumatic fever
- Erythematous annular papules and plaques occurring as polycyclic lesions in waves over trunk, proximal extremities; evolving and resolving within hours.
- Pharyngitis preceding polyarthritis, carditis, subcutaneous nodules, and chorea.

## ERYTHRASMA

**Definition:** Erythrasma is a mild, chronic, localized superficial infection of the skin caused by a group of closely related aerobic coryneform bacteria, usually known as *Corynebacterium minutissimum.*

- Particularly common in obese, middle-aged black women.
- Diabetes was found to coexist.
- **Clinical features**
  - ➤ Erythrasma, as detected by Wood's light examination, involves the toe clefts more frequently than any other site.
  - ➤ It occurs most commonly in the groins, axillae and the intergluteal and submammary flexures.
  - ➤ The patches are of irregular shape and sharply marginated, at first red, but later becoming brown. New lesions are smooth, but older lesions tend to be finely creased or obviously scaly (Fig. 16.3).
- **Differential diagnosis**
  - ➤ Pityriasis versicolor is most commonly confused with erythrasma, but it occurs predominantly on the upper trunk, and the individual lesions are small and are not erythematous.
  - ➤ On the thighs, groins and pubic area, *tinea cruris* and candidiasis.

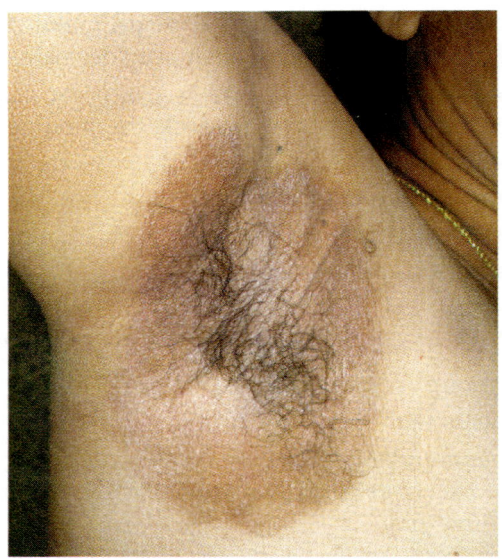

**Fig. 16.3:** Hyperpigmented irregular well demarcated patch of erythrasma

➤ It is difficult to differentiate erythrasma of the toe clefts from *tinea pedis* or Candida infection, but, as in all varieties of erythrasma, the presence of coral-red fluorescence under Wood's light is diagnostic.

• **Treatment**

| | |
|---|---|
| Most respond to | Topical antifungals—clotrimazole and miconazole (2 wks) |
| For extensive lesions | Erythromycin (the most effective approach) |
| Alternatives | Topical fusidin and oral tetracycline |

## TRICHOMYCOSIS AXILLARIS

• Superficial infection of axillary and pubic hairs with the formation of adherent granular nodules—yellow, black or red—on the hair shaft. These may be hard, or soft and nodular, or more diffuse.
• Caused by corynebacteria
• Asymptomatic.
• Differential diagnosis: Pediculosis pubis and piedra
• Diagnosis is by KOH preparation
• Clipping the affected hairs and the application of an antimicrobial ointment, such as benzoic acid compound ointment or 1% aqueous formalin, are effective.

## PITTED KERATOLYSIS

- Recent work suggests that *Dermatophilus congolensis, Micrococcus sedentarius,* a Corynebacterium or a combination of these organisms, may be responsible for pitted keratolysis.
- There are numerous superficial erosions of the horny layer of the soles and the undersurfaces of the toes. All parts of both soles may be affected, but pressure bearing or friction areas are most commonly affected.
- Conspicuous, discrete, shallow, circular lesions with a punched-out appearance coalesce in places to produce irregular erosions.
- Hyperhidrosis is often associated.
- Diagnosis is by Gram staining or culture on brain–heart infusion agar.
- Treatment is by topical antibiotics or imidazoles. Hyperhidrosis should be controlled.

## ECTHYMA GANGRENOSUM

- Caued by Pseudomonas areuginosa.
- Indurated plaque evolving into hemorrhagic bulla or pustule that sloughs, resulting in eschar formation; erythematous halo.
- Most common in axillary, groin, perianal regions
- Usually affects neutropenic patients; occurs in up to 28% of individuals with pseudomonas bacteremia

## *N. MENINGITIDIS*

- It is a gram-positive coccus
- It colonizes human upper respiratory tract
- It is transmitted by droplet from patients or healthy carriers
- It causes meningitis, conjunctivitis, otitis media, and fatal disease with septicemia.
- Acute meningococcal septicemia and meningitis present as fulminating illness.
- Rash is a very useful diagnostic clue
- The lesions are not always hemorrhagic and take form of discrete pink macules and papules.
- Transient erythematous, morbiliform or urticarial eruptions are occasionally seen.
- **Treatment:** IV benzyl penicillin in high doses is Rx of choice.

## ERYSIPELOID

- It is caused by *Erysipelothrix rhusiopathiae* and *Bacillus erysipelas.*
- *Erysipelothrix rhusiopathiae* is a rod-shaped, nonmotile, gram-positive organism.
- It is most often associated with fish and swine.
- It causes cellulitis primarily in fishmongers and bone renderers; veterinarians and those who handle pork products.
- Transmitted by contact with animals.
- *Erysipelothrix rhusiopathiae* is present on dead matter of animal origin.
- **Swine** is more frequently infected that any other animals.
- Turkeys are also infected and disease may arise from handling contaminated dressed Turkeys.
- It is also present in the slime of saltwater fish, on crabs and on other shellfish.
- **Treatment**
  - ➤ **Penicillin** 1 g/day for 5–10 days
  - ➤ Ciprofloxacin
  - ➤ Clindamycin
  - ➤ Imipenem

## "HOT-TUB" FOLLICULITIS

- Caused by *Pseudomonas aeruginosa*
- Pruritic, erythematous, follicular, papular, vesicular, or pustular lesions that may involve axillae, buttocks, abdomen, and especially areas occluded by bathing suits; can manifest as tender isolated nodules on palmar or plantar surfaces (the latter designated "Pseudomonas hot-foot syndrome").
- Affects bathers in hot-tubs or swimming pools; occurs in outbreaks. Earache, sore eyes and/or throat; generally self-limited.

## BACILLARY ANGIOMATOSIS

- Bacillary angiomatosis, a treatable opportunistic infection, was initially reported as atypical subcutaneous infection in patients with advanced HIV disease.
- The agents causing this infection, initially designated as Rocha-limaea, have been reclassified as Bartonella.
- The term bacillary angiomatosis is being replaced by Bartonella infection because the infectious agents causing this condition have been identified as two species of Bartonella—*B. henselae* and *B. quintana.*

## ERYTHEMA MIGRANS

- It is the cutaneous manifestation of Lyme disease, which is caused by the spirochete *Borrelia burgdorferi*.
- In the initial stage (3–30 days after tick bite), a single annular lesion is usually seen, which can expand to 10 cm in diameter. Within several days, approximately half the patients develop multiple smaller erythematous lesions at sites distant from the bite.
- Associated symptoms include fever, headache, photophobia, myalgias, arthralgias, and malar rash.

## QUESTIONS FROM PREVIOUS EXAMINATIONS

1. Lyme's disease
2. *Corynebacterium minutissimum* infection of skin
3. Atypical Mycobacterium
4. Blistering distal dactylitis
5. Pinna hair sign
6. Bacillary angiomatosis
7. Lupus vulgaris
8. Cutaneous infection of Staphylococcus
9. Pastia's lines
10. Price curve—moschella—normal bacterial flora
11. Scrofuloderma
12. Genital sore
13. Erysipeloid
14. Rhinosporidiosis
15. Cutaneous manifestations of Streptococcus
16. Ponarited histiocyte (infectious granuloma)
17. *Pityrosporum folliculitis*
18. Perianal staphylococcal cellulitis
19. Normal flora of skin
20. Cutaneous TB
21. Skin opportunistic infections
22. Echthyma
23. Botryomycosis
24. *Pseudofolliculitis barbae*
25. Remel body

26. Pseudomonas
27. Diphtheroids
28. Pillsbury occlusion triad
29. Bacteroids
30. Tuberculids
31. Intertrigo
32. Chronic paronychia
33. Necrotizing fasciitis
34. Secondary pyoderma
35. Pyoderma vegetans
36. Buruli's ulcer
37. SSSS

## MULTIPLE CHOICE QUESTIONS

1. **Coral-red fluorescence in Wood's lamp is seen with:** *(AIIMS 99)*
   (a) Porphyria cutanea tarda   (b) Erythrasma
   (c) Livedo reticularis   (d) Hypomelanosis

2. **Erythrasma is caused by:** *(MH 2001; Delhi 06)*
   (a) *Corynebacterium minutissimum*
   (b) *Corynebacterium diphtheriae*
   (c) *Corynebacterium ulcerans*
   (d) *Corynebacterium vaginale*

3. **Commonest skin infection in children:** *(AI 92)*
   (a) Scabies   (b) Impetigo contagiosa
   (c) Molluscum contagiosum   (d) Warts

4. **Following are the types of pyoderma** *except:* *(AP 92)*
   (a) Impetigo   (b) Folliculitis
   (c) Erythrasma   (d) Ecthyma

5. **Honey-colored crusts are characteristic of:** *(Manipal 2001)*
   (a) Nummular eczema   (b) Impetigo
   (c) Herpes zoster   (d) Cutaneous TB

6. **Ecthyma gangrenosum is seen in:** *(Manipal 99)*
   (a) Pseudomonas septicemia   (b) Lepromatous leprosy
   (c) Ulcerative colitis   (d) All of the above

7. **Morbilliform rash in a patient of meningitis suggest in which of the following infection?**
   (a) *Staphylococcus aureus*   (b) *Streptococcus pneumoniae*
   (c) *N. meningitidis*   (d) *H. influenzae*

8. **Erysipeloid is transmitted by:**    *(PGI 99)*
   - (a) Droplet
   - (b) Feco-oral
   - (c) Mosquito bite
   - (d) Contact with animal

9. **Staphylococcus can cause following** *except:*    *(PGI 99)*
   - (a) Scarlet fever
   - (b) TSS
   - (c) Carbuncle
   - (d) Sycosis barbae

10. **False about impetigo:**    *(PGI 09)*
    - (a) Caused by Staphylococcus or Streptococcus or both
    - (b) Predisposes to glomerulonephritis
    - (c) Produces scar on healing
    - (d) Erythromycin in DOC
    - (e) It is contagious disease

11. **Toxic shock syndrome is caused by:**    *(AI 93)*
    - (a) Staphylococcus
    - (b) Streptococcus
    - (c) Pseudomonas
    - (d) *E. coli*

12. **Following are staphylococcal infections** *except:*    *(AI 97)*
    - (a) Impetigo
    - (b) Erysipelas
    - (c) Ecthyma
    - (d) Scalded skin syndrome

13. **A 3-month-old male infant developed otitis media for which he was given a course of cotrimoxazole. A few days later he developed extensive peeling of skin. However, there were no mucosal lesions and the baby was not toxic. The likely diagnosis is:**    *(AIIMS 04)*
    - (a) Toxic epidermal necrolysis
    - (b) SSSS
    - (c) Stevens-Johnson syndrome
    - (d) Infantile pemphigus

14. *Corynebacterium minutissimum* **causes:**    *(MH 2002)*
    - (a) Erysipelas
    - (b) Erythrasma
    - (c) Erythema ab igne
    - (d) Erythroplasia

15. **Bacillary angiomatosis is caused by:**    *(JIPMER 07)*
    - (a) *B. henselae*
    - (b) *B. pertussis*
    - (c) *R. conorii*
    - (d) *A. actinomycetemcomitans*

16. **Cutaneous larva migrans is caused by:**    *(Delhi 08)*
    - (a) Strongyloides
    - (b) Ankylostoma
    - (c) Ascaris
    - (d) Toxocara

17. **Most common organism associated with necrotizing fasciitis:**    *(TN 99)*
    - (a) Group A streptococci
    - (b) Group B streptococci
    - (c) *S. aureus*
    - (d) *E. coli*

18. **Cutaneous manifestation of Lyme disease:**    *(PGI 08)*
    (a) Erythema gyratum repens
    (b) Erythema migrans
    (c) Erythema marginatum
    (d) Necrolytic migratory erythema

19. **"Hot-tub" folliculitis is caused by:**    *(JIPMER 09)*
    (a) Group A streptococci    (b) Group B streptococci
    (c) *S. aureus*    (d) *Pseudomonas aeruginosa*

20. **Forschheimer spots are seen in:**    *(Delhi 08)*
    (a) Measles    (b) Rubella
    (c) Erythema infectiosum    (d) Erythema subitum

21. **Pastia's lines seen in:**    *(DNB 2013)*
    (a) Scarlet fever    (b) Erythrasma
    (c) Rubella    (d) Typhoid

## Answers

1. **Ans. (b)** Erythrasma
   *(Ref. Harrison's Medicine, 17th edn/312, 326; Rook's Textbook of Dermatology, 7th edn/27.38)*

2. **Ans. (a)** *Corynebacterium minutissimum*

3. **Ans. (b)** Impetigo contagiosa *(Ref. IADVL, 2nd edn/193)*

4. **Ans. (c)** Erythrasma *(Ref. IADVL, 2nd edn/197)*

5. **Ans. (b)** Impetigo *(Ref. IADVL, 2nd edn/194)*

6. **Ans. (a)** Pseudomonas septicemia *(Ref. Harrison's Medicine, 17th edn, Table 18–1)*

7. **Ans. (c)** *N. meningitidis (Ref. Harrison's Medicine, 17th edn/ Table 54–13; Rook's Textbook of Dermatology, 7th edn/27.44)*

8. **Ans. (d)** Contact with animals *(Ref. Rook's Textbook of Dermatology, 7th edn/27.8–40)*

9. **Ans. (a)** Scarlet fever *(Ref. Rook's Textbook of Dermatology, 7th edn, 27. 8–40; Harrison's Medicine, 17th edn, Table 129–1)*

10. **Ans. (c, d)** *(Ref. Rook's Dermatology, 7th edn/27. 8–40)*

11. **Ans. (a)** Staphylococcus *(Ref. Andrew's Diseases of Skin, 10th edn, 257)*

12. **Ans. (b)** Erysipelas *(Ref. Harrison's Medicine, 17th edn/Table 18–1)*

13. **Ans. (b)** SSSS *(Ref. Rook's Dermatology, 7th edn/27.8–40)*

14. **Ans. (b)** Erythrasma *(Ref. Harrison, Principles of Medicine, 17th edn, Table 119–1; Ananthanarayan, 7th edn, 204)*

15. **Ans. (a)** *B. henselae*

16. **Ans. (b)** Ankylostoma

17. **Ans. (a)** Group A streptococci *(Ref. Rook's Dermatology, 7th edn/ 14.47)*

18. **Ans. (b)** Erythema migrans *(Ref. Harrison's Internal Medicine, 17th edn/ Chapter 54; Table 54–6)*

19. **Ans. (d)** *Pseudomonas aeruginosa (Ref. Harrison, 17th edn/Table 18–1)*

20. **Ans. (b)** Rubella *(Ref. Harrison, 17th edn/ Table 18–1).*

    Forschheimer's spots refers to an enanthem of red macules or petechiae confined to the soft palate in patients with rubella. The sign presents in up to 20% of patients during the prodromal period or on the first day of the exanthem.

21. **Ans. (a)** Scarlet fever.

    Pastia's lines refer to pink or red transverse lines found in the antecubital fossae and axillary folds. The lines are produced from confluent petechiae and are seen in patients with the pre-eruptive stage of scarlet fever.

# 17  Skin Tuberculosis

Tuberculosis of skin is caused by *Mycobacterium tuberculosis, M. hominis* and *M. bovis*.

## Classification of Skin Tuberculosis

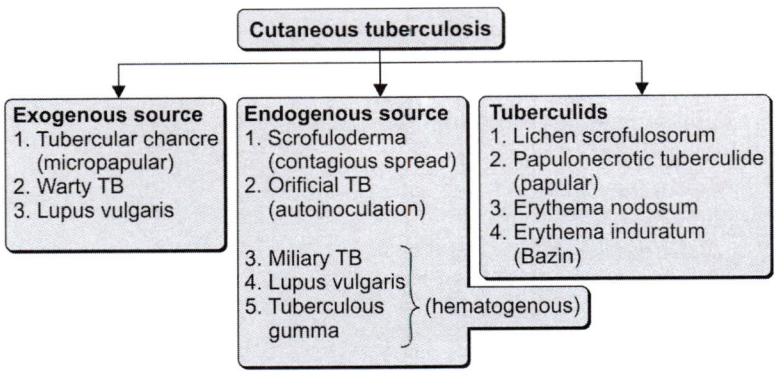

Cutaneous tuberculosis

**Exogenous source**
1. Tubercular chancre (micropapular)
2. Warty TB
3. Lupus vulgaris

**Endogenous source**
1. Scrofuloderma (contagious spread)
2. Orificial TB (autoinoculation)
3. Miliary TB
4. Lupus vulgaris
5. Tuberculous gumma
} (hematogenous)

**Tuberculids**
1. Lichen scrofulosorum
2. Papulonecrotic tuberculide (papular)
3. Erythema nodosum
4. Erythema induratum (Bazin)

## TUBERCULOSIS VERRUCOSA CUTIS (WARTY TUBERCULOSIS)

- This type occurs mainly in adults and in individuals with high resistance due to external inoculation of tubercle bacilli.
- The lesion appears mainly on the extremities, on the dorsum of the fingers, hands, ankles and buttocks as an indolent warty plaque. The verrucous surface shows fissures from which pus can be expressed (Fig. 17.1).
- This is characterized by a very chronic course that may be accompanied by lymphangitis, lymphadenitis and rarely by skin gangrene.

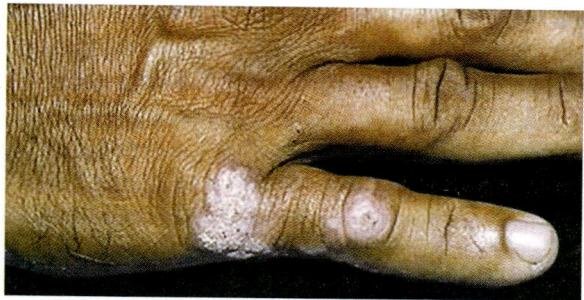

**Fig. 17.1:** Warty plaque over dorsum of a little finger

## TUBERCULOSIS CUTIS ORIFICIALIS

- Young adults and children with complete energy are affected by this type, which is usually accompanied by visceral TB.
- The lesions involve the mucous membranes of the mouth, palate, larynx, intestinal and lung mucous membranes. Lesions are painful shallow ulcers with undermined bluish edges.
- Lesions occur particularly in the mouth, on the genitalia and around the anus.

## PRIMARY TUBERCULOUS COMPLEX (TUBERCULOUS CHANCRE)

- Primary complex lesions involve the skin and lymph nodes mainly that of infants and young children.
- Cutaneous reaction at the site of inoculation of tubercle bacilli in an individual not previously exposed to the bacillus.
- Analogous to Ghon's complex in lungs.
- Lesions arise within 2–4 weeks after inoculation
- Asymptomatic ulcer covered with crust. Regional lymph nodes become enlarged and tender. They may suppurate producing draining sinuses.
- The common sites involved are the face and extremities. Usually heals spontaneously.

## MILIARY TUBERCULOSIS

- Miliary tuberculosis of the skin:
  - Occurs in association with generalized miliary tuberculosis
  - Due to hematogenous dissemination of mycobacteria into the skin.

- It is rare and usually affects young children or immunosuppressed. patients such as those with concurrent HIV infection or following viral infections such as measles.
- Profuse crops of minute bluish papules, vesicles, pustules or hemorrhagic lesions in a patient who is obviously ill. The vesicles may become necrotic to form small ulcers.
- The diagnosis is sometimes only made by the biopsy of a skin lesion showing acid-fast bacilli.
- Antituberculosis therapy should be started immediately
  - ➢ The tuberculin test is negative.
  - ➢ The prognosis is poor.

## LUPUS VULGARIS

- Lupus vulgaris is the most common type of cutaneous TB.
- Acquired from exogenous source, although may arise from hematogenous dissemination of bacilli.
- Patients have a moderate or high degree of immunity against tubercle bacilli.
- In India, buttocks, thighs, and legs are common site of involvement. In European cases, the lesions occur on face particularly about the nose and on the cheek with frequent involvement of the mucous membrane of then nose and the lips.
- Initial lesion is erythematous nodule slightly elevated above the surface. A few surrounding nodules appear and coalesce to form plaque. There is irregular extension of plaque.
- Ultimately healing may occur, with thin superficial scarring—a characteristic feature.
- Presence of "apple jelly" nodules at the edge of a plaque is may be seen, but their presence is not pathognomonic of lupus vulgaris. They do not exhibit this color on Indian skin.
- Rarely squamous cell carcinoma may arise in the scar.
- **Histology**
  Tubercles are often found in the dermis, but bacilli are difficult to demonstrate.

## SCROFULODERMA

- **Earlier known as** tuberculosis cutis colliquativa.
- It develops as infection into the skin from an underlying focus, usually lymph nodes and occasionally the bone.
- The commonest site of involvement is cervical region with the infected cervical lymph nodes breaking down into the skin.

- Linear or serpiginous ulcers and dissecting fistulas and subcutaneous tracts studded with soft nodules may develop. They are soft and their edges are undermined.
- Spontaneous healing may take years, eventuating in cord-like keloid scars; lupus vulgaris may also develop. They are soft and their edges are undermined.
- Scrofuloderma of a cervical lymph node often originates in the larynx and was linked in the past to ingestion of milk containing *M. bovis.*
- Lesions may also originate from an underlying infected joint, tendon, bone, or epididymis.
- The differential diagnosis includes syphilitic gumma, deep fungal infections, actinomycosis, and hidradenitis suppurativa.
- The course is indolent, and constitutional symptoms are typically absent.
- Antituberculous therapy is usually effective.

## TUBERCULIDS

- The tuberculids, first described by Darier in 1896, represent a form of cutaneous hypersensitivity reaction to tuberculosis (TB) antigens.
- Tuberculids form a group of eruptions usually symmetrical distributed, as a result of internal focus of TB.
- They are cured by anti-TB therapy.
- The probable cause is hematogenous dissemination of bacilli in a person with high degree of immunity.
- The tuberculin test is always positive in tuberculids.
- There is absence of tubercular bacilli in biopsy specimen.
- The internal TB may not be clinically active and patient's health is good.

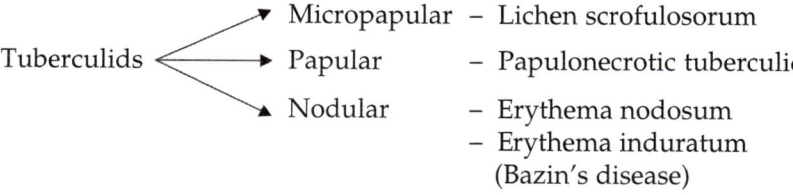

Tuberculids
- Micropapular  – Lichen scrofulosorum
- Papular  – Papulonecrotic tuberculid
- Nodular  – Erythema nodosum
          – Erythema induratum (Bazin's disease)

## Lichen Scrofulosorum

It is an uncommon lichenoid eruption ascribed to hematogenous spread of mycobacteria in an individual strongly sensitive to *M. tuberculosis.*
- Usually associated with chronic tuberculosis of the lymph nodes, bones, or pleura, it has also been observed after BCG vaccination and in association with *M. avium intracellulare* infections.

- Associated pulmonary or extrapulmonary tuberculosis is common.
- Lichenoid eruption of minute papules occurring in children and adolescents with TB.
- Strongly positive tuberculin reaction.
- Skin-colored, symptom less, 0.5 to 3 mm closely grouped lichenoid papules occur in perifollicular distribution, mainly found on abdomen chest back and proximal limbs.
- HPE—superficial dermal granulomas surrounds hair follicles and sweat ducts and may occupy several dermal papillae, foreign body granuloma without caseation.
- Mycobacteriums are not seen and cannot be cultured from biopsy material.
- Differential diagnosis
  - Lichen nitidus
  - Keratosis spinulosa
  - Keratosis pilaris
  - Drug eruptions
- **Treatment**
  - Anti-tuberculosis therapy
  - Lesions clear in 4–8 wks without scarring

## Papulonecrotic Tuberculids

- Most common tuberculid
- A chronic, recurrent, and symmetric eruption of necrotizing skin papules arising in crops, involving primarily the arms and the legs.
- Lesions are capped by pustules and ulcerate forming crusts.
- A **hallmark** of this condition is that lesions heal with varioliform scarring.
- The eruption is believed to represent a hypersensitivity reaction to TB antigens released from a distant focus of infection.

## Erythema Induratum

- Subcutaneous nodules and plaques.
- Located on calves of young adult females.
- Involves overlying skin with ulceration and heal with atrophic scars
- Bilaterally symmetrical
- Chronic and recurrent
- Males almost never affected

## Erythema Nodosum (Table 17.1)

| Table 17.1: Erythema nodosum | | | | |
|---|---|---|---|---|
| Disease | Etiology | Description | Group affected | Clinical syndrome |
| Erythema nodosum (septal panniculitis) | Infections (e.g. streptococcal, fungal, mycobacterial, yersinial); Drugs (e.g. sulfas, penicillins, oral contraceptives); Sarcoidosis; Idiopathic causes | Large, violaceous, nonulcerative, subcutaneous nodules; exquisitely tender; usually on lower legs (shin) but also on upper extremities | More common in females 15–30 years old | Arthralgias (50%); features vary with associated condition |

### Diagnosis of TB

- **Absolute criteria**
  - ➢ The positive culture of *M. tuberculosis* from the lesion
  - ➢ Successful guinea pig inoculation
  - ➢ Mycobacterial DNA identification by PCR.
- **Relative criteria**
  - ➢ The presence of active, proven tuberculosis elsewhere in the body
  - ➢ The presence of acid-fast bacilli in the lesion itself—this will also be seen in infections with other mycobacteria
  - ➢ The histopathology
  - ➢ A positive reaction to tuberculin
  - ➢ The clinical history and physical signs
  - ➢ The effect of specific therapy

### Management

- A standard 6-month regimen for adults is now recommended by the British and American Thoracic Societies.
- It includes four drugs (doses for adults only are given here):
  - ➢ Isoniazid (300 mg daily) for the full 6 months
  - ➢ Rifampicin (450 mg daily for those weighing less than 50 kg and 600 mg daily above this weight) for the full 6 months
  - ➢ Pyrazinamide for the first 2 months (1.5 g daily for those weighing less than 50 kg; 2.0 g daily for those weighing over 50 kg)

> Ethambutol for the first 2 months (dosage 15 mg/kg body weight daily).
- All drugs are taken on an empty stomach once daily.
- **Multidrug-resistant (MDR) tuberculosis:** This is defined as resistance to rifampicin and isoniazid with or without resistance to other antituberculous drugs, and is now a worldwide problem.

  **Extremely drug-resistant (XDR) tuberculosis:** Multidrug-resistant strains with resistance to at least three of the main six classes of second-line drugs, first reported from South Africa in patients with HIV.

## Atypical Mycobacterial Infections

- **Swimming pool granuloma**
  > It is caused by *M. marinum.*
  > Infection is often acquired from swimming pools or acquaria (fishtank granuloma).
  > Chlorination of water does not seem to be effective prophylactic measure.
- **Buruli ulcer**
  > It is caused by *Mycobacterium ulcerans.*
  > The tissue reaction is not tuberculoid.
  > Ulcers may be very deep and involve muscle and bone.
  > Skin test with burulin gives positive response.

### QUESTIONS FROM PREVIOUS EXAMINATIONS

1. Scrofuloderma
2. Erythema induratum
3. Lichen scrofulosorum
4. Lupus vulgaris
5. Buruli ulcer
6. Swimming pool granuloma
7. Tuberculids
8. Tuberculosis verrucosa cutis
9. Skin and TB
10. Tuberculin test
11. Management of TB

# MULTIPLE CHOICE QUESTIONS

1. **Forms of skin tuberculosis include all** *except:*
   *(Maharashtra 2006)*
   (a)  Lupus vulgaris          (b)  Scrofuloderma
   (c)  Erythema nodosum        (d)  Erythema annulare

2. **Skin TB from an underlying structure is called:**    *(AI 99)*
   (a)  Scrofuloderma           (a)  Lupus vulgaris
   (c)  Erythema nodosum        (d)  Erythema gangrenosum

3. **Apple jelly nodules are seen in:**    *(MH 2003; NEET 2012)*
   (a)  Scrofuloderma           (b)  Lupus vulgaris
   (c)  Lichen scrofulosorum    (d)  Tuberculosis verrucosa cutis

4. **Swimming pool granuloma is caused by:**    *(PGI 99)*
   (a)  *M. marinum*            (b)  *M. ulcerans*
   (c)  *M. avium*              (d)  *M. kansasii*

5. **Buruli ulcer is caused by:**    *(TN 2002)*
   (a)  *M. marinum*            (b)  *M. ulcerans*
   (c)  *M. avium intracellulare*  (d)  *M. tuberculosis*

6. **Which of the following is/are tuberculids?**    *(PGI 2000)*
   (a)  Lichen scrofuloderma    (b)  Lichen nitidus
   (c)  Lichen aureus           (d)  Erythema nodosum

7. **Which of the following is tuberculid?**    *(AIIMS Nov 06)*
   (a)  Lichen scrofulosorum    (b)  Erythema nodosum
   (c)  Lupus vulgaris          (d)  Scrofuloderma

8. **Erythema nodosum is seen in:**    *(AIIMS 94)*
   (a)  Salicylate poisoning    (b)  Nontyphoid fever
   (c)  TB                      (d)  Leprosy

9. **Most common type of cutaneous TB:**    *(PGI 06)*
   (a)  Lupus vulgaris          (b)  Scrofuloderma
   (c)  TB verruca cutis        (d)  Erythema induratum

10. **Which of the following is a skin manifestation of TB?**
    (a)  Lupus vulgaris         (b)  Lupus pernio
    (c)  Scrofuloderma          (d)  Butcher's warts

11. **An 8-year-old boy presented with well-defined annular lesion over the buttock with central scaring that is gradually progressive over the last 8 months. What is the diagnosis?**
    *(AIIMS 2001)*
    (a)  Annular psoriasis      (b)  Lupus vulgaris
    (c)  *Tinea corporis*       (d)  Chronic granulomatous disease

12. **A young boy presented with a lesion over his right buttock, which had peripheral scaling with central clearing and scarring. The investigation of choice would be:**
    - (a) Tzanck smear
    - (b) KOH preparation
    - (c) Biopsy
    - (d) Sabourad's agar

13. **Scrofuloderma is:**                                      *(MH 05)*
    - (a) Chronic infection by *Staphylococcus epidermidis*
    - (b) Tubercular sinus with discharge
    - (c) Rupture of a lymph node with involvement of skin
    - (d) Lesion in lupus vulgaris

14. **Forms of skin tuberculosis include all *except:***      *(MH 06)*
    - (a) Lupus vulgaris
    - (b) Scrofuloderma
    - (c) Erythema nodosum
    - (d) Erythema annulare

15. **Involvement of sweat glands and hair follicles is typically seen in which *tuberculid?***                *(AI 09)*
    - (a) Lichen scrofulosorum
    - (b) Miliary TB
    - (c) Papulonecrotic type
    - (d) Lupus vulgaris

16. **Most common type of tuberculid:**                        *(MP 09)*
    - (a) Lichen scrofulosorum
    - (b) Miliary TB
    - (c) Papulonecrotic type
    - (d) Lupus vulgaris

17. **Erythema nodosum can be seen with:**            *(Jharkhand 04)*
    - (a) OC pills
    - (b) Barbiturates
    - (c) Penicillin
    - (d) Sulfonylureas

18. **False about erythema nodosum:**                         *(MP 04)*
    - (a) Considered a hypersensitivity reaction
    - (b) Overlying skin is red, smooth and shiny
    - (c) Usually non-tender
    - (d) Can be seen in TB

## Answers

1. **Ans. (d)** Erythema annulare *(Ref. Harrison's Medicine, 17th edn, Table 18–1)*
2. **Ans. (a)** Scrofuloderma *(Ref. IADVL, 2nd edn/208)*
3. **Ans. (b)** Lupus vulgaris *(Ref. IADVL, 2nd edn/209)*
4. **Ans. (a)** *M. marinum* *(Ref. IADVL, 2nd edn/210)*
5. **Ans. (b)** *M. ulcerans*
6. **Ans. (a)** Lichen scrofuloderma and **(d)** Erythema nodosum *(Ref. IADVL, 2nd edn/207–209)*
7. **Ans. (a)** Lichen scrofulosorum and **(b)** Erythema nodosum *(Ref. IADVL, 2nd edn/207–209)*

8. **Ans. (c)** TB *(Ref. Andrew's Diseases of Skin, 10th edn/488)*
9. **Ans. (a)** Lupus vulgaris *(Ref. Rook's Textbook, 7th edn/28.14–28.16; IADVL, 2nd edn/208)*
10. **Ans. (a)** Lupus vulgaris; **(c)** Scrofuloderma *(Ref. IADVL Textbook of Dermatology, 2nd edn/208)*
11. **Ans. (b)** Lupus vulgaris *(Ref. Rook's Textbook, 7th edn/28.10–30)*
12. **Ans. (c)** Biopsy *(Ref. Rook's Textbook, 7th edn/28.10–30)*
13. **Ans. (c)** Rupture of a lymph node with involvement of skin *(Ref. Nelson's Textbook of Pediatrics, 17th edn, 2228)*
14. **Ans. (d)** Erythema annulare
15. **Ans. (a)** Lichen scrofulosorum *(Ref. Rook's Textbook of Dermatology, 7th edition/28.20).*
16. **Ans. (c)** Papulonecrotic type *(Ref. Rook's Textbook of Dermatology, 7th edition/28.20).*
17. **Ans. (a)** OC pills *(Ref. Harrison, 17th edn/ Table 18–1)*
18. **Ans. (c)** Usually non-tender *(Ref. Harrison, 17th edn/ Table 18–1).*

# 18  Leprosy

- **Leprosy** is a chronic infectious disease caused by *M. leprae,* whose clinical manifestations are largely confined to the skin, peripheral nerves, upper respiratory tract, eye and testis.
- Lepra bacillus was discovered by Hansen in 1873.
- Leprosy affects all ages and both sexes.
- Incubation period varies from 3 to 5 years.
- *M. leprae* is an **obligate intracellular bacillus**.
- The organism is acid-fast, indistinguishable microscopically from other mycobacteria, and ideally detected in tissue sections by a **modified Fite stain**.
- *M. leprae* produces no known toxins and is well adapted to penetrate and reside within macrophages, yet it may survive outside the body for months.
- The multiplication of *M. leprae* in mouse footpads (albeit limited, with a **doubling time of ~2 weeks**) has provided a means to evaluate antimicrobial agents, monitor clinical trials, and screen vaccines.
- *M. leprae* **grows best in cooler tissues** (the skin, peripheral nerves, anterior chamber of the eye, upper respiratory tract, and testes), sparing warmer areas of the skin (the axilla, groin, scalp, and midline of the back).
- Contact, inhalation, ingestion, and transmission through insects are considered as possible methods of transmission of leprosy.
- Although it is possible that infants could acquire infection through breast milk, there is no direct evidence to show that leprosy is transmitted through ingestion.
- *M. leprae* have special affinity for nerves.
- Nerves are more severely affected where they lie superficially just under skin. Although any peripheral nerve may be enlarged

(including small digital and supraclavicular nerves), those **most commonly** affected are the ulnar, posterior auricular, peroneal, and posterior tibial nerves.

## RIDLEY-JOPLING CLASSIFICATION

- Lepromatous leprosy
- Borderline lepromatous leprosy
- Mid-borderline leprosy
- Borderline tuberculoid leprosy
- Tuberculoid leprosy (Table 18.1)

**Table 18.1:** Comparison between tuberculoid and lepromatous leprosy

|  | *Tuberculoid* | *Lepromatous* |
|---|---|---|
| **Number of lesions** | 1–10 | Hundreds, confluent |
| **Distribution** | Asymmetrical, anywhere | Symmetrical, avoiding 'spared' areas |
| **Definition and clarity** | Defined, edge, markedly hypopigmented | Vague edge, slight hypopigmentation |
| **Anaesthesia** | Early, marked, defined, localized to skin lesions or major peripheral nerve | Late, initially slight, ill-defined, but extensive, over 'cool' areas of body |
| **Autonomic loss** | Early in skin and nerve lesions | Late, extensive as for anesthesia |
| **Nerve enlargement** | Marked, in a few nerves | Slight but widespread |
| **Mucosal and systemic** | Absent | Common, severe during type 2 reactions |
| **Number of *Mycobacterium leprae*** | Not detectable | Numerous in all affected tissues |

### Indeterminate Leprosy

- One or a few hypopigmented nonscaly macules
  - ➤ Slightly erythematous
  - ➤ Shiny due to epidermal atrophy
- Doubtful sensory loss
- Nerves not enlarged
- Resident of endemic areas

### Tuberculoid

- One or a few lesions with well-defined margins
- Hypopigmented macules or erythematous plaques (Fig. 18.1).

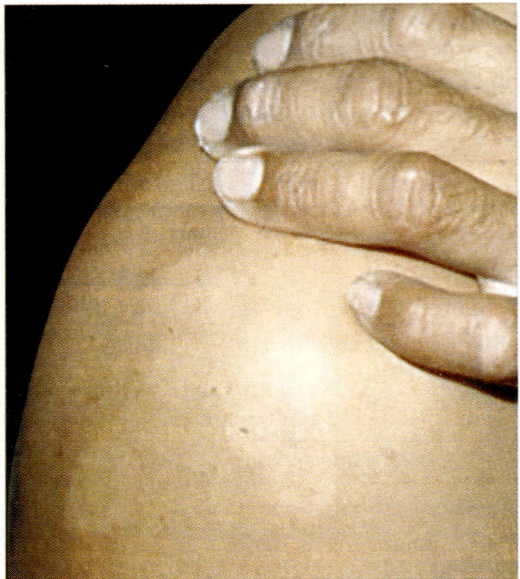

**Fig. 18.1:** Well-defined hypopigmented macules

- Nerve to the patch may be thickened
- Anesthetic and hairless
- Peripheral nerves may be thickened
- Most common in India and Africa

### Borderline Tuberculoid (BT)

- BT is commonest presenting form of leprosy in Southeast Asia
- Lesions are well-defined infiltrated plaques varying from 3 to 10 in number.
- Lesions may have well-defined margins and margin may be raised in one and flat and vague in another part of the lesion.
- Lesions have tendency for break in borders.
- Lesions have tendency for development of satellite lesions.
- Surface is dry and anhidrotic.
- Pain and temperature sensations are usually lost/impaired.
- Nerves in vicinity are enlarged.
- Lepromin test is weakly positive.
- AFB may be found on serial sections.
- Type 1 reactions are common in BT.

### Mid-borderline

- Inverted saucer lesions (annular plaque-like lesions where the margins slope towards normal skin)
- Macules, papules or plaques are bilateral with a tendency to symmetry.

### Borderline Lepromatous

- Numerous less well-defined and almost symmetrical lesions.

### Lepromatous Leprosy

- **Skin lesions in the patients with lepromatous leprosy** include macules, papules, nodules, or with all the three, but macules are likely to appear first (Fig. 18.2).
- Skin lesions are multiple and have a bilateral symmetrical distribution.
- Macules are erythematous on light skins and coppery on dark skins.
- Papules and nodules are firm on palpation.
- In untreated patients leonine facies may be seen.
- Sensations are unimpaired in early stages. Later glove and stocking anesthesia and bilateral symmetrical thickening of peripheral nerve trunks is seen.
- Early involvement of face common

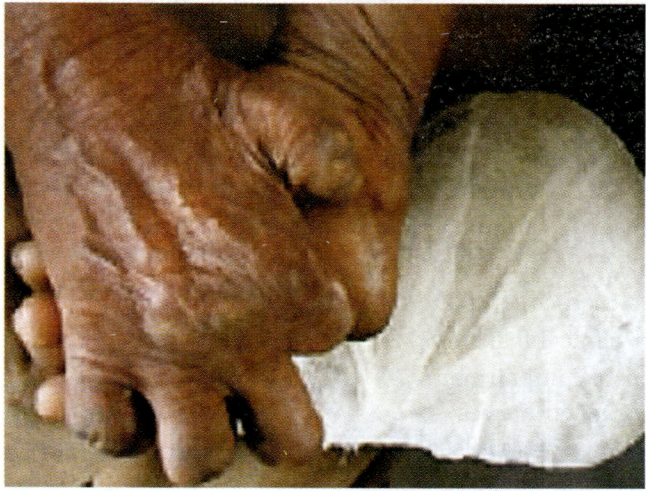

**Fig. 18.2:** Deformity of hand and loss of phalanges in a lepromatous leprosy patient

- Diffuse erythema becoming worse on exposure to sun; tingling, nasal stuffiness or epistaxis and edema of lower legs are the earliest manifestations.
- Nodules with predilection for external ears.
- Superciliary and ciliary madarosis (loss of hair on outer half of eyebrows)
- Mucous membrane involvement and ulceration.
- Saddle nose
- Regurgitation due to perforation of palate.
- Conjunctivitis and episcleritis.
- Hoarseness or difficulty in breathing (larynx involvement)
- Loss of testicular sensations, loss of libido, impotence and gynecomastia.
- Perforating/neuropathic ulcer is a complication of lepromatous leprosy because sensory impairment appears before motor weakness and patient continues to misuse his feet and hands.
- Swollen macrophages; packed with bacilli seen in lepromatous leprosy are **known as lepra cells or virchow cells.** Bacilli packed within macrophages appear in dense round collections known as globi.
- Lepra cell is a histiocyte with multiple lepra bacilli in it, arranged in bundle of cigarrete like manner.

### Pure Neuritic Leprosy

- The Indian classification of leprosy and its modified version have recognized **pure neuritic leprosy** as a distinct group (Table 18.2).
- 4.3–10.7% of cases
- Males > females
  20–40 yrs of age
- Presenting symptoms:
  - ➤ Sensory symptoms > nerve pain > deformity.
  - ➤ Rarely nerve abscess
- Ulnar, median, and lateral popliteal nerves commonly involved. Other clinical features:
  - ➤ Sensory impairment
  - ➤ Thickened nerves
  - ➤ Absence of skin lesions
  - ➤ Slit smear negative
- Nerve biopsy diagnostic
- 35% of cases develop skin lesions over 3–5 yrs with or without Rx.

| Table 18.2: Various types of leprosy | |
|---|---|
| *Leprosy type* | *Features* |
| Neural/neuritic leprosy | • Only nerve trunk involvement, no skin lesions<br>• Noninfectious<br>• Slit smear negative |
| Tuberculoid (TT) | • Most common type in India<br>• Can be either one large red patch with well-defined raised borders or a large hypopigmented asymmetrical spot<br>• Lesions become dry and hairless<br>• Loss of sensation may occur at site of some lesions<br>• Tender, thickened nerves with subsequent loss of function are common<br>• Spontaneous resolution may occur<br>• Only type in which histological involvement of epidermis and superficial dermis occurs<br>• Not associated with lepra reaction |
| Borderline tuberculoid (BT) | • Most common type in Southeast Asia<br>• Similar to tuberculoid type except that lesions are smaller and more numerous<br>• Does not heal spontaneously<br>• Disease may stay in this stage or convert back to tuberculoid form, or progress<br>• Satellite lesions<br>• Associated with type 1 lepra reaction but not with ENL. |
| Borderline borderline (BB) | • Numerous, red, irregularly shaped plaques<br>• Sensory loss is moderate<br>• Punched out lesions are characteristic<br>• Disease may stay in this stage, improve or worsen |
| Borderline lepromatous (BL) | • Numerous lesions of all kinds, plaques, macules, papules and nodules<br>• Hair growth and sensation are usually not impaired over the lesions |
| Lepromatous leprosy (LL) | • Early nerve involvement may go unnoticed<br>• Numerous lesions of all kinds, plaques, macules, papules and nodules<br>• Early symptoms include nasal stuffiness, discharge and bleeding, and swelling of the legs and ankles |

*Contd.*

| Table 18.2: Various types of leprosy *(Contd.)* | |
|---|---|
| *Leprosy type* | *Features* |
| | • Madarosis (loss of eyelashes) |
| | • Globi (bacilli 109/gm in clumps) |
| | • Left untreated, the following problems may occur: |
| |   – Skin thickens over forehead (leonine facies), eyebrows and eyelashes are lost, nose becomes misshapen or collapses (saddle nose), ear lobes thicken, upper incisor teeth fall out |
| |   – Eye involvement causing photophobia (light sensitivity), glaucoma and blindness |
| |   – Skin on legs thickens and forms ulcers when nodules break down |
| |   – Testicular atrophy and gynecomastia |
| |   – Internal organ infection causing enlarged liver and lymph nodes |
| |   – Voice becomes hoarse due to involvement of the larynx |
| |   – Slow scarring of peripheral nerves resulting in nerve thickening and sensory loss. Fingers and toes become deformed due to painless repeated trauma |
| |   – **Lazarine leprosy** |

## DIAGNOSIS OF LEPROSY

The following tests are used in diagnosis of leprosy:

- Clinical examination
  - ➢ Sensory testing
  - ➢ Peripheral nerve palpation
- Slit skin smear
  - ➢ Ziehl-Neelsen staining
- Nasal smears and nose blows
  - ➢ Negative in most
- Skin biopsy
  - ➢ Virchow cells and globi
  - ➢ Periappendiceal lymphocytosis
- Nerve biopsy
- Histamine test (histamine flare)
  - ➢ Delayed and feeble—borderline indeterminate

- Phenolic glycolipid antigen (PGL-1)
- Food pad culture
- PCR

## Lepromin Test

- Nonspecific test
- Positive in majority of individuals in regions where leprosy is endemic
- Mitsuda first described lepromin test.
  - ➤ Intradermal injection in lepromin antigen is typically biphasic in reaction, early Fernandez reaction characterized by erythema and induration in 24–48 hours and lasting for 3–5 days, analogous to tuberculin test, but of no significance, late is Mitsuda reaction in 4 weeks (peak) and subsides with ulceration, it is the measure of CMI.
- **Principle of the test**: Delayed hypersensitivity reaction
- **Lepromin used**
  - ➤ Human type
  - ➤ Armadillo type
  - ➤ Dharmendra antigen
- **Purpose of the test**
  - ➤ For classification of leprosy
  - ➤ For assessment of prognosis and response to treatment (not used for diagnosis).
  - ➤ To assess resistance of the individual
  - ➤ To verify the identity of candidate lepra bacillus
- Strongly positive in typical tuberculoid case and positivity getting weaker as one pass through the spectrum to lepromatous end.
- Typical lepromatous case is lepromin negative.

## NERVE ABSCESS IN LEPROSY

- **Nerve abscess** is most commonly seen in tuberculoid leprosy.
- Granuloma softens and develops into abscess.
- Usually occurs during active disease.
- Most common nerve trunk affected is **ulnar.**
- **Rarely** affected are popliteal and median nerve.
- Three times more common in males.
- Rarely, may lead to calcification and stone formation.
- In LL, multiple bilateral and involves more than 2 nerves.
- **Treatment:** Corticosteroids or simple drainage

- **Management of cold abscess of nerve trunk**
  - ➤ It depends on the state of nerve.
  - ➤ **If nerve shows no recent functional deficit,** patient can be kept under observation. Usually abscess subsides in a few months.
  - ➤ **If nerve is completely and irreversibly paralyzed** no need to intervene except for cosmetic purpose.
  - ➤ **When the paralysis is incomplete or recurrent,** the abscess should be explored and drained.

## REACTIONS IN LEPROSY

### Type 1: Reaction

- Type 4 hypersensitivity reaction.
- Seen in borderline patients because of immunological instability.
- Upgrading/reversal reaction:
  - ➤ Increase in CMI as in patients under Rx
  - ➤ LLs (subpolar) → BL → BB → BT → TT
  - ➤ Downgrading reaction
  - ➤ Reduction is immunity
  - ➤ BT → BB → BL → LLs
- **Clinical features**
  - ➤ Lesions become erythematous, prominent, shiny, and warm.
  - ➤ Pain, swelling, tenderness of nerves noted.
  - ➤ Motor disturbance (claw hand, drooped feet and facial palsy)
  - ➤ Rarely nerve abscess
  - ➤ Edema of hand, feet, or face
  - ➤ Tenderness of palms and soles
  - ➤ Fever and malaise (unusual)
- T cell activation in reversal reaction (type 1) is indicated by demonstration of a 10-fold increase of interferon-$\alpha$ in the lesions.
- Reversal reactions are typified by a TH1 cytokine profile, with an influx of CD4+ helper cells and increased levels of IFN gamma and IL-12. In addition, type 1 reactions are associated with large numbers of T cells bearing/receptors—a unique feature of leprosy.
- Nerve enlargement (common)—rapid swelling of one or more nerves with pain and tenderness at the site of swelling, usually where the nerve is most superficial.
- Motor involvement of nerve may occur:
  - ➤ Ulnar (claw hand)
  - ➤ Lateral popliteal (foot drop)
  - ➤ Facial palsy

➤ The cause of nerve pain is increased intra-neural pressure from edema and cellular reaction.

➤ Rarely nerve abscess may form, mostly ulnar nerve is affected, but great auricular or common peroneal can also be involved.

## Type 2: Lepra Reaction (Erythema Nodosum Leprosum)

• It is a type 3 hypersensitivity reaction occurring exclusively in BL, LL which usually follows therapy but may precede therapy.

• **Predisposing factors for type 2 lepra reaction**
  ➤ Infection
  ➤ Injury
  ➤ Surgery
  ➤ Physical stress
  ➤ Mental stress
  ➤ Immunization
  ➤ Pregnancy
  ➤ Parturition
  ➤ Ingestion of potassium iodide and anti-leprosy drugs.

• **Clinical features**
  ➤ No change in appearance of existing leprosy lesions.
  ➤ Crops of brightly erythematous tender papules and nodules which come and go seen mainly over face and extremities.
  ➤ Lesions may break down to form ulcers: Erythema necroticans (ENL) (Fig. 18.3).
  ➤ Systemic disturbances seen.
  ➤ Occurs in later course of Rx when skin lesions are quiescent and all or most of the bacilli are granular.
  ➤ The clinical manifestations of liver, tissue damage, etc. in ENL can be explained by the role of TNF-α.

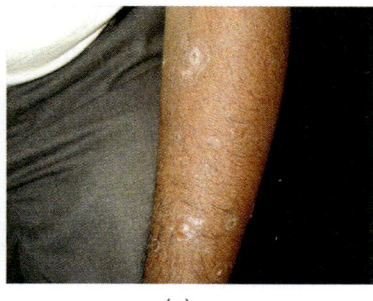
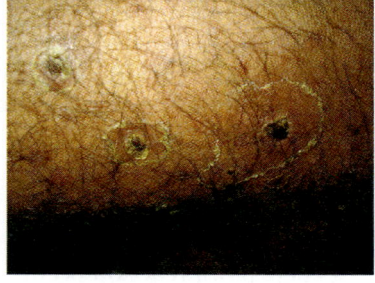

(a)                                    (b)

**Figs 18.3 a and b:** Ulcerated lesions with crusting in ENL

- ➢ ENL is thought to be a consequence of immune complex deposition, given its TH2 cytokine profile and its high levels of IL-6 and IL-8.
- ➢ Skin biopsy of ENL papules reveals vasculitis or panniculitis, sometimes with many lymphocytes but characteristically with polymorphonuclear leukocytes as well.

Type 2 lepra reaction (ENL) occurs exclusively in patients near the lepromatous end of the leprosy spectrum (BL-LL).

- • The term "ENL" reaction has been in use for a long time. Actually, type 2 lepra reaction includes ENL and various other symptoms.
- • **Other infestations of type 2 reaction**
  - ➢ Fever
  - ➢ Malaise
  - ➢ Nerve pain
  - ➢ Periosteal pain
  - ➢ Muscle pain
  - ➢ Pain and swelling in joints
  - ➢ Rhinitis
  - ➢ Epistaxis
  - ➢ Acute iritis
  - ➢ Painful dactylitis
  - ➢ Acute epididymoorchitis
  - ➢ Proteinuria and glomerulonephritis
  - ➢ Swollen tender lymph nodes (femoral)
  - ➢ Anemia, leucocytosis, raised ESR
  - ➢ Abnormal LFT ($\uparrow$ aminotransferases)
- • Steroid therapy is well-established method of controlling the worst aspects of lepra reaction like:
  - ➢ Neuritis
  - ➢ Neuritis when muscle paralysis is threatened
  - ➢ Iritis not responding to steroid eye drops
  - ➢ Epididymoorchitis
  - ➢ Erythema necroticans

## LUCIO PHENOMENON

- • Type 2 lepra reaction occurring in Lucio leprosy. Lesions are seen mostly over the extremities. Lesions undergo infarction and heal with ulceration and scarring.

- Neither glucocorticoids nor thalidomide is effective against this syndrome.
- Optimal wound care and therapy for bacteremia are indicated. Ulcers tend to be chronic and heal poorly.
- Respond to dapsone and rifampicin.
- In severe cases, exchange transfusion may prove useful.

## Treatment of Lepra Reaction

Continue the antileprosy treatment.

- **Type 1**
  - ➤ **Mild:** Chloroquine and aspirin.
  - ➤ **Severe:** Steroid + large doses of clofazimine (if patient is of MB group) + splinting of affected nerve (acute stage).
- **Type 2**
  - ➤ **Mild/ moderate** (fever with a few skin lesions):
    - – Rest
    - – Chloroquine
    - – Aspirin
    - – Antimonials (when associated with bone and joint problem)
  - ➤ **Severe ENL** (neuritis/arthritis/uveitis/orchitis):
    - – Steroid
    - – Clofazimine (in large doses)
    - – Thalidomide: Thalidomide is of no value in type 1 reaction. It is used in management of type 2 reaction in dosage of 3–4 tablets of 100 mg daily, tailing off as the reaction subsides and continuing one tablet daily or alternate day to prevent outbreaks. It is teratogenic hence contraindicated in women of childbearing age.

## TREATMENT OF LEPROSY

- *Single lesion paucibacillary leprosy:* Includes indeterminate and tuberculoid leprosy.
- *Paucibacillary leprosy:* Clinically 2–5 lesions or only one nerve trunk being involved. It includes indeterminate leprosy, tuberculoid leprosy and most BT leprosy cases. SSS should be negative.
- *Multibacillary leprosy:* Clinically more than 5 lesions or more than one nerve trunk is involved. Consists of LL, BL, BB and some BT leprosy cases. SSS is positive (Table 18.3).

**Table 18.3:** Antimicrobial regimens recommended for the treatment of leprosy in adults

| Form of leprosy | More intensive regimen | WHO recommended regimen (1982) |
|---|---|---|
| **Tuberculoid (paucibacillary)** | Dapsone (100 mg/d) for 5 years | Dapsone (100 mg/d, unsupervised) plus rifampin (600 mg/month, supervised) for 6 months |
| **Lepromatous (multibacillary)** | Rifampin (600 mg/d) for 3 years plus dapsone (100 mg/d) indefinitely | Dapsone (100 mg/d) plus clofazimine (50 mg/d), unsupervised; and rifampin (600 mg) plus clofazimine (300 mg) monthly (supervised) for 1–2 years |

- **For adults** with body weight <35 kg the dose of rifampicin should be 450 mg once monthly and dapsone 50 mg daily.
- **Children**
  - ➤ 0–5 yrs    – Rifampicin monthly 300 mg
    Dapsone daily 25 mg
  - ➤ 6–14 yrs    – Rifampicin monthly 300 mg
    Dapsone daily 50 mg
- **Single lesion leprosy** → ROM
  - ➤ Rifampicin (600 mg) + Ofloxacin (400 mg) + Minocycline (100 mg) → single dose. Released from Rx on the same day and kept under surveillance for 2 yrs.
- **Rifampicin**
  - ➤ It is a semi-synthetic derivative of rifamycin B produced by *Streptomyces mediterranei*.
  - ➤ It is highly potent bacteriocidal drug.
  - ➤ It inhibits RNA synthesis.
  - ➤ **Side-effects** (Table 18.4)
    - – Daily intermittent administration:
      *Mild*
      - o Discoloration (red) of urine
      - o Transient rash
      - o GIT symptoms
      - o Drowsiness
      - o Weakness
      - o Dizziness

| Table 18.4: Side-effects of drugs | |
|---|---|
| **Dapsone** | Anemia: Give iron and continue treatment |
| | Abdominal pain: Symptomatic treatment |
| | Exfoliative dermatitis: Stop dapsone and refer to higher level |
| | Jaundice: Stop dapsone and refer to higher level |
| | Kidney damage: Stop dapsone and refer to higher level |
| **Rifampicin** | Red discoloration of urine, saliva and sweat: Reassure, continue treatment |
| | Jaundice: Stop rifampicin and refer to higher level |
| | Flu-like illness: Symptomatic treatment |
| | Skin rash: Stop rifampicin |
| **Clofazimine** | Brown–red discoloration of skin, urine: Reassure, continue treatment. |
| | Dryness, abdominal pain: Symptomatic treatment |

*Serious (uncommon)*
- o Hepatitis
- o Thrombocytopenia
- o Psychosis
- o Osteomalacia
- o Hypersensitivity reaction
- o Stevens-Johnson syndrome
- o Porphyria cutanea tarda
- o Pemphigus vulgaris
- – Confined to intermittent administration:
  - o Occurs with once weekly or twice weekly administration
  - o Flu-like syndrome: Fever and malaise which begin 1–2 hrs after each Rx and last up to 8 hrs.
  - o Shock, dyspnea, hemolytic anemia and renal failure.

- **Dapsone**
  - ➤ *The first effective Rx* for leprosy was a sulphone named promin (glucosulphone sodium) and this pioneer work was reported from Carville, USA in 1943.
  - ➤ *Dapsone* was introduced later in the 1940s by Cochrane and Muir in India.
  - ➤ Dapsone (4,4'-diaminodiphenylsulfone) inhibits bacterial folic acid synthesis.
  - ➤ It is now considered the second most active drug (after rifampin) in the treatment of leprosy because of its ready availability, low cost, and low toxicity and the susceptibility of untreated strains of *M. leprae* to low concentrations.

> *Pharmacology*
  - Dapsone is well absorbed orally and distributes well throughout the body.
  - The usual daily dosage is 100 mg for adults and 0.9–1.4 mg/kg for children.
  - Plasma concentrations peak within 1–3 hours.
  - The median elimination half-life is 22 hours.
  - Dapsone is cleared by acetylation in the liver.
  - The drug is 70% bound to plasma protein.
  - Usual daily doses produce serum concentrations of 10–15 g/ml, which far exceed the MIC for *M. leprae* (0.01–0.001 g/ml).

> *Adverse effects*
  - Hemolysis and methemoglobinemia are common untoward reactions to dapsone.
  - Patients should be screened for glucose-6-phosphate dehydrogenase deficiency to prevent serious drug-induced hemolysis.
  - However, most patients tolerate dapsone therapy well with adequate clinical and laboratory supervision:
  - Other side effects include:
    o Gastrointestinal intolerance
    o Headache
    o Pruritus
    o Peripheral neuropathies
    o Psychosis
    o Nephrotic syndrome
    o Fever
    o Rash (SJS, TEN, exfoliative dermatitis and dapsone syndrome)

- **Clofazimine**
  > Synthetic iminophenothiazine dye
  > Mild bactericidal on *M. leprae*
  > Not water soluble
  > Micronized crystals in oilwax base and encapsulated in soft gelatin for oral administration.
  > Stored in macrophages and cells of RES.
  > Special role in management of patients with ENL (anti-inflammatory).
    - It is very useful in chronic recurrent ENL.
  > If given alone, *M. leprae* develop resistance, hence should be used a part of MDT.
  > Clofazimine's mode of action is not well understood. Its serum half-life is ~60–70 days; only a small proportion of the dose is excreted daily into the urine or bile.

➤ Bactericidal activity is very slow and is evident for ~50 days after administration.

➤ The usual adult dosage is 50–100 mg/d, 100 mg three times a week, or (for treatment of ENL) 300 mg/d.

➤ *Adverse effects of clofazimine*

   – Brownish-red discoloration
   – Xerosis and later ichthyosis (extensors)
   – Abdominal pain, diarrhea, malabsorption, and cachexia.
   – Hypokalemia and death in severe cases.
   – Splenic infarcts and steroid congestion of small intestine.
   – Crosses placenta and affects complexion of fetus.

   **Higher doses** (200–300 mg)

➤ No teratogenic effect known.

• **Thiacetazone**

➤ Thiacetazone had been in use in the Rx of TB and leprosy.

➤ It is bacteriostatic.

➤ It is cheap (advantage).

➤ Serious side-effects may occur (disadvantage).

➤ Further *M. leprae* resistant to thiacetazone shows cross resistance to thiomides.

➤ Hence, it is no longer considered in Rx of leprosy.

• **Causes of nerve hypertrophy**

➤ **Dejerine-Sottas disease (HMSN type 3)**

➤ **Refsum's disease (HMSN type 4)**

➤ **Charcot-Marie-Tooth syndrome (hereditary motor and sensory neuropathy (HMSN) type 1)**

➤ **Chronic relapsing neuropathies**

➤ **Multiple sclerosis (very rarely)**

➤ **Isolated peripheral nerve lesions**

➤ **Leprosy**

➤ **Diabetes mellitus**

➤ **Neurofibromatosis**

➤ **Amyloidosis**

➤ **Sarcoidosis**

➤ **Hypothyroidism**

➤ **Acromegaly.**

## QUESTIONS FROM PREVIOUS EXAMINATIONS

1. Leprosy and eye
2. Side-effects of the drugs used in leprosy
3. Lepra reactions
4. Morphological index
5. Histoid leprosy
6. Newer drugs in leprosy
7. Type 1 reaction
8. Borderline spectrum leprosy
9. Dapsone
10. ENL
11. Vaccines in leprosy
12. Immunology of leprosy
13. LEAP (lower extremity amputation prevention)
14. HPE of histoid leprosy
15. Ape thumb
16. Nine-banded armadillos
17. Trophic lesions in leprosy
18. Polyneuritic leprosy
19. HPE of skin lesions in leprosy
20. Diferential diagnosis of hypopigmented patches
21. Microcellulose rubber
22. Immunoprophylaxis
23. Molluscum leprosum
24. Mechanism of claw hand in leprosy
25. Classification of leprosy merits/demerits
26. Lab diagnosis
27. Persisters
28. Mouse foot pad inoculation
29. Eradication of leprosy by 2000
30. Leprosy: Systemic disease
31. SFG ratio
32. Histoid habitus
33. Pathogenesis of chronic pedal edema in LL
34. Lepromin test
35. AFB
36. Significance of negative Mitsuda in indeterminate leprosy
37. Corrective surgeries in management (mx) of leprosy

38. Falia leprosy
39. Trpohic ulcers and mx
40. Bone lesions in leprosy
41. Factors for spread of leprosy
42. Gynecomastia
43. Berhardt's syndrome
44. Lucio phenomenon
45. Repository sulphones
46. Current concepts in leprosy
47. Drug recurrences in leprosy

## MULTIPLE CHOICE QUESTIONS

1. **Lesion not seen in lepromatous leprosy:**           *(AI 97)*
   (a) Macule              (b) Papule
   (c) Nodule              (d) Vesicle
2. **Virchow's cells are seen in:**           *(Orissa 99)*
   (a) Henoch-Schönlein purpura
   (b) Toxic epidermal necrolysis
   (c) Congenital syphilis
   (d) Leprosy
3. **Lepra cell is a:**           *(Maharashtra 2001)*
   (a) Plasma cell          (b) Neutrophill
   (c) Lymphocyte           (d) Histiocyte
4. **Commonest nerve involved in leprosy:**           *(AIIMS 94)*
   (a) Ulnar nerve          (b) Median nerve
   (c) Radial nerve         (d) Musculocutaneous
5. **In leprosy, nerve abscess most commonly affects:**           *(AP 96)*
   (a) Ulnar nerve          (b) Radial nerve
   (c) Great auricular      (d) Posterior tibial
6. **Type 2 lepra reaction is seen in:**    *(AP 97; Maharashtra 2002)*
   (a) TT                   (b) LL
   (c) Indeterminate        (d) Borderline
7. **Erythema nodosum leprosum occurs in:**           *(AIIMS 92)*
   (a) Lepromatous leprosy  (b) Tuberculoid leprosy
   (c) Borderline lepromatous (d) Borderline tuberculoid
8. **Drug of choice for type 1 lepra reaction with severe neuritis:**
                                                          *(AIIMS 94)*
   (a) Systemic steroids    (b) Clofazimine
   (c) Thalidomide          (d) Chloroquine

9. **Who was the first person to use DDS in India?**    *(Kerala 98)*
   (a) Jopling                (b) Shepard
   (c) Kirchheimer            (d) Cochrane

10. **Commonest side-effect of dapsone:**    *(PGI 97)*
    (a) Hemolytic anemia      (b) Thrombocytopenia
    (c) Cyanosis              (d) Bone marrow depression

11. **Earliest sensation lost in Hansen's disease:**    *(TN 99)*
    (a) Pain                  (b) Touch
    (c) Vibration             (d) Temperature

12. **Satellite lesions are seen in:**    *(MH 14)*
    (a) Tuberculoid           (b) BT
    (c) LL                    (d) Histoid leprosy

13. **Slit smear negative leprosy:**    *(AI 97)*
    (a) Neuritic type         (b) TT
    (c) Indeterminate         (d) Lepra reaction

14. **Duration of Rx in paucibacillary leprosy:**    *(AI 93)*
    (a) 6 months              (b) 9 months
    (c) 2 yrs                 (d) Till symptoms subside

15. **The most preferred regimen for paucibacillary leprosy:** *(AI 96)*
    (a) Dapsone 100 mg OD for 6 months
    (b) Dapsone 100 mg OD and rifampicin 300 mg OD for 6 months
    (c) Dapsone 100 mg OD and rifampicin 300 mg for 6 months
    (d) Dapsone 100 mg OD and rifampicin 600 mg 6 monthly

16. **In leprosy, neural involvement occurs in what % of patients:**
    (a) 30%                   (b) 60%
    (c) 90%                   (d) 100%

17. **Following are adverse effects of clofazimine** *except:*    *(PGI 93)*
    (a) Skin staining         (b) Icthyosis
    (c) GI problems           (d) Gastritis

18. **Which one of the following is side-effect of clofazimine?**
    *(AI 96)*
    (a) Hyperpigmentation
    (b) Erythema
    (c) Discoloration of body secretion
    (d) Macular rash

19. **The first line anti-leprosy drugs include the following** *except:*
    *(Delhi 93)*
    (a) Dapsone               (b) Thiacetazone
    (c) Clofazimine           (d) Rifampicin

20. **Rx of choice for nerve abscess in case of a tuberculoid leprosy:**
    *(AIIMS 96)*
    (a) Incision and drainage
    (b) High dose clofazimine
    (c) Steroids
    (d) Thalidomide

21. **Following are used in Rx of lepra reaction** *except:*    *(AP 92)*
    (a) Steroids
    (b) Clofazimine
    (c) Cyclophosphamide
    (d) Thalidomide

22. **Reversal lepra reaction shows no response to:**    *(JIPMER 95)*
    (a) Clofazimine
    (b) Chloroquine
    (c) Steroids
    (d) Thalidomide

23. **Leprosy affects the following** *except:*    *(AI 2007)*
    (a) Skin
    (b) Ovary
    (c) Eye
    (d) Nerves

24. **Which of the following is not true about lepromin test?**
    *(AIIMS 2006, AI 2007)*
    (a) Helpful in classifying leprosy
    (b) Negative in most of the children in first 6 months of life
    (c) It is a diagnostic test
    (d) BCG vaccination converts lepra reaction from negative to positive

25. **Following are the mode of transmission of leprosy** *except:*
    *(AI 2004)*
    (a) Breast milk
    (b) Insect bite
    (c) Transplacental spread
    (d) Droplet infection

26. **In the management of leprosy, the lepromin test is most useful for:**    *(AI 2003)*
    (a) Herd immunity
    (b) Prognosis
    (c) Treatment
    (d) Epidemiological investigations

27. **Under leprosy eradication programme, the management of single lesion is:**    *(AIIMS 2000)*
    (a) Single dose of rifampicin and dapsone
    (b) Rifampicin and dapsone for 6 months
    (c) Rifampicin, ofloxacin, and minocycline single dose
    (d) Rifampicin and minocycline for 6 months

28. **In paucibacillary leprosy, single dose regimen for single lesion include:**    *(PGI 2000)*
    (a) Rifampicin, ofloxacin, clarithromycin
    (b) Dapsone, rifampicin, clofazimine
    (c) Rifampicin, ofloxacin, minocycline
    (d) Dapsone, clofazimine

29. **Multidrug therapy is given for Rx of:**    *(AI 94)*
    - (a) Syphilis
    - (b) Leprosy
    - (c) Herpes
    - (d) Icthyosis vulgaris

30. **Most potent anti-leprotic drug:**
    - (a) Rifampicin
    - (b) Dapsone
    - (c) Clofazimine
    - (d) Norflox

31. **Which of the following is an anti-leprosy drug also used in Rx of lepra reaction?**    *(AIIMS 97)*
    - (a) Rifampicin
    - (b) Dapsone
    - (c) Ciprofloxacin
    - (d) Clofazimine

32. **Leromin test is positive in:**    *(AIIMS 2000)*
    - (a) Lepromatous
    - (b) Indeterminate
    - (c) Histoid
    - (d) Tuberculoid

33. **Skin pigmentation and icthyosis like side-effects are seen with:**    *(AI 96)*
    - (a) Clofazimine
    - (b) Rifampicin
    - (c) Dapsone
    - (d) Steroids

34. **Leprosy does not involve:**    *(PGI 98)*
    - (a) CNS
    - (b) Testis
    - (c) Skin
    - (d) Cornea

35. **Most common type of leprosy in India:**    *(PGI 97)*
    - (a) BT
    - (b) TT
    - (c) LL
    - (d) BL

36. **The following is not used for diagnosis of leprosy:**    *(AIIMS May 06)*
    - (a) Lepromin test
    - (b) Slit skin smear
    - (c) FNAC
    - (d) Skin biopsy

37. **A 16-year-old student reported for the evaluation of multiple hypopigmented macules on the trunk and limbs. All of the following tests are useful in making a diagnosis of leprosy *except*:**    *(AIIMS Nov 03)*
    - (a) Sensation testing
    - (b) Lepromin test
    - (c) Slit smears
    - (d) Skin biopsy

38. **The main cytokine involved in ENL:**    *(AIIMS May 06)*
    - (a) IL2
    - (b) Interferon γ
    - (c) TNF-α
    - (d) Macrophage CSF

39. **Manifestations of ENL include the following *except*:**
    - (a) Pancreatitis
    - (b) Fever
    - (c) Hepatitis
    - (d) Arthritis
    - (e) Cutaneous nodules

40. A 27-year-old patient was diagnosed to have borderline leprosy and started on multibacillary multidrug therapy. About 6 wks latter, he developed pain in the nerves and redness and swelling of skin lesions. Management of his illness include the following except: *(AIIMS 04)*
   - (a) Stop anti-leprosy drugs
   - (b) Systemic corticosteroids
   - (c) Rest to limbs affected
   - (d) Analgesics

41. All are features of lepromatous leprosy except: *(AIIMS 94)*
   - (a) Gynecomastia
   - (b) Madarosis
   - (c) Saddle nose
   - (d) Perforating ulcer

42. CMI is maximum suppressed in: *(AIIMS 93)*
   - (a) BT
   - (b) LL
   - (c) TT
   - (d) Indeterminate

43. Skin biopsy in leprosy is characterized by: *(AI 97)*
   - (a) Periappendiceal bacilli
   - (b) Periappendiceal lymphocytosis
   - (c) Perivascular lymphocytosis
   - (d) All of the above

44. Erythema nodosum is seen in the following except: *(AP 05)*
   - (a) RA
   - (b) TB
   - (c) Enteric fever
   - (d) Aspirin therapy

45. "Inverted saucer shaped" lesion is found in: *(DNB 07)*
   - (a) LL
   - (b) TT
   - (c) Borderline leprosy
   - (d) Indeterminate leprosy

46. Symmetrical multiple lesions are seen in which type of leprosy? *(MH 2001)*
   - (a) Border line
   - (b) Neuritic
   - (c) Lepromatous
   - (d) Tubercular

47. Type 2 lepra reaction is not seen in: *(MH 2003)*
   - (a) Borderline leprosy
   - (b) Lepromatous leprosy
   - (c) Tuberculoid leprosy
   - (d) Molluscum contagiosum

48. Exacerbation of existing skin lesions is a characteristic of: *(Kar 07)*
   - (a) Lucio reaction
   - (b) Erythema nodosum leprosum
   - (c) Type 1 lepra reaction
   - (d) Jarisch-Herxheimer reaction

49. Thickened peripheral nerves are seen in all the following conditions except: *(Kar 07)*
   - (a) Hansen's neuropathy
   - (b) Amyloid polyneuropathy
   - (c) Diabetic neuropathy
   - (d) Refsum's disease

**50. Leprosy affects all the following organs** *except*:    *(AIIMS 2006)*
- (a) Bone
- (b) Liver
- (c) Ovary
- (d) Nails

**51. Best treatment for borderline tuberculoid leprosy with severe ulnar neuritis:**    *(AIIMS 06)*
- (a) Multidrug therapy with chloroquine
- (b) Multidrug therapy with steroids
- (c) Single drug therapy with thalidomide
- (d) Single drug therapy only

**52. Treatment of choice for type 2 lepra reaction:**    *(AI 08)*
- (a) Steroids
- (b) Thalidomide
- (c) Clofazimine
- (d) Chloroquine

**53. A 45-year-old male had multiple hypoasthetic mildly erythematous large plaques with elevated margins, on the trunk and extremities. His ulnar and popliteal nerves on the both sides were enlarged. The most probable diagnosis:**
*(AIIMS Nov 03)*
- (a) Lepromatous leprosy
- (b) Borderline leprosy
- (c) Borderline tuberculoid leprosy
- (d) Borderline lepromatous lepsrosy

**54. Grading of which of the following disease is done with the use of bacterial index, Dharmendra's scale, and Ridley's scale:**
*(AI 08)*
- (a) Leprosy
- (b) Syphilis
- (c) Tuberculosis
- (d) Cholera

**55. The main cytokine, involved in erythema nodosum leprosum (ENL) reaction, is:**    *(AIIMS May 2006; Orissa 08)*
- (a) Interleukin-2
- (b) Interferon-gamma
- (c) Tumor necrosis factor-alpha
- (d) Macrophage colony-stimulating factor

**56. The following drug is not used for the treatment of type 2 lepra reaction:**    *(AIIMS May 2006)*
- (a) Chloroquine
- (b) Thalidomide
- (c) Cyclosporine
- (d) Corticosteroids

## Answers

1. **Ans. (d)** Vesicle *(Ref. Handbook of Lepros by Jopling, 5th edn/23)*
2. **Ans. (d)** Leprosy *(Ref. Handbook of Leprosy by Jopling, 5th edn/19)*
3. **Ans. (d)** Histiocyte *(Ref. Robbin's, Pathologic Basis of Disease, 6th edn, 385)*
4. **Ans. (a)** Ulnar nerve *(Ref. IADVL, 2nd edn/1588)*
5. **Ans. (a)** Ulnar nerve *(Ref. IADVL, 2nd edn/1590)*
6. **Ans. (b)** LL *(Ref. Handbook of Leprosy by Jopling, 5th edn/84)*
7. **Ans. (a)** Lepromatous leprosy *(Ref. Handbook of Leprosy by Jopling, 5th edn/84)*
8. **Ans. (a)** Systemic steroids *(Ref. Handbook of Leprosy by Jopling, 5th edn, 118)*
9. **Ans. (d)** Cochrane *(Ref. Handbook of Leprosy by Jopling, 5th edn/102)*
10. **Ans. (a)** Hemolytic anemia *(Ref. Handbook of Leprosy by Jopling, 5th edn/102)*
11. **Ans. (d)** Temperature *(Ref. Clinical Methods in Dermatology and Venerology by JS Pasricha, page 75)*
12. **Ans. (b)** Borderline tuberculoid (Ref. IADVL, 2nd *edn* / 1582)
13. **Ans. (a)** Neuritic type *(Ref. IADVL, 2nd edn/1582)*
14. **Ans. (a)** 6 months *(Ref. IADVL, 2nd edn/ 1617)*
15. **Ans. (d)** Dapsone 100 mg OD and rifampicin 600 mg monthly for 6 months *(Ref. IADVL, 2nd edn/1617)*
16. **Ans. (d)** 100% *(Ref. IADVL, 2nd edn/ 1588)*
17. **Ans. (d)** Gastritis *(Ref. IADVL, 2nd edn/1588)*
18. **Ans. (a)** Hyperpigmentation *(Ref. IADVL, 2nd edn/1615)*
19. **Ans. (b)** Thiacetazone *(Ref. IADVL, 2nd edn/1616)*
20. **Ans. (a)** Incision and drainage *(Ref. IADVL, 2nd edn/1644)*
21. **Ans. (c)** Cyclophosphamide *(Ref. IADVL, 2nd edn/1623)*

### Rx of lepra reaction

22. **Ans. (a) and (d)** Clofazimine and thalidomide *(Ref. Handbook of Leprosy by Jopling, 5th edn/120)*
23. **Ans. (b)** Ovary
24. **Ans. (c)** It is a diagnostic test *(Ref. Park PSM, 20th edn/158, 258)*
25. **Ans. (c)** Transplacental spread *(Ref. IADVL, 2nd edn/1546; 1547)*
26. **Ans. (a)** Prognosis *(Ref. Ananthanarayan Microbiology, 4th edn/365)*
27. **Ans. (c)** Rifampicin, ofloxacin, and minocycline single dose *(Ref. IADVL, 2nd edn/ 1546; 1547)*
28. **Ans. (c)** Rifampicin, ofloxacin, and minocycline *(Ref. Park PSM, 20th edn/158, 258)*

29. **Ans. (b)** Leprosy *(Ref. Rook's Textbook of Dermatology, 29.1–29.19)*
30. **Ans. (a)** Rifampicin *(Ref. Handbook of Leprosy by Jopling, 5th edn/ 106)*
31. **Ans. (d)** Clofazimine *(Ref. Handbook of Leprosy by Jopling, 5th edn/106)*
32. **Ans. (d)** Tuberculoid *(Ref. Rook's Textbook of Dermatology, 29.1–29.19)*
33. **Ans. (a)** Clofazimine *(Ref. IADVL, 2nd edn/1615)*

*Rifampin*

34. **Ans. (a)** CNS *(Ref. Rook's Textbook of Dermatology, 29.1–29.19)*
35. **Ans. (b)** TT *(Ref. Rook's Textbook of Dermatology, 29.1–29.19)*
36. **Ans. (a)** Lepromin test *(Ref. Handbook of Leprosy by Jopling, 5th/59)*
37. **Ans. (b)** Lepromin test *(Ref. Handbook of Leprosy by Jopling, 5th/59)*
38. **Ans. (c)** TNF-α *(Ref. IADVL, 2nd edn/ 1574)*
39. **Ans. (a)** Pancreatitis *(Ref. Handbook of Leprosy by Jopling, 5th edn/84)*
40. **Ans. (a)** Stop anti-leprosy drugs *(Ref. Rook's Dermatology, 7th edn/29. 1–29.19)*
41. **Ans. (d)** Perforating ulcer *(Ref. Rook's Dermatology, 7th edn/29. 1–29.19)*
42. **Ans. (b)** LL *(Ref. Rook's Dermatology, 7th edn/29. 1–29.19)*
43. **Ans. (d)** All of the above *(Ref. Handbook of Leprosy by Jopling, 5th/16–19)*
44. **Ans. (a) and (d)** rheumatoid arthritis and aspirin therapy *(Ref. Andrew's Diseases of Skin, 10th edn/488)*
45. **Ans. (c)** Borderline leprosy *(Ref. Rook's Dermatology, 7th edn/29. 1–29.19)*
46. **Ans. (c)** Lepromatous *(Ref. Robbin's Pathologic Basis of Disease, 6th edn, 30)*
47. **Ans. (c)** Tuberculoid leprosy
48. **Ans. (c)** Type 1 lepra reaction *(Ref. Harrison's Internal Medicine, 17th edn, Chapter 57)*
49. **Ans. (c)** Diabetic neuropathy *(Ref. http://bjr.birjournals.org/cgi/ reprint/65/772/344.pdf)*
50. **Ans. (c)** Ovary *(Ref. Rook's Textbook of Dermatology, 29.1–29.19)*
51. **Ans. (b)** Multi-drug therapy with steroids *(Ref. Rook's Textbook of Dermatology, 29.1–29.19)*
52. **Ans. (a)** Steroids
53. **Ans. (d)** Borderline lepromatous lepsrosy
54. **Ans. (a)** Leprosy
55. **Ans. (c)** Tumor necrosis factor-alpha.
56. **Ans. (c)** Cyclosporine

# 19 Viral Infections

## MOLLUSCUM CONTAGIOSUM ('WATER BLISTERS')

- Molluscum contagiosum is a common cutaneous infection of childhood caused by molluscum contagiosum virus belonging to poxvirus family.
- Restriction endonuclease and PCR analyzes of MCV DNA have identified two main types, MCV-1 and MCV-2, with two much rarer types, MCV-3 and MCV-4.
- The incubation period is variously estimated at 14 days to 6 months.
- The individual lesion is a shiny, pearly white, hemispherical, umbilicated papule which may show a central pore. Enlarging slowly it may reach a diameter of 5–10 mm in 6–12 weeks (Fig. 19.1).
- Lesions exhibit **Köbner's phenomenon**.
- They can occur at any body site including the genitalia.

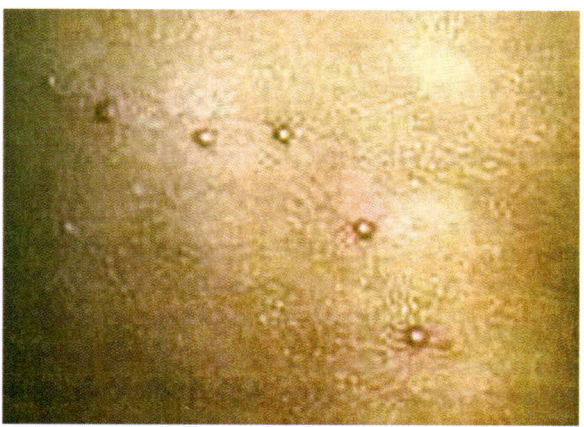

**Fig. 19.1:** Multiple skin-colored umbilicated papules

- Transmission is by direct contact. In adults, sexual contact is common.
- Plaques composed of many small lesions ('agminate'form or giant molluscum) occur rarely. Common in HIV infection.
- After trauma, or spontaneously after several months, inflammatory changes result in suppuration, crusting and eventual destruction of the lesion.
- Most cases are self-limiting within 6–9 months.
- More common in children with atopic eczema.
- Common in HIV infection and immunosuppression.
- **HPE**: The virus seems first to enter the basal epidermis where an early increase in cell division extends into the suprabasal layer. The cellular proliferation produces lobulated epidermal growths which compress the papillae until they appear as fibrous septa between the lobules, which are pear-shaped with the apex upwards. The basal layer remains intact. Cells at the core of the lesion show the greatest distortion and are ultimately destroyed, and appear as large hyaline bodies (molluscum bodies/Henderson-Patterson bodies) some 25 μm in diameter, containing cytoplasmic masses of virus material.
- The diagnosis can be confirmed by direct microscopy or electron microscopy of the papule contents, by histopathology or by molecular analysis.
- **Treatment**
  - ➤ Curettage
  - ➤ Cryotherapy
  - ➤ Trichloroacetic acid, cantharidin, diluted liquefied phenol, 10% KOH application
  - ➤ Imiquimod cream
  - ➤ Intralesional interferon
  - ➤ Topical or IV cidofovir
  - ➤ Carbon dioxide and pulsed dye lasers
  - ➤ Photodynamic therapy
  - ➤ Oral cimetidine

## WARTS

- Human papillomaviruses are small 50 to 55 nm diameter DNA viruses that infect squamous epithelia, causing cell proliferation. They belong to Papovavirus family.
- The commonest effect of HPV infection is the development of warts (verrucae).

- These can affect a wide variety of sites, principally skin of extremities, genital skin and mucosa, larynx and oral mucosa.
- HPVs can infect and cause disease at any site in stratified squamous epithelium, either keratinizing (skin) or non-keratinizing mucosa.
- The incubation period has been estimated to range between a few weeks and more than a year.
- Warts are spread by direct or indirect contact.
- *Common warts*
  - ➢ These are due mainly to HPV-2, but also to the closely related types 27, 57 and types 1 and 4.
  - ➢ Firm papules with a rough, horny surface, they range in size from less than 1 mm to over 1 cm in diameter, and by confluence can form large masses.
  - ➢ They are most commonly situated on the backs of the hands and fingers, and in children under 12 years of age, on the knees, but may occur anywhere on the skin.
  - ➢ New warts may form at sites of trauma, though this Köebner-like isomorphic phenomenon is usually less marked than in plane warts.
- *Periungual warts*
  - ➢ Common warts around the nails, especially at the nail folds or beneath the nail, can disturb nail growth.
  - ➢ Nail biting may increase the risk of infection at this site.
- *Plantar warts*
  - ➢ Plantar warts are caused by HPV-1, 2, 4, 27 or 57. The deep 'myrmecia' form is due to HPV-1.
  - ➢ Smaller lesions may contain HPV-2, 4, 27 or 57, while mosaic warts are commonly caused by HPV-2.
  - ➢ A plantar wart at first appears as a small shining 'sago-grain' papule, but soon assumes the typical appearance of a sharply defined, rounded lesion, with a rough, keratotic surface surrounded by a smooth collar of thickened horn.
  - ➢ If the surface is gently pared with a scalpel the abrupt separation between the wart tissue and the protective horny ring becomes more obvious, as the epithelial ridges of the plantar skin are not continued over the surface of the wart.
  - ➢ If the paring is continued, small bleeding points, the tips of the elongated dermal papillae, are evident.
  - ➢ Dermoscopy can also help to distinguish a plantar wart from a corn or a callosity.

➢ Most plantar warts are beneath pressure points, the heel or the metatarsal heads.

➢ Individuals may be affected by single or numerous lesions.

➢ Mosaic warts are so described from the appearance presented by a plaque of closely grouped small warts. The angular outlines of the tightly compressed individual warts are seen when the surface is pared. Pain is a common but variable symptom.

- *Plane warts (flat warts)*
  ➢ Plane warts, due mainly to HPV-3 and 10, are smooth, flat or slightly elevated and are usually skin-colored or greyish-yellow, but may be pigmented.

  ➢ They are round or polygonal in shape and vary in size from 1 to 5 mm or more in diameter.

  ➢ The face and the backs of the hands and the shins are the sites of predilection and the number present ranges from two or three to many hundreds.

  ➢ Contiguous warts may coalesce and a linear arrangement in scratch marks is a characteristic feature.

- *Filiform and digitate warts*
  ➢ Filiform and digitate warts occur commonly in the male, on the face and neck, irregularly distributed, and often clustered.

  ➢ Digitate warts, often in small groups, also occur on the scalp in both sexes, where they are occasionally confused with epidermal naevi.

- *Anogenital warts*
  ➢ Anogenital warts are common and are caused in 75% by HPV-6.

  ➢ The remainder is caused by HPV-11 or more unusual, low-risk HPVs.

  ➢ They are often asymptomatic, but may cause discomfort, discharge or bleeding. The typical anogenital wart is soft, pink, elongated and sometimes filiform or pedunculated.

  ➢ The lesions are usually multiple especially on moist surfaces, and their growth can be enhanced during pregnancy or in the presence of other local infections.

  ➢ Large malodorous masses may form on vulvar and perianal skin. This classical 'acuminate' (sometimes called papillomatous, or hyperplastic) form constitutes about two-thirds of anogenital warts.

  ➢ The commonest sites, the area of frenulum, corona and glans in men, and the posterior fourchette in women, correspond to the likely sites of greatest coital friction.

- **HPE**
  - ➢ Viral warts show acanthosis and hyperkeratosis, usually with the characteristic feature of koilocytosis of upper keratinocytes.
  - ➢ In most warts there is also papillomatosis.
  - ➢ In koilocytes and other granular layer cells, there may be basophilic nuclear inclusion bodies, which are seen ultrastructurally to be composed of arrays of viral particles.
  - ➢ These upper epidermal cells have eosinophilic inclusions representing irregular, clumped keratohyaline granules.
- **Diagnosis**
  - ➢ Clinical diagnosis of warts is often sufficient, but atypical, subclinical or dysplastic lesions may need laboratory confirmation of HPV infection. Methods available are:
    - – Histology
    - – Detection of virus particles by electron microscopy—this method would not be helpful for those types of warts which have a few virus particles, for example genital warts, or in high grade
    - – Neoplasia or invasive cancer
    - – Immunohistochemistry or immunocytochemistry using type-common or type-specific antibodies
    - – DNA hybridization on tissue extracts or *in situ*
    - – PCR for HPV DNA.
- **Treatment**
  - ➢ Topical salicylic acid (12–26%) and glutaraldehyde (20%)
  - ➢ Podophyllin (10–25%) and podophyllotoxin (0.5%)
  - ➢ Formalin soaks with 2–3% formalin in water for 15 to 20 min daily are useful for plantar warts.
  - ➢ Topical 5-fluorouracil (5%) and retinoic acid (0.05%)
  - ➢ Photodynamic therapy
  - ➢ Cryotherapy
  - ➢ Topical trichloroacetic acid
  - ➢ Intralesional interferon
  - ➢ 5% imiquimod cream
  - ➢ Carbon dioxide laser and pulsed dye laser
  - ➢ Oral cimetidine, retinoids, zinc
  - ➢ Topical or oral cidofovir
  - ➢ Intralesional bleomycin

# HERPESVIRUSES

- The herpesvirus group consists of relatively large, enveloped DNA viruses.
- They replicate within the nucleus and produce typical intranuclear inclusion bodies detectable in stained preparations.
- They are sub-grouped according to genome similarities into the α, β and γ herpesviruses.
- A feature of infection by members of the herpesvirus group is the absence of virus elimination following clinical recovery.
- Virus persists throughout the person's life as a latent infection in the cells for which the strain is specific.
- Under certain conditions, especially immune suppression, the virus may become reactivated and produce an acute infective episode with cellular damage.

## Herpes Simplex Infections

- Herpes simplex is caused by the herpes simplex virus (HSV) or herpesvirus hominis.
- There are two major antigenic types: Type 1, which is classically associated with facial infections; and type 2, which is typically genital, although there is considerable overlap in disease manifestations.
- Both type 1 and type 2 HSV are acquired by direct contact with, or droplets from, infected secretions entering via skin or mucous membrane, where primary infection may become evident.
- The establishment of latent infection is common with the virus persisting in ganglia of sensory nerves innervating the primary infection site.
- From this condition of latency, the virus may travel peripherally along the nerve fiber, and, if it replicates in the skin or mucous membrane, may cause recurrent disease.
- Primary type 1 infections occur mainly in infants and young children.
- Type 2 infections occur mainly after puberty, and are often transmitted sexually.
- **Clinical features**
  *Primary infection*
  ➤ Primary infection occurs in a previously seronegative individual and is often subclinical.
  ➤ When clinical lesions develop, the severity is generally greater than in recurrences.

> Genital primary disease is more commonly symptomatic than oral.

> *Herpetic gingivostomatitis*
>   - This is the most common clinical manifestation of primary infection by type 1 although the sites infected by the two HSV types are not mutually exclusive.
>   - Most cases occur in children between 1 and 5 years of age. After an incubation period of approximately 5 days, the stomatitis begins with fever, which may be high, malaise, restlessness and excessive dribbling.
>   - Drinking and eating are very painful and the breath is foul-smelling.
>   - The gums are swollen, inflamed and bleed easily.
>   - Vesicles presenting as white plaques are present on the tongue, pharynx, palate and buccal mucous membranes. The plaques develop into ulcers with a yellowish pseudomembrane.
>   - The regional lymph nodes are enlarged and tender. Encephalitis is a rare complication. After 3–5 days, the fever normally subsides and recovery is usually complete in 2 weeks.

> *Herpes genitalis*
>   - Infection in the genital area is usually sexually transmitted. HSV-2 has been the most common type in this area.
>   - The ulcers, which may be preceded by a general malaise, are most frequent on the glans, prepuce and shaft of the penis.
>   - They are sore or painful and last for 2–3 weeks if untreated.
>   - In male homosexuals, herpes simplex is common in the perianal area and may extend into the rectum. In HIV infection, ulceration may become chronic.
>   - In the female, similar lesions occur on the external genitalia and mucosae of the vulva, vagina and cervix. Pain and dysuria are common. Infection of the cervix may progress to a severe ulcerative cervicitis.

> *Keratoconjunctivitis*
>   - Primary herpes infection of the eye causes a severe and often purulent conjunctivitis with opacity and superficial ulceration of the cornea.
>   - The eyelids are grossly edematous and there may be vesicles on the surrounding skin.
>   - The pre-auricular gland is enlarged and tender.

> *Inoculation herpes simplex*
  - Direct inoculation of the virus into an abrasion or into normal skin gives rise to indurated papules, large bullae or irregularly scattered vesicles after an incubation period of 5–7 days.
  - The regional nodes are enlarged but fever and constitutional symptoms are usually mild.
  - Inoculation of the fingertips results in a 'herpetic whitlow', in which painful, deep vesicles coalesce to give a honeycombed appearance or to form a large bulla.
  - Multiple crops of vesicles and pustules on plaques or erythema and edema on the face, scalp and upper trunk, simulating impetigo and lasting some 10–12 days have occurred in wrestlers (herpes gladiatorum).
  - Facial contact during rugby is another recognized means of acquiring herpes simplex virus infection commonly called 'scrumpox'.

> *Neonatal herpes*
  - Primary genital herpes infection or active recurrent infection in the mother at the time of delivery makes the risk of transmission to the baby during vaginal delivery very high.
  - A symptomatic viral shedding between attacks or contact with acute infection in the neonatal period may also result in neonatal herpes.
  - The effects on the baby range in severity and may be due to disseminated disease, predominantly central nervous system, or limited to skin, eyes and mouth.
  - If the infection is disseminated, there is likely to be lethargy, seizures, respiratory distress, hepatosplenomegaly with hepatitis and thrombocytopenia.
  - Disseminated or systemic infection may occur in the immunodeficient and in those neonates not protected by maternally acquired antibody.

## Recurrent Infection

- After the first infection, whether symptomatic or subclinical, there may be no further clinical manifestations throughout life.
- Recurrences occur in 30–50% of cases of oral herpes, but are more frequent after genital herpes infection, developing in 95% of those with type 2 HSV compared with 50% in individuals with type 1 infection.

- Recurrences may be triggered by minor trauma, or by infections including febrile illnesses but also trivial, non-febrile, upper respiratory tract infections, by ultraviolet radiation , by trigeminal neuralgia and especially after intracranial operations for that disease, by dermabrasion or laser resurfacing.
- Recurrent infections differ from primary infections in the smaller size of the vesicles and their close grouping, and in the usual absence of constitutional symptoms. Itching or burning precedes by an hour or two the development of small, closely grouped vesicles on an inflamed base. They usually become pustular and crusted before healing in 7–10 days without scarring. The eruption may be painful just at the onset or pain may last for a few days. They occur most frequently on the face, particularly around the mouth.
- *Herpes genitalis:* Recurrences are fairly common, occurring two to six times per year with clusters of small vesicles which produce non-indurated ulcers on the glans or shaft of the penis. They are of shorter duration than the initial infection. Similar lesions may occur on the labia, vagina or cervix and can cause distressingly painful symptoms.
- *Subclinical viral shedding:* Asymptomatic shedding of HSV-2 is more frequent than of HSV-1 and correlates with the frequency of symptomatic recurrences.
- *Herpes encephalitis*
    A. HSV is the most commonly identified cause of recurrent lymphocytic meningitis ("Mollaret's **meningitis**"). HSV accounts for 10 to 20% of all cases of sporadic viral encephalitis.
    B. Cases are distributed throughout the year, and the age distribution appears to be biphasic, with peaks at 5 to 30 and >50 years of age.
    C. Subtype 1 virus causes >95% of cases of HSV encephalitis.
    D. The clinical hallmark of HSV encephalitis has been the acute onset of fever and focal neurologic symptoms and signs, especially in the **temporal lobes**.
    E. The most sensitive noninvasive method for early diagnosis of HSV encephalitis is the demonstration of HSV DNA in cerebrospinal fluid (CSF) by PCR.
    F. Intravenous acyclovir is more effective than vidarabine.
- **HPE**
    ➢ In the cutaneous lesions, the cytoplasm of the infected epithelial cells becomes edematous and the cells swell, producing the so-called 'ballooning degeneration'.

➤ Thick-walled vesicles are formed by the combination of intra-
and intercellular edema.
➤ Giant cells containing two to 15 or more nuclei are almost
invariably present.
➤ Intranuclear inclusions are seen.

- **Diagnosis**
  ➤ Tzanck smear:Shows multinucleated giant cells
  ➤ Culture: Takes 1–5 days
  ➤ Serological diagnosis: Seroconversion or rising antibody titres
  ➤ Detection of antigen by immunofluoroscence
  ➤ Electron microscopy
  ➤ PCR

- **Treatment**
  ➤ *Primary infection*
    - Acyclovir systemically is the treatment of choice for severe
      or potentially severe primary herpes simplex infection.
      Treatment should be started as soon as possible. The usual
      dose is 5 mg/kg 8-hourly intravenously.
    - For less severe infections and when swallowing is not
      impaired, oral treatment is adequate. The usual oral dose is
      200 mg five times daily for 7–10 days.
    - In children, the oral suspension given at 15 mg/kg five times
      per day for 7 days reduces the duration of symptoms and
      virus shedding.
    - Famciclovir 500 mg twice daily and valaciclovir, 1000 mg
      twice daily for 10 days, are of similar efficacy to acyclovir.
    - Neonatal herpes is treated with high-dose intravenous
      acyclovir (60 mg/kg/day in three-divided doses for 2 to
      3 weeks)
  ➤ *Recurrent infection*
    - Oral acyclovir 200 mg five times daily started as soon as
      possible after onset of symptoms and given for 5 days can
      shorten the duration and decrease the intensity of an episode.
    - If recurrences are frequent, long-term prophylactic acyclovir
      at a dose of 200–400 mg twice daily for 4–6 months may
      increase the time between episodes.

## Varicella Zoster Virus

- The varicella zoster virus (VZV) is the cause of both varicella
  (chickenpox) and zoster (shingles).

## Varicella (Chickenpox)

- Occurs usually in childhood.
- The virus is transmitted by droplet infection from the nasopharynx.
- Patients are infectious to others from about 2 days before to 5 days after the onset of the rash.
- The incubation period is usually 14–17 days (range 9–23 days).
- After a day or two of fever and malaise an inconstant and fleeting scarlatiniform or morbilliform erythema is followed by the development of papules which very rapidly become tense, clear, unilocular vesicles.
- Within a few hours the contents become turbid and the pustules are surrounded by red areolae (dew drop on a rose petal). In 2–4 days a dry crust forms and soon separates, to leave a shallow, pink depression which, in the absence of secondary infection, heals without scarring.
- The vesicles appear in three to five crops over 2–4 days. They are most numerous on the trunk, then on the face and scalp and on the limbs.
- Their distribution is centripetal, and on the limbs the eruption is more profuse on thighs and upper arms than on lower legs and forearms.
- A characteristic feature is the presence of lesions at different stages in each site.
- Mucous membranes are involved.
- Fever is variable in severity and duration and roughly parallels the extent of the eruption.
- Hyper- or hypopigmentation may persist for weeks and small, round, depressed scars can occur.
- **Complications**
  - Encephalitis
  - Varicella pneumonia
  - Hepatitis
  - Secondary infection
  - Cutaneous gangrene ('varicella gangrenosa')
  - Thrombocytopenic purpura, beginning on the fifth to 10th day and usually recovering spontaneously after 3 or 4 months, occasionally follows otherwise benign varicella.
  - Reye's syndrome has been associated with preceding varicella

## Zoster

- The primary infection of varicella includes viraemia and a widespread eruption, after which the virus persists in nerve ganglion cells, usually sensory.
- Zoster is the result of reactivation of this residual latent virus.
- It is uncommon in childhood and the incidence increases with age.
- The sexes are equally affected.
- The first manifestation of zoster is usually pain, which may be severe, and may be accompanied by fever, headache, malaise and tenderness localized to areas of one or more dorsal roots. It usually precedes the eruption by 3–4 days.
- Closely grouped red papules, rapidly becoming vesicular and then pustular, develop in a continuous or interrupted band in the area of one, occasionally two, and rarely, more contiguous dermatomes.
- Mucous membranes within the affected dermatomes are also involved.
- The lymph nodes draining the affected area are enlarged and tender.
- The pain and the constitutional symptoms subside gradually as the eruption disappears.
- In uncomplicated cases recovery is complete in 2–3 weeks in children and young adults, and 3–4 weeks in older patients.
- Occasionally the pain is not followed by the eruption ('zoster sine eruptione').
- The thoracic (53%), cervical (usually C 2, 3, 4, 20%), trigeminal, including ophthalmic (15%) and lumbosacral (11%) dermatomes are most commonly involved at all ages, but the relative frequency of ophthalmic zoster increases in old age.
- In patients with lymphomas or who are otherwise immuno-compromised, generalized varicella ('disseminated zoster') develops and may be hemorrhagic.
- **Motor involvement:** This occurs overall in 5% of cases and is commoner in older patients and in those with malignancy, and in cranial compared with spinal nerve involvement. The motor weakness usually follows the pain and the eruption, by a few days to a few weeks, but occasionally precedes or accompanies them.
- **Trigeminal nerve zoster:** In ophthalmic nerve zoster the eye is affected in two-thirds of cases, especially when vesicles on the side of the nose indicate involvement of the nasociliary nerve (Hutchinson's sign).

- Ocular complications include uveitis, keratitis, conjunctivitis, conjunctival edema (chemosis), ocular muscle palsies, proptosis, scleritis (which may be acute or delayed for 2–3 months), retinal vascular occlusion, and ulceration, scarring and even necrosis of the lid.
- Involvement of the ciliary ganglia may give rise to Argyll–Robertson pupil.
- Zoster of the maxillary division of the trigeminal nerve produces vesicles on the uvula and tonsillar area, whilst with involvement of the mandibular division, the vesicles appear on the anterior part of the tongue, the floor of the mouth and the buccal mucous membrane.
- **Ramsay Hunt syndrome**
- **Post-herpetic neuralgia**
  - ➤ The commonest and most intractable sequel of zoster is post-herpetic neuralgia, generally defined as persistence or recurrence of pain more than a month after the onset of zoster, but better considered after 3 months.
  - ➤ Increases in incidence and severity with age.
  - ➤ Most frequent when the trigeminal nerve is involved.
  - ➤ The pain has two main forms, a continuous burning pain with hyperesthesia, and a spasmodic shooting type, but a pruritic 'crawling' paresthesia may also occur.
  - ➤ Allodynia, pain caused by normally innocuous stimuli, is often the most distressing symptom and occurs in 90% of people with post-herpetic neuralgia.
- **Other complications**
  - ➤ Scar sarcoid
  - ➤ Secondary infection
  - ➤ Encephalitis or meningoencephalitis
  - ➤ Acute retinal necrosis syndrome
  - ➤ Guillain-Barré syndrome and transverse myelitis

## Pregnancy and Varicella Zoster Infection

- Maternal varicella in the first 20 weeks of pregnancy is associated with an approximate 2% risk of fetal damage, including skin lesions, central nervous system and ocular defects, and limb hypoplasia, with a 30% mortality within the first year of life.

- Maternal zoster in pregnancy is not associated with intrauterine infection.
- Zoster in infancy has followed maternal varicella, the baby's primary infection having occurred *in utero*.
- If the mother has varicella within 4 days before to 2 days after term, the neonate would have no maternal antibody and is at risk of severe varicella with a mortality rate up to 30% in the absence of treatment.
- **HPE**
  - Cells of the Malpighian layer show ballooning of their cytoplasm by intracellular edema, and distinctive nuclear changes, comprising eosinophilic inclusions and marginated chromatin.
  - The multinucleate giant cells with up to 15 nuclei, which are a characteristic feature of infections with herpesvirus varicellae and herpesvirus hominis, are produced mainly by cell fusion.
  - Intracellular edema combined with intercellular edema forms the vesicle, the roof of which consists of the upper malpighian and horny layers.
  - A mild inflammatory reaction is seen in the dermis.
- **Diagnosis**
  - Tzanck smear: Multinucleated giant cells
  - Viral culture
  - Electron microscopy of vesicle fluid
  - Detection of VZV antigen by direct fluorescent-antibody staining of a smear.
  - Detection of VZV DNA by PCR in a scraping from the base of a vesicle.
- **Treatment**
  - Varicella in the otherwise healthy child requires only symptomatic treatment.
  - Rest and analgesics are sufficient. Soothing antiseptic applications may be helpful and secondary bacterial infection will require antibiotics.
  - An antiviral is indicated for varicella in adults and for severe varicella or zoster infections at any age in the immuno-compromised. Treatment should be started as early as possible, preferably within the first 1 or 2 days.
  - Acyclovir 800 mg five times a day for 7–10 days or with valaciclovir 1 g or famciclovir 250 or 500 mg three times a day for 7 days.

> **Post-herpetic neuralgia**
  – A tricyclic antidepressant such as amitriptyline or nortriptyline (or clomipramine or doxepin) is useful, especially for hyperesthesia and constant burning pain.
  – For stabbing pain, sodium valproate (or other anticonvulsant, e.g. clonazepam or carbamazepine) is of value.
  – Gabapentin or pregabalin can be useful analgesics for the pain.
  – Topical capsaicin 0.025%, a substance P depleter, may relieve pain in some patients.
  – Topical anesthetic applied as a cream or a patch can also give relief.

• **Prevention**
  > *Pre-exposure prophylaxis:* A live attenuated vaccine developed from the Oka strain of VZV is effective in preventing varicella in healthy children. The vaccine is given in two doses, 3 months apart. Its efficacy persists for 10 years.
  > *Post-exposure prophylaxis*
  – Specific zoster immune globulin (ZIG) administered within 10 days of contact reduces the severity of varicella but does not always prevent it.
  – It should be given to neonates whose mothers develop varicella within the period from 7 days before to 7 days after delivery.
  – Zoster immune globulin is also indicated for healthy neonates in contact with active chickenpox or zoster, and for immunocompromised children and adults, for example organ-transplant recipients and patients who have taken oral steroids for at least 14 days within the previous 3 months who have not had previous chickenpox, if exposed to varicella or zoster (Tables 19.1 and 19.2).

| Table 19.1: HHV 6 7 8 and associated diseases | |
|---|---|
| *Type of HHV* | *Associated disease* |
| HHV-8 or KSHV | – Kaposi's sarcoma |
| HHV-7 | – Exanthema subitum |
| | – Other childhood febrile illnesses |
| | – Some neurologic syndromes |
| | – Pityriasis rosea |
| HHV-6 | – Exanthema subitum (roseola infantum) |

**Table 19.2:** Diseases caused by different viruses

| Disease | Causative agent | Clinical features |
|---------|-----------------|-------------------|
| Rubeola (measles, first disease) | Paramyxovirus | • Seen in nonimmune individuals<br>• Discrete lesions that become confluent as rash spreads from hairline downward, sparing palms and soles; lasts ≥3 days; Koplik's spots<br>• Cough, conjunctivitis, coryza, severe prostration can be associated features |
| Rubella (German measles, third disease) | Togavirus | • Seen in nonimmune individuals<br>• Spreads from hairline downward, clearing as it spreads<br>• Forschheimer spots<br>• Adenopathy, arthritis |
| Erythema infectiosum (fifth disease) | Human parvovirus B19 | • Most common in children aged 3–12 years; occurs in winter and spring<br>• Bright-red "slapped-cheek" appearance followed by lacy reticular rash that waxes and wanes over 3 weeks; rarely, papular-purpuric "gloves-and-socks" syndrome on hands and feet<br>• Mild fever; arthritis in adults; rash following resolution of fever |
| Exanthema subitum (roseola, sixth disease) | Human herpesvirus 6 | • Usually affects children <3 years old<br>• Diffuse maculopapular eruption (sparing face); resolves within 2 days<br>Rash following resolution of fever; similar to Boston exanthem (echovirus 16). |

## PARVOVIRUS

• **Erythema infectiosum**
  ➢ Erythema infectiosum is the most common manifestation of B19 infection and occurs predominantly in children (Table 19.2).
  ➢ This entity is also called fifth disease because it was classified in the late nineteenth century as the fifth in a series of six exanthems of childhood.

➢ Normally a mild illness, erythema infectiosum typically presents as a facial rash with a "slapped-cheek" appearance that is sometimes preceded by low-grade fever (Table 19.3).

➢ The trunk, palms, and soles are less commonly involved.

➢ The typical rash resolves in about a week but can recur intermittently.

➢ Arthralgia and arthritis are uncommon among children but are frequent among adults.

- Arthropathy
- Transient aplastic crisis in sicle cell disease
- Chronic anemia in immunodeficient patients: Some cases of idiopathic pure red cell aplasia probably are caused by persistent B19 infection.
- Fetal and congenital infection

| **Table 19.3:** Erythemas | |
|---|---|
| Erythema chronicum migrans | Lyme's disease |
| Erythema necrolyticum migrans | Glucagonoma causes |
| Erythema marginatum | Rheumatic fever |
| Erythema infectiosum | Parvovirus |
| Erythema multiformis | Stevens-Johnson syndrome |
| Erythema nodosum | Drugs and infections |
| Erythema arthriticum epidemicum | Haverhill fever, streptobacillus moniliformis |
| Erythema gyratum repens | Internal malignancy |
| Erythema ab igne | A reticulated, pigmented, macular |
| Erythema caloricum (toasted shins) | eruption that occurs mostly on the shins, of bakers, stokers, and others exposed to radiant heat |

## QUESTIONS FROM PREVIOUS EXAMINATIONS

1. Etiology clinical features complications and management of herpes simplex
2. Herpes zoster
3. HPV + epidermodysplasia verruciformis classify
4. Koplik spots
5. Treatment of plantar warts
6. Kaposi's varicelliform eruption
7. Fever with joint pains with erythematous rash in 30-year-old patients

8. Milker's nodules
9. Eczema herpeticum
10. Ramsay Hunt syndrome
11. Common viral infections
12. CMV infection
13. HPE of common warts
14. Smallpox
15. Mycoplasma
16. MC
17. Hand-foot-mouth disease
18. TORCH infections
19. Measles
20. Roseola infantum
21. Herpetic whitlow
22. DNA virus-skin
23. Motor complications of herpes zoster

## MULTIPLE CHOICE QUESTIONS

1. **True about erythema infectiosum:**
   (a) Usually affects children <3 years old
   (b) Causative agent is human herpesvirus 6
   (c) Fifth disease
   (d) Forschheimer spots are characteristically seen

2. **In a 7-year-old child with two small lesions of molluscum contagiosum, the ideal treatment is:**
   (a) Surgery              (b) Radiation
   (c) Cryotherapy          (d) Observation

3. **The following viral diseases are characterized by maculopapular rash except one:**
   (a) Measles              (b) Rubella
   (c) Erythema infectiosum (d) Herpangina

4. **The following statements regarding varicella and zoster are true except one:**
   (a) They are two diseases caused by one virus
   (b) Varicella is the primary illness, whereas zoster is the recurrent form of the disease
   (c) They have the same clinical picture
   (d) Varicella is a disease of children, whereas zoster is a disease of elderly and immunosuppressed patients.

## Answers

1. **Ans. (c)** Fifth disease
2. **Ans. (d)** Observation (molluscum contagiosum lesions spontaneously resolve on their own. Most treatment end up cause scarring).
3. **Ans. (d)** Herpangina
4. **Ans. (c)** They have the same clinical picture.

## Phakomatoses (Neurocutaneous Syndromes/Neuroectodermal Dysplasias)

- **Autosomal dominant**
  - ➢ Neurofibromatosis (von Recklinghausen)
  - ➢ Tuberous sclerosis (Bourneville)
  - ➢ Retinocerebellar hemangioblastoma (von Hippel-Lindau)
  - ➢ Neurocutaneous melanosis
- **Not autosomal dominant**
  - • Encephalotrigeminal angiomatosis (Sturge-Weber-Dimitri)
  - • Ataxia-telangiectasia

## TUBEROUS SCLEROSIS (BOURNEVILLE'S DISEASE/EPILOIA)

- Incidence: 1:10,000–50,000
- Inheritance: Autosomal dominant (low penetrance)
- Chromosomes 9 and 16
- Clinical features: Classic **triad of** epilepsy, low IQ and adenoma sebaceum.
- **Major features** (Table 20.1)
  - ➢ **Facial angiofibromas** or forehead plaque
  - ➢ Non-traumatic ungual or **periungual fibroma** (Koenen's tumors)
  - ➢ **Shagreen patch** (connective tissue nevus)—usually in the lumbosacral region (Fig. 20.1)
  - ➢ Multiple retinal nodular hamartomas
  - ➢ Cortical tuber
  - ➢ Subependymal nodules
  - ➢ Subependymal giant cell astrocytoma
  - ➢ Cardiac rhabdomyoma, single or multiple
  - ➢ Lymphangioleiomyomatosis
  - ➢ Renal angiomyolipoma

| Table 20.1: Features of tuberous sclerosis | |
|---|---|
| **CNS lesion** | – Cortical tubers<br>– Benign white matter lesions<br>– Subependymal nodules (95%) typically located in lateral ventricles along striothalamic groove, often calcified (increases with age)<br>– Subependymal giant cell astrocytoma **(SEGA)** typically located at foramen of Monro. Unique brain tumor of tuberous sclerosis<br>Miscellaneous lesions:<br>– Retinal phakomas<br>– Aneurysms<br>– Nonatheromatous vascular stenosis<br>– Mild nonspecific ventricular enlargements |
| **Cutaneous lesions** | – Shagreen patch<br>– Adenoma sebaceum (angiofibromas of face)<br>– Subungual fibromas (Koenen's tumor)<br>– Ash leaf macules (earliest cutaneous feature)<br>– Café au lait spots, poliosis |
| **Renal lesions** | – Bilateral multiple asymptomatic renal angiomyolipomas<br>– Multiple bilateral cortical cysts<br>– Angiomyolipomas are also seen in liver, adrenals, and pancreas |
| **Cardiopulmonary lesions** | – Cardiac rhabdomyoma<br>– Interstitial lung disease indistinguishable from lymphangioleiomyomatosis |
| **Musculoskeletal lesions** | – 'Flame shaped' sclerotic bone islands especially affecting pelvis (osteosclerosis). |

- **Hypomelanotic macules/ash leaf macules** (more than three)— alone their presence is not indicative of TSC (Fig. 20.2).

  Suggestive features requiring further investigation (minor features)

  ➢ Multiple randomly distributed pits in dental enamel
  ➢ Hamartomatous rectal polyps
  ➢ Bone cysts
  ➢ Cerebral white matter radial migration lines
  ➢ Gingival fibromas
  ➢ Non-renal hamartoma
  ➢ Retinal achromic patch

> 'Confetti' skin lesions
> Multiple renal cysts
> Skin tags
- **Positive family history in first-degree relative**
  - Definite tuberous sclerosis complex—either 2 major features or one major plus two minor features
  - Probable tuberous sclerosis complex—one major feature plus one minor feature
  - Possible tuberous sclerosis complex—either one major feature or two or more minor features.

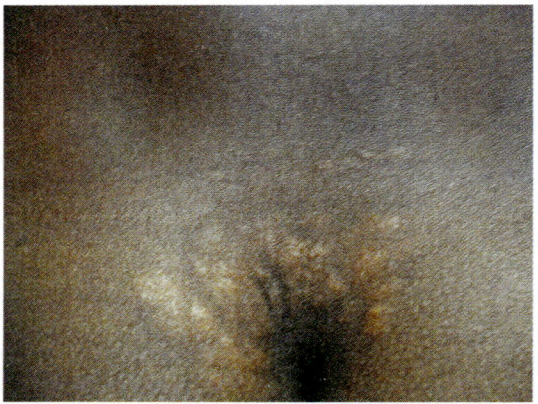

**Fig. 20.1:** Shagreen patch in lumbosacral area of a patient with tuberous sclerosis

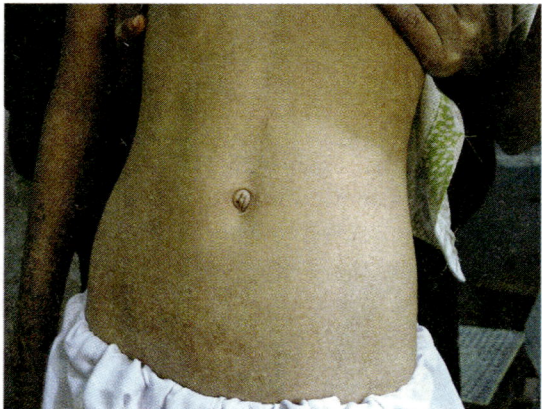

**Fig. 20.2:** Multiple hypopigmented macules over abdomen (ash leaf macules)

## STURGE-WEBER (ENCEPHALOTRIGEMINAL ANGIOMATOSIS)

- Angiomas involving the leptomeninges and skin of the face
- Typically involves the ophthalmic and maxillary distributions of the trigeminal nerve.
- **Classical triad**
  - ➢ Facial portwine stain in the distribution of first branch of the trigeminal nerve.
  - ➢ Mental retardation
  - ➢ Seizures
- Usually sporadic
- Developmental defect of certain ectodermal and mesodermal elements closely approximated in the brain and meninges at 4 to 8 weeks.
- Portwine stain is present at birth and unilateral, but may cross midline and also involve mucosae. They are not neoplasms but instead exhibit normal endothelial turnover and are errors of vascular morphogenesis which manifest as various vascular channel abnormalities.
- They are congenital vascular malformations composed of a superficial collection of ectatic vessels that grow commensurably with the child. A PWS may appear as a pale, erythematous macule or patch that darkens in color with age.
- Convulsions of grandmal type generally appear during the first year of life.
- Behavioral problems, subnormal intelligence, contralateral hemiparesis and EEG abnormalities may be seen.
- **Ocular features**
  - ➢ Ipsilateral *glaucoma*
  - ➢ Buphthalmos
  - ➢ Strabismus
  - ➢ Loss of vision
- **CT scan:** Tram-track or S-shaped intracranial calcifications are found in the leptomeninges within first few months of life. On X-rays seen after the age of 2 years. Ipsilateral choroid plexus and venous angiomas with leptomeningeal angiomatoses usually over the posterior parietal and occipital lobes of the cerebral cortex.
- **Treatment**: Laser for portwine stain.
  - ➢ A variety of lasers has recently been developed for the treatment of congenital and acquired vascular lesions. These includes **pulsed dye** (FPDL, APDL) lasers (577 nm, 585 nm and 595 nm), KTP lasers (532 nm), long pulsed alexandrite lasers (755 nm),

pulsed diode lasers (in the range of 800 to 900 nm), long pulsed 1064 Nd:YAG lasers and intense pulsed light sources (IPLS, also called flash-lights or pulsed light sources).

➤ Several vascular lasers (such as argon, tunable dye, copper vapor, krypton lasers), which were used in the past are no longer useful as they pose a higher risk of complications such as dyschromia (hypopigmentation or hyperpigmentation) and scarring.

➤ Any PWS should be treated as they turn darker and thicker with age. PWS on the head and neck respond more favorably to treatment than lesions elsewhere on the body. Choice of the laser for PWS—first choice: FPDL, IPLS, Nd:YAG, KTP (large spot).

## VON HIPPEL-LINDAU DISEASE

• Autosomal dominant with incomplete penetrance
• Affects males and females equally
• **Associated tumors**
  ➤ Hemangioblastomas—cerebellum, retina, medulla, spinal cord
  ➤ Pheochromocytoma (NIH type 2a or 2b)
  ➤ Renal cysts 60%
  ➤ Renal cell carcinoma 45%
  ➤ Pancreatic, epididymis, or liver cysts
  ➤ Islet cell tumors
  ➤ Endolymphatic sac tumors (ELSTs)
  ➤ Serous adenomas
  ➤ Portwine stains and café au lait macules
• Erythropoietin produced by hemangioblastomas may result in polycythemia.
• Mutation of the von Hippel-Lindau (vHL) gene on chromosome 3p, a tumor-suppressor gene, causes this disorder.

### Neurofibromatosis Type 1 (von Recklinghausen's Disease)

• Autosomal dominant
• Mutation of the NF1 gene on chromosome 17 causes von Recklinghausen's disease. The NF1 gene is a tumor-suppressor gene; it encodes a protein, neurofibromin, which modulates signal transduction through the ras GTPase pathway.
• NF1 is characterized by cutaneous neurofibromas, pigmented lesions of the skin called café au lait spots, freckling in non-sun-

exposed areas such as the axilla and other intertriginous areas, hamartomas of the iris termed Lisch nodules, and pseudoarthrosis of the tibia.

- **Neurofibromas** (benign Schwann cell tumors) are soft papules or nodules that exhibit the **"button-hole" sign**, that is, they invaginate into the skin with pressure in a manner similar to a hernia.
- **CALMs** (café au lait macules) are discrete, well circumscribed, round or oval, uniformly pigmented patches seen over the trunk and limbs.
- Neurofibromas are benign peripheral nerve tumors composed of proliferating Schwann cells and fibroblasts. They present as multiple, palpable, rubbery, cutaneous tumors. They are generally asymptomatic; however, if they grow in an enclosed space, e.g. the intervertebral foramen, they may produce a compressive radiculopathy or neuropathy.
- Aqueductal stenosis with hydrocephalus, scoliosis, short stature, hypertension, epilepsy, and mental retardation may also occur.
- Patients with NF1 are at increased risk of developing nervous system neoplasms, including plexiform neurofibromas, **optic pathway gliomas**, ependymomas, meningiomas, astrocytomas, and pheochromocytomas. Neurofibromas may undergo secondary malignant degeneration and become sarcomatous.

    Café au lait spots are the first feature of the disease to appear in all children.
- **Lisch nodules**
    - ➤ Lisch nodules are melanocytic hamartomas, usually clear yellow to brown, that appear as well defined, dome-shaped elevations projecting from the surface of the iris.
    - ➤ They may be seen without magnification but a slit lamp examination may be necessary to distinguish them from nevi on the iris.
    - ➤ Lisch nodules are the most common clinical finding in adults over 20 years of age with type I neurofibromatosis.

**A diagnosis of NF1, according to the national institutes of health consensus development conference statement, is based on two or more of the following criteria:**

1. Six or more café au lait macules of over 5 mm in greatest diameter in prepubertal individuals and over 15 mm in greatest diameter in postpubertal individuals (Fig. 20.3).
2. Two or more neurofibromas of any type or one plexiform neurofibroma.

3. Freckling in the axillary or inguinal regions (Fig. 20.4).
4. Optic glioma
5. Two or more Lisch nodules
6. Distinctive osseous lesion such as sphenoid dysplasia or thinning of the long bone cortex with or without pseudoarthrosis.
7. A first-degree relative (parent, sibling, offspring) with NF1 by the above criteria.

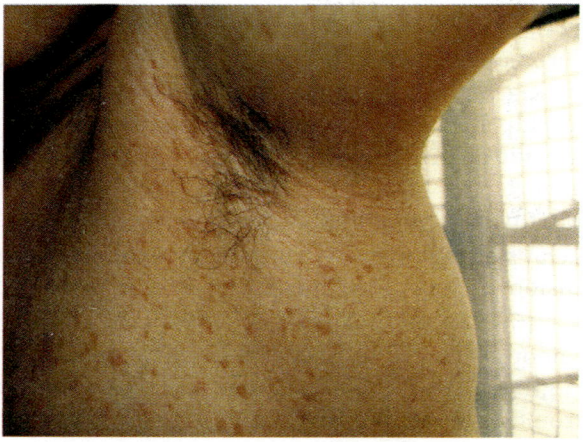

**Fig. 20.3:** Axillary freckling with multiple café au lait macules

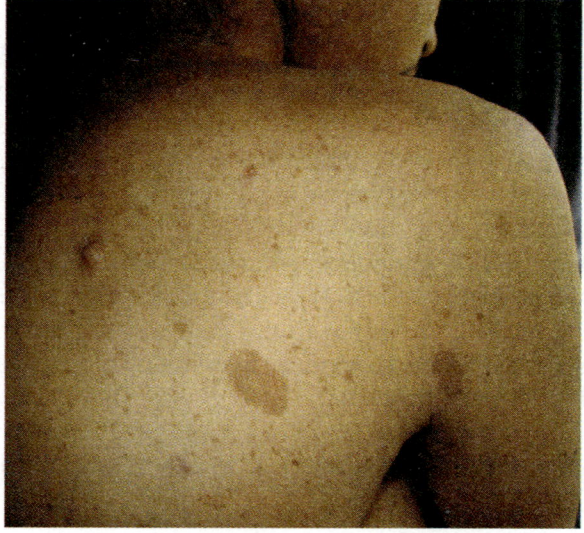

**Fig. 20.4:** Café au lait macules with neurofibroma

## Neurofibromatosis Type 2

- NF2 is characterized by the development of bilateral vestibular schwannomas in >90% of individuals who inherit the gene.
- Patients with NF2 also have a predisposition for the development of meningiomas, gliomas, and schwannomas of cranial and spinal nerves.
- In addition, a **characteristic type of cataract**, juvenile posterior subcapsular lenticular opacity, occurs in NF2.
- Multiple café au lait spots and peripheral neurofibromas occur rarely. Crowe's sign, also known as axillary freckling, is one of the defining features of type 2 neurofibromatosis.
- In patients with NF2, vestibular schwannomas usually present with progressive unilateral deafness early in the third decade of life.
- This syndrome is caused by mutation of the NF2 gene on chromosome 22q; NF2 encodes a protein called neurofibromin 2, schwannomin, or merlin, with homology to a family of cytoskeletal proteins that includes moesin, ezrin, and radixin.

## QUESTIONS FROM PREVIOUS EXAMINATIONS

1. Neurofibroma
2. X chromatid
3. Barr bodies
4. Lyon hypothesis
5. Incontinentia pigmenti
6. Mode of inheritance in the genodermatosis
7. Prenatal diagnosis
8. Mucocutaneous syndromes
9. Neurofibromatosis
10. Tuberous sclerosis
11. Bloom's syndrome
12. Red urine in dermatological patient
13. Genetic counseling
14. Phakomatosis
15. Adenoma sebaceum
16. Aplasia cutis
17. Biotrophy
18. Trisomy 21
19. Familial tumor syndromes
20. Apert syndrome
21. Oro-occulogenital syndrome

## MULTIPLE CHOICE QUESTIONS

1. Classical skin lesion of tuberous sclerosis is:        *(MH 2006)*
   - (a) Adenoma
   - (b) Angiofibroma
   - (c) Angiokeratoma
   - (d) Fibrolipoma

2. Port wine stain, seizures, hemiparesis, intracranial calcification and glaucoma are features of which of the following neuro-cutaneous syndrome?        *(MH 2009)*
   - (a) Neurofibromatosis
   - (b) Tuberous sclerosis
   - (c) Sturge-Weber syndrome
   - (d) vHL

3. Koenen's tumor in tuberous sclerosis represents:     *(DNB 05)*
   - (a) Angiofibroma
   - (b) Lipofibroma
   - (c) Subungual fibroma
   - (d) Adenoma sebaceum

4. Koenen's periungual fibromas are seen in >50% of cases of:
   *(JIPMER 02)*
   - (a) Tuberous sclerosis
   - (b) Encephalotrigeminal angiomatosis
   - (c) Neurofibromatosis
   - (d) Ataxia-telangiectasia

5. In neurofibromatosis, the first feature of the disease to appear in all children is:
   - (a) Café au lait macules
   - (b) Axillary freckling
   - (c) Lisch nodules (pigmented iris hamartomas)
   - (d) Mollusca fibrosa

6. A patient had seven irregular hyperpigmented macules on the trunk and multiple small hyperpigmented macules in the axillae and groins since childhood. There were no other skin lesions. Which is the most likely investigation to support the diagnosis?
   *(AI 06)*
   - (a) Slit lamp examination of eye
   - (b) Measurement of intraocular tension
   - (c) Examination of fundus
   - (d) Retinal artery angiography

7. A child has erythematous non-blanching bosselated lesion on the right side of the face. Which of the following would be most appropriate Rx?        *(AIIMS 2011)*
   - (a) Q ruby laser
   - (b) Erbium laser
   - (c) Nd:YAG laser
   - (d) Flash light pumped pulsed dye laser

## Answers

1. **Ans. (b)** Angiofibroma
2. **Ans. (c)** Sturge-Weber syndrome *(Ref. IADVL, 2nd edition 168)*
3. **Ans. (c)** Subungual fibroma
4. **Ans. (a)** Tuberous sclerosis *(Ref. Rook's Dermatology, 7th edition, Table 12.3)*
5. **Ans. (a)** Café au lait macules *(Ref. Rook's Dermatology, 7th edn/12.28)*
6. **Ans. (a)** Slit lamp examination of eye *(Ref. Roxburgh's Skin Diseases, 17th edn/199, 301).*
7. **Ans. (d)** Flash light pumped pulsed dye laser.

# 21 Connective Tissue Disorders and Skin Manifestations

## LUPUS ERYTHEMATOSUS

- Lupus erythematosus is divided into three groups—cutaneous LE (DLE), intermediate LE (SCLE) and SLE.

### Discoid Lupus Erythematosus

- DLE is a benign disorder of the skin, most frequently involving the face, and characterized by well-defined, red scaly patches of variable size, which heal with atrophy, scarring and pigmentary changes.
- The disease affects twice as many females as males, with a peak age of onset in the fourth decade.
- Genetic predisposition and exacerbation of disease by ultraviolet light.
- **Pathology**
  - ➢ Hyperkeratosis with follicular plugging.
  - ➢ Liquefaction degeneration of the basal cell layer of the epidermis.
  - ➢ Degenerative changes in the connective tissue, consisting of hyalinization, edema and fibrinoid change, most marked immediately below the epidermis.
  - ➢ A patchy dermal lymphocytic infiltrate with a few plasma cells and histiocytes, particularly around the appendages.
- **Types**
  - ➢ *Localized DLE:* Disease limited to the head and neck
  - ➢ *Disseminated DLE:* Lesions below chin over the trunk and extremities.
    - – *Localized DLE*
      - o The face is most commonly affected, and the scalp, ears, nose, arms, legs and trunk to a lesser extent.

- o The circumscribed or discoid type is the most frequent and occurs particularly on the cheeks, the bridge of the nose, the ears, the side of the neck and the scalp.
- o Lesions may be bilateral, although not necessarily symmetrical, or unilateral. Usually, lesions occur as well-defined erythematous patches, varying in size from a few millimeters to 10–15 cm.
- o There is adherent scale in many cases, and when this is removed its undersurface shows horny plugs which have occupied dilated pilosebaceous canals. This so-called **'Carpet-tack' sign**/'tin-tack' sign.
- o The plaques expand centrifugally with a raised erythematous hyperpigmented margin and central depigmentation and atrophy with loss oh hair (Fig. 21.1).
  - – *Disseminated DLE (DDLE)*
    - o Characteristic lesions of DLE may occur in a widespread pattern on the trunk and limbs, or may be localized to other body sites. This occurs almost always in women, and they are usually cigarette smokers.

- **Chilblain lupus**
  - ➤ Approximately 6% of patients, predominantly female, develop chilblain-like lesions chiefly on the toes and fingers, but also on the heels, calves, knees, knuckles, elbows, nose and ears.
  - ➤ Some patients may have cryofibrinogenemia or cold agglutinins.
  - ➤ Patients are usually Ro antibody positive.
  - ➤ They are also either smokers, or have markedly abnormal peripheral circulation with low resting blood flow.

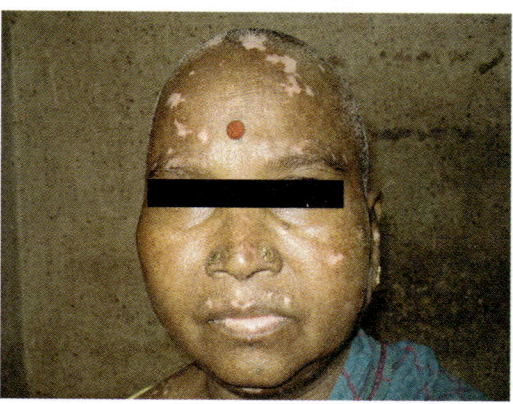

**Fig. 21.1:** Depigmented atrophic plaques over scalp and face in a case of chronic DLE

- *Lupus erythematosus and erythema multiforme-like syndrome (Rowell's syndrome)*
  - ➤ The distinctive syndrome of cutaneous LE, either discoid or systemic, occurring with lesions resembling erythema multiforme on the face, neck, hands, chest and in the mouth.
  - ➤ They show a characteristic pattern of serological abnormality, in that the speckled type of antinuclear factor is associated with rheumatoid factor and anti-La (SS-B).
- *Lupus erythematosus profundus (panniculitis)*
  - ➤ This is an unusual clinical variety of LE in which the cutaneous infiltrate occurs primarily (but not always exclusively) in deeper portions of the corium, with only microscopic epidermal changes, giving rise to firm, sharply defined nodules from one to several centimeters in diameter, lying beneath clinically normal skin.
- *LE hypertrophicus et profundus*
  - ➤ Starts as a violaceous, scaly, tender lesion, which rapidly enlarges, developing a warty hypertrophic surface with coarse adherent scales, which form a hard brown-black tar-like plaque.
- **Diagnosis**
  - ➤ Hemogram: Anemia, leukopenia or thrombocytopenia
    Raised erythrocyte sedimentation rate (ESR)
  - ➤ Urine analysis
  - ➤ Skin biopsy
  - ➤ LE cell phenomenon
  - ➤ Antinuclear antibodies (ANA ) are found in between 5 and 60% of cases: The 'homogeneous' type of antinuclear factor being twice as frequent as the 'speckled' type. Antinuclear antibodies (ANA) are more common in older patients, in those who have had the disease for a long time and when there is extensive skin involvement. They are also more common in patients with chilblains, Raynaud's phenomenon and joint pains.
  - ➤ Raised serum globulin
  - ➤ Positive Coombs' test
  - ➤ Positive cryoglobulins and cold agglutinins
  - ➤ False-positive syphilis serology
  - ➤ Positive anticardiolipin antibodies (mainly IgM)
  - ➤ Positive rheumatoid factor
  - ➤ Other autoantibodies: Anti-DNA ab, antibodies to single-stranded DNA, anti-La/SS-B

- **Treatment**
  - ➤ *Strict photoprotection:* Use of sunscreens, protective clothing, umbrella and hat.
  - ➤ *Topical therapy:* Steroids
  - ➤ *Systemic therapy:* Steroids, antimalarials, cyclophosphamide, thalidomide, biologicals.
  - ➤ *Carbon dioxide laser:* Argon laser and pulsed dye laser have been tried.

## Subacute Cutaneous Lupus Erythematosus

- Non-scarring papulosquamous (two-thirds) or annular polycyclic (one-third) lesions.
- The disease predominantly affects adults. Common in females.
- Lesions usually occur above the waist and particularly around the neck, on the trunk and on the outer aspects of the arms.
- Follicular plugging and hyperkeratosis are not prominent, and the lesions resolve leaving grey–white hypopigmentation and telangiectases.
- The pigmentary changes usually resolve completely.
- Diffuse non-scarring alopecia and photosensitivity occur in approximately half of patients.
- Other features include mouth ulceration (especially of the palate), reticular livedo, periungual telangiectasia and Raynaud's phenomenon.
- Approximately half of patients fulfil the criteria for SLE of the American Rheumatism Association (ARA), with arthritis the most frequent feature.
- Fever, malaise and central nervous system involvement occur, but renal disease is mild and infrequent.
- Histopathologically, SCLE can be differentiated from DLE by the presence of more epidermal atrophy and less hyperkeratosis, basement-membrane thickening, follicular plugging and inflammatory infiltration. Dust-like particles of inter- and intracellular IgG in the basement layers of the epidermis may be a specific feature.
- Homogeneous antinuclear antibodies are found in approximately 60% and anti-Ro/SS-A antibodies in approximately 80% of patients. Anticardiolipin antibodies occur in 16%.
- **Treatment**
  - ➤ Photoprotection
  - ➤ Topical steroids

- Topical tacrolimus and pimecrolimus
- Oral antimalarials
- Oral steroids
- Cyclophosphamide, thalidomide, retinoids, dapsone
- Intravenous immunoglobulins
- Biologicals

## Systemic Lupus Erythematosus (SLE)

- A systemic disease characterized by multisystem organ inflammation, most commonly the skin, joints and vasculature, and associated immunological abnormalities.
- The main clinical features include fever, rashes and arthritis, but renal, pulmonary, cardiac and neurological involvement may occur.
- Condition tends to occur in early adult life.
- Common in females.
- Genetic predisposition is seen.
- Exacerbated by ultraviolet light.
- Bacterial infection, mental or physical stress may trigger onset of SLE.
- The role of viruses is suspected.
- SLE may be precipitated by drugs especially hydalazine.
- **Cutaneous manifestations**
  - The cutaneous changes may be broadly divided between:
    - Those specific for LE, and showing the characteristic histopathological appearances of LE;
    - Those that are less specific in their origin and not showing LE histological changes.

*Specific changes*

- Cutaneous erythema is the most common feature, particularly on light-exposed areas.
- A butterfly blush or discrete maculopapular eruption with fine scaling on the butterfly area of the cheeks or elsewhere is also frequently found.

*Non-specific changes*

- *Reticulate telangiectatic erythema* seen on the thenar and hypothenar eminences of the palms, on the pulps and dorsum of the fingers, and to a lesser extent, on the toes and over the lateral borders of the feet and heels.
- The nail folds may show hyperkeratotic and ragged cuticles. Splinter hemorrhages may sometimes be seen in the nails, and

other changes include pitting, ridging, onycholysis, striate leukonychia and red lunulae.

➢ *Hair changes:* Alopecia occurs in over 50% of patients, especially in the active phase of the disease. This takes the form of diffuse loss of hair with a reddish scalp, or less frequently, permanent scarring alopecia, similar to that found in DLE. The hair is usually coarse, dry and fragile, especially on the frontal margin. This leads to an unruly appearance with short, broken-off hair, the so-called 'lupus hair'.

➢ SLE may present as hypocomplementemic urticarial vasculitis.

➢ Widespread purpura, resulting from thrombocytopenia or cutaneous vasculitis, is a common finding.

➢ Leukocytoclastic vasculitis may lead to purpuric macules, up to 1 cm in diameter, and in certain cases purpuric urticarial lesions may be found.

➢ Livedo reticularis, a mottled or bluish red discoloration, which blanches on pressure and is not affected by temperature changes, may develop, especially on the outer aspects of the arms.

➢ Atrophie blanche and lesions similar to those of malignant atrophic papulosis (Degos' disease) are other features of vasculitis.

➢ Chronic pyoderma gangrenosum occurs

➢ Leg ulcers occur in approximately 10% of patients, usually near the malleoli but sometimes on the feet and elsewhere, from breakdown in reticular livedo and in areas of cutaneous vasculitis.

➢ Erythromelalgia (pain in the feet aggravated by heat and dependence and relieved by cooling and elevation) may be a presenting feature.

➢ *Mucinosis:* Papular or nodular lesions resulting from mucinous deposits in the dermis without microscopic features of LE have been reported.

➢ Pigmentary changes. Pigmentary disturbances are not uncommon.

➢ *Mucous membrane lesions:* Mucous membrane lesions occur in 26% of cases, usually on the palate buccal mucosa or gums, in active phases of the disease. Lesions start as small erythematous or purpuric areas, which break down to form shallow and sometimes painful ulcers, with a dirty yellowbase and surrounding reddish halo. There may be difficulty in swallowing. Patients may present with vulval and vaginal ulceration.

- **Bullous SLE**
  - Blistering is uncommon in SLE. In the classic disease, separation of the epidermis and dermis occurs as a result of severe liquefaction degeneration of the basal layer and dermal edema.
  - A separate subset called bullous SLE has been defined, with distinct clinical and histopathological features, the latter resembling dermatitis herpetiformis.
  - Subepidermal vesicles contain neutrophils with microabscesses, and nuclear 'dust' and fibrin at the tips of dermal papillae.
  - Immunohistology, however, shows linear deposition of IgA, IgG and IgM, and to a lesser extent, C3 at the basement membrane, resembling bullous pemphigoid and unlike the IgA seen in the dermal papillae in dermatitis herpetiformis.
  - Electron microscopy shows the immunoreactants to be in the sublamina densa and not in the lamina lucida as in pemphigoid.
  - Clinically, the bullous lesions are predominantly on the face, neck and upper trunk, but may be more widespread, and may heal with milia formation.
  - One-thirds have mouth lesions.
  - Photosensitivity may occur.
  - Dapsone alone or in combination with prednisone is the treatment of choice.
- **Pemphigus erythematosus**
  - Erythematous, scaly, hyperkeratotic or crusted lesions, sometimes adversely affected by the sun, occur in a butterfly distribution on the cheeks and in a seborrheic distribution on the trunk of patients with Senear-Usher syndrome.
  - This combines the immunological features of pemphigus and LE.
  - Direct immunofluorescence shows immunoglobulin and complement in the intercellular substance and at the dermal–epidermal junction of perilesional, and to a lesser extent, of light-exposed and non-exposed skin.
  - Circulating pemphigus-like antibodies and antinuclear factor occur in 80–100%, but anti-DNA and ENA antibodies are not found.
  - Antidesmoglein antibodies have also been demonstrated.
  - The condition occurs spontaneously, but has been induced by penicillamine, propranolol, captopril, pyritinol and thiopronine.
  - Topical steroids alone may control the condition, but systemic steroids, immunosuppressives or dapsone may be required.

- **ARA criteria for SLE**
  1. Malar rash
  2. Discoid rash
  3. Photosensitivity (by history or observation)
  4. Oral ulcers, usually painless, observed by physician
  5. Arthritis—nonerosive, involving two or more joints
  6. Serositis—pleuritis or pericarditis
  7. Renal disorder—proteinuria (>500 mg/day) or cellular casts
  8. Central nervous system disorder-seizures or psychosis (absence of known cause)
  9. Hematologic disorder—hemolytic anemia, leukopenia ($<4000/mm^2$) or thrombocytopenia ($<100,000/mm^2$)
  10. Immunologic disorder—positive LE prep, abnormal titers of antinative (n) DNA, and anti-Sm, false-positive VDRL
  11. Antinuclear antibody
- If four or more criteria are present serially or simultaneously during any period of observation, the patient is considered to have SLE.
- **Treatment**
  - ➤ Photoprotection: Protective clothing, umbrella, hat, physical and chemical sunscreens.
  - ➤ Oral Antimalarials: Chloroquine and hydroxychloroquine
  - ➤ Oral steroids: Prednisolone 1–2 mg/kg body wt/day
  - ➤ Cyclophosphamide, azathioprine, methotrexate, thalidomide, retinoids, dapsone
  - ➤ Intravenous immunoglobulins
  - ➤ Biologicals

## LOCALIZED MORPHEA

- A disorder of unknown cause in which there is localized sclerosis of the skin.
- All ages are affected, the peak incidence occurring between 20 and 40 years of age.
- The female to male ratio is around 3 : 1
- Round or oval localized indurated plaques are seen. Most common on trunk. Loss of hair and sweating with depigmented atrophic shiny depressed skin are final sequelae of the disease.
- The condition has traditionally been subdivided clinically into the following types:
  - ➤ Circumscribed plaques
  - ➤ Morphea profundus/subcutaneous (deep)

- ➢ Bullous morphea
- ➢ Linear morphea
- ➢ Frontoparietal lesions (en coup de sabre), with or without hemiatrophy of the face.
- **Pathology**
  - ➢ The epidermis may be normal, or flattened and atrophic with loss of the rete ridges.
  - ➢ At first the dermis is edematous, with swelling and degeneration of the collagen fibrils, which become homogeneous and eosinophilic.
  - ➢ There may be a scanty perivascular lymphocytic infiltrate.
  - ➢ Later, the dermis is markedly thickened, with dense collagen and relatively a few recognizable fibroblasts.
  - ➢ The elastic tissue is reduced.
  - ➢ The dermal appendages and dermal and subcutaneous fat are progressively lost. Some sweat glands may survive, deep in the dense sclerotic mass.
- **Laboratory abnormalities**: ESR and serum protein assays are usually normal, but eosinophilia may occur.
- **Autoantibodies:** Anti-single-stranded DNA antibodies, antihistone antibodies, antinuclear antibodies. The presence of ANA (with homogeneous and nucleolar patterns), antibodies to single-stranded DNA and the presence of eosinophilia may indicate disease activity and the late development of systemic complications.
- Ultrasound scanning has been reported as being helpful in diagnosing morphea, in differentiating morphea from lichen sclerosus et atrophicus, and in monitoring the course of localized morphea.
- **Treatment**
  - ➢ As the expected natural history is towards spontaneous resolution, the condition may be allowed to take its natural course, if uncomplicated.
  - ➢ Topical and intralesional steroids
  - ➢ Topical calcipotriol, topical tacrolimus and 5% imiquimod cream.
  - ➢ PUVA therapy
  - ➢ Hydroxychloroquine
  - ➢ Physical therapy in the form of physiotherapy may be helpful in preventing joint deformities and contractures, and in maintaining joint movement and muscle strength.
  - ➢ Surgical intervention for the relief of contractures, the lengthening of limbs and the correction of deformities may have to be carried out in certain cases.

## PROGRESSIVE SYSTEMIC SCLEROSIS (SYSTEMIC SCLERODERMA/ ACROSCLEROSIS)

- Systemic sclerosis is a multisystem disorder characterized by vascular abnormalities, connective tissue sclerosis and atrophy, and autoantibodies.
- Common in females.
- Present between ages 20–60 yrs.
- **Classification of systemic sclerosis**
  - ➢ Diffuse cutaneous systemic sclerosis
    - – Short interval (<1 year) between the onset of Raynaud's phenomenon
    - – Development of skin changes
    - – Truncal and peripheral skin involvement
    - – Tendon friction rubs
    - – Pulmonary fibrosis, renal failure, gastrointestinal disease, myocardial involvement
    - – Capillary dropout visible in nail folds
    - – Scl-70 antibody-positive
    - – Anticentromere antibody-negative
  - ➢ Limited cutaneous systemic sclerosis
    - – Long history of Raynaud's phenomenon
    - – Limited skin involvement (peripheral only)
    - – Calcification, telangiectasia, late onset of pulmonary hypertension
    - – Capillary dilatation visible in nail folds
    - – Anticentromere antibody-positive.
- **Cutaneous features**
  - ➢ The earliest feature is usually, but not invariably, Raynaud's phenomenon.
  - ➢ The hands and face are the most frequently involved, but the changes may extend proximally to involve the forearms and upper arms.
  - ➢ The fingers may be edematous and swollen, and the skin feels tight and has a shiny appearance. With increasing severity, the skin becomes immovable or hidebound.
  - ➢ The facial appearance in a well-developed case is characteristic. The forehead is smooth and shiny, the skin is bound down and hard, the lines of expression are smoothed out and the nose becomes small and pinched. The mouth opening is constricted and radial furrows appear, giving a pursed appearance.

> The lower eyelids cannot be depressed by the fingers to show the conjunctivae, because of atrophy of the tissues. Small mat-like telangiectases are frequently found on the face.

> Atrophy occurs first in the pulps of the fingers, and small painful ulcers are formed, which heal leaving depressed scars.

> Pitted scars occur in over one-third of patients, not only on the tips of the fingers but also in a linear distribution on the ulnar border of the thumb and radial borders of the index and middle fingers, as well as the dorsa of the fingers over the joints.

> Later, sclerosis of the overlying skin of the fingers develops, giving the fingers a smooth shiny tapered appearance, with the nails curving over the atrophic phalanges. Later still, the nails become very small and the whole of the distal part of the finger atrophies.

> The nail folds may show ragged cuticles. Pterygium inversum unguis-like changes are sometimes found. Using wide-field microscopy, the capillaries are enlarged and distorted. There is loss of capillaries with disruption of the capillary bed in approximately 90% of patients.

> Telangiectases varying from 2 to 20 mm are found mainly on the face, lips, mouth, upper trunk and hands, but may extend as far as the upper thighs.

• The criteria for diagnosis have been established by the subcommittee for scleroderma criteria of the ARA . Patients should have either:

1. Scleroderma proximal to the digits, affecting limbs, face, neck or trunk—this is the single major criterion; or

2. At least two minor criteria, consisting of:

    (a) sclerodactyly

    (b) digital pitted scarring

    (c) bilateral basal pulmonary fibrosis.

• Crest syndrome: Calcinosis, Raynaud's phenomenon, esophageal dysmotility, sclerodactyly  and telangiectasia.

• Systemic features include:

> Arthritis

> Dysphagia

> Alternate constipation and diarrhea

> Pulmonary fibrosis

> Cardiac and renal involvement.

- **Diagnosis**
  - ➤ HPE shows atrophic epidermis, hyalinization of dermal collagen, replacement of subcutaneous tissue with collagen and intimal thickening of blood vessels.
  - ➤ Autoantibodies: ANA, anti-Scl-70 and anticentromere antibodies
  - ➤ Radiography of chest, hand and soft tissues
  - ➤ Barium studies of gastrointestinal tract
  - ➤ Pulmonary function tests.
- **Treatment**
  - ➤ Drugs used are:
    - **Vasodilators for Raynaud's phenomenon:** Nifedipine, prazosin, prostacyclins, low molecular wt dextran IV, IV pentoxifylline.
    - **Immunosuppressives:** Corticosteroids, cyclophosphamide, methotrexate, ciclosporine, azathioprine, chlorambucil.
    - **Antifibrotic agents:** d-Penicillamine.

## DERMATOMYOSITIS

- A distinctive entity identified by a characteristic rash accompanying, or more often preceding, muscle weakness.
- When only muscle inflammation is present in the absence of skin manifestations, it is called polymyositis.
- Females are more commonly affected.
- Both children and adults are affected.
  Up to 50% of the cases may be a paraneoplastic phenomenon, indicating the presence of cancer.
- **Cutaneous manifestations**
  - ➤ Periorbital violaceous erythema with associated edema of eyelids and periorbital tissues  (heliotrope rash) (Fig. 21.2).

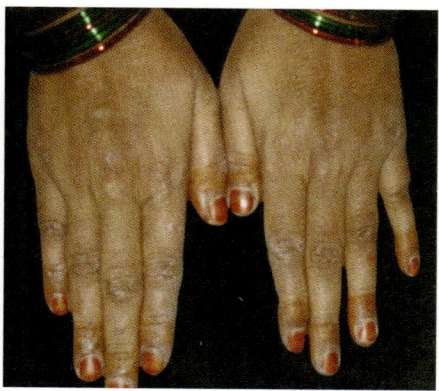

**Fig. 21.2:** Flat topped papules over dorsum of hand (Gottron's papules)

➢ Heliotrope sign is seen in patients with dermatomyositis as a violaceous erythema involving the periorbital skin. The term refers to the purplish color of the flowers of the heliotrope plant, so named because its flowers rotate to face the sun. Similar to Gottron's sign, the heliotrope sign is strongly suggestive of dermatomyositis.

➢ *Gottron's papules:* Violaceous flat topped papules on the interphalangeal joints and knuckles. Similar lesions may occur over other bony prominences such as knees, elbows and medial malleoli (Fig. 21.3).

➢ *Gottron's sign:* Symmetric macular violaceous erythema with or without edema in the above mentioned sites.

➢ Macular violaceous erythema overlying the dorsal hands, extensor forearms and arms, deltoids, posterior shoulder, nape of the neck, "V" area of neck, upper chest and forehead (Shawl sign and V sign) (Fig. 21.4).

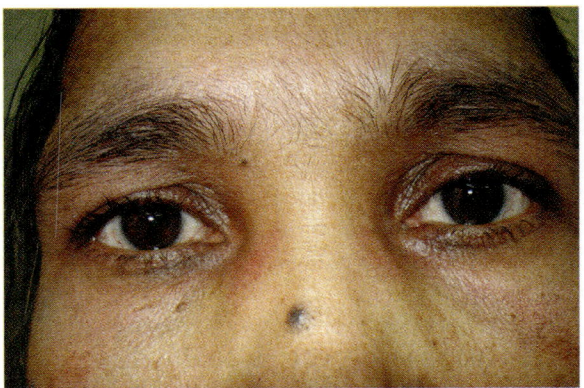

**Fig. 21.3:** Periorbital erythema and edema (heliotrope rash)

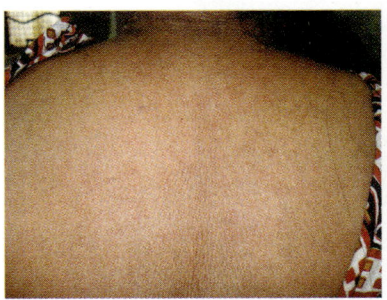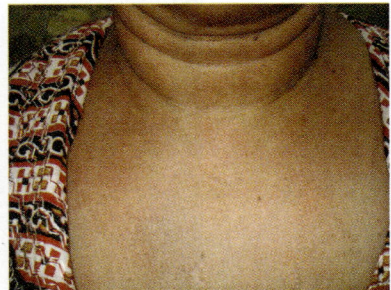

**Fig. 21.4:** Erythema over upper back and front of chest (Shawl sign and V sign)

> ➤ Palmar hyperkeratosis (or "mechanic's hands")
> ➤ Priapism may occur
> ➤ Poikiloderma atrophicans vasculare.
> ➤ Holster sign is found in dermatomyositis. Pruritic, macular, violaceous erythema affects the lateral aspects of hips and thighs.
> ➤ *Nail changes*
>   – Capillary loop dilatation (telangiectasia)
>   – Periungual erythema and ragged cuticles
> ➤ Symmetrical proximal muscle weakness is seen especially of the hips and thighs. Patient has difficulty in rising from chair, combing hair, climbing steps.

- **Bohan and Peter criteria for diagnosis**
  > ➤ Symmetric proximal muscle weakness
  >   – Most common symptom
  > ➤ Typical rash
  > ➤ Elevated serum muscle enzymes (CPK, SGOT, SGPT, LDH)
  > ➤ Myopathic changes on EMG
  > ➤ Characteristic muscle biopsy abnormalities and absence of histopathologic signs of other myopathies.
- **Complications**
  > ➤ Interstitial lung disease
  > ➤ Esophageal disease
  > ➤ Myocarditis
  > ➤ Malignancy (adenocarcinoma of the cervix, lung, ovaries, pancreas, bladder and stomach make up about 70% of associated cancers)
- **Gottron's papules show features of lichenoid reaction such as:**
  > ➤ Basal cell degeneration
  > ➤ "Colloid bodies"
  > ➤ Upper dermal lymphocytic infiltrate
  > ➤ PAS positive thick basement membrane zone
- **There are two classic microscopic findings of dermatomyositis:**
  > ➤ A mixed B and T cell perivascular inflammatory infiltrate
  > ➤ Perifascicular muscle fiber atrophy
- The diagnosis of dermatomyositis can be confirmed by muscle biopsy (perivascular and perimysial inflammation is often seen).
- **Treatment**
  > ➤ Systemic steroids
  > ➤ Methotrexate

> IVIg
> Azathioprine
> Cyclophosphamide
> Rituximab and other biologicals

## OVERLAP SYNDROME

- Patient manifests symptoms of more than one connective tissue disease.
- Systemic sclerosis with dermatomyositis is the most frequently seen overlap syndrome.

## MIXED CONNECTIVE TISSUE DISEASE

- First described by Sharp and colleagues in 1972.
- Patients are predominantly female.
- Show features of SLE, systemic sclerosis, dermatomyositis and polymyositis.
- Raynaud's phenomenon, arthritis and arthralgia, sausage-shaped fingers and swelling of the dorsa of the hands, abnormal esophageal motility, impaired pulmonary diffusing capacity and myositis are frequent.
- The incidence of clinical renal disease is approximately 5%, but renal histology is abnormal in 20%.
- Aseptic meningitis, trigeminal neuropathy, transverse myelitis and psychosis are prominent neurological features.
- Speckled type of antinuclear antibody is seen.
- High titre of antibodies to $U_1 RNP$.
- The response to treatment with corticosteroids is good.
- Mixed connective tissue disease may be more severe in children, in whom cardiac and renal disease and arthritis are common, and thrombocytopenia may be marked, although the overall prognosis may be quite good.

## LICHEN SCLEROSUS ET ATROPHICUS

- Chronic disease of skin and mucous membranes.
- Common in females.
- This frequently involves the perineal skin in the female, and the penis and foreskin in the male.
- The condition occurs particularly around and after the menopause, but also occurs in girls between the ages of approximately 1 and 13 years.

- **Etiology:** Unknown. Following factors are suspected.
  - ➤ Hormonal cause
  - ➤ Autoimmune cause
  - ➤ Infection
  - ➤ Trauma
- **Clinical features**

*Non-genital lesions*

  - ➤ The lesions on the skin are symptomless and occur on the trunk, particularly on the upper part and around the umbilicus, around the neck, in the axillae, on the flexor surfaces of the wrists, around the eye, and very rarely, on the scalp, palms and soles.
  - ➤ Lesions can occur at sites of pressure (e.g. underneath bra straps or belts). The lesions are small, ivory or porcelain-white, shiny, round macules or papules, a few millimeters in diameter, but occasionally, they are semitranslucent and resemble mother-of-pearl.
  - ➤ They are slightly raised, or level with the surface of the skin, and typically their surface shows prominent dilated pilosebaceous or sweat duct orifices, which often contain yellow or brown horny plugs.
  - ➤ In the later stages, atrophy occurs, and the surface of the lesions becomes wrinkled, and may actually be depressed.

*Anogenital lesions in women*

  - ➤ The condition most commonly starts between 45 and 60 years of age but is not uncommon in childhood.
  - ➤ Lesions occur on the vulva and around the anus, and may extend to the skin of the inner side of the thighs.
  - ➤ The ivory-colored atrophic papules with follicular hyper-keratosis and plugging can often be identified on the vulva but, owing to friction and moisture, the lesions frequently break down to form a red raw surface, resembling macerated intertrigo.
  - ➤ Sometimes, particularly in children—the condition is symptomless.
  - ➤ Patients often complain of soreness rather than pruritus, and dyspareunia may be considerable.
  - ➤ Atrophy is a feature, and there may be gross shrinkage of the vulva, especially of the clitoris and labia minora.
  - ➤ Labial fusion, clitoral burial and labial resorption can all occur. The vaginal introitus may become as small as 1 cm in diameter (figure of eight or hourglass appearance).

*Mouth lesions*
➢ Occasionally, lesions are found in the mouth. They consist of bluish-white plaques, usually on the inner surface of the cheek or on the palate. There may be superficial ulceration.

*Lichen sclerosus in the male (balanitis xerotica obliterans)*
➢ Acquired phimosis or recurrent balanitis is the presenting features, together with itching and soreness, and erection may be painful.
➢ The prepuce becomes sclerotic and cannot be retracted. Ulceration of the foreskin can occur.
➢ The glans and undersurface of the prepuce are shining and bluish white, and there can be considerable telangiectasia.
➢ The condition is most common between the ages of 15 and 50 years.
- **Complications**: Malignancy can occur.
  ➢ *Treatment:* Topical steroids, testosterone and tretinoin have been used. Surgical intervention is needed.

## SJÖGREN'S SYNDROME

- The onset occurs most frequently in the fourth, fifth and sixth decades, and 90% of the patients with the primary form are women.
- The disease is caused by an immune-mediated inflammation of exocrine glands, and involves salivary, lacrimal and sweat glands.
- It may be primary, in which case the exocrine dysfunction occurs alone, or as secondary Sjögren's syndrome in association with a connective tissue disease (rheumatoid arthritis is most common).
- The most common features of the condition are dryness and atrophy of the conjunctiva and cornea (keratoconjunctivitis sicca), and a dry mouth (xerostomia).
- **Cutaneous manifestations**
  ➢ Xeroderma, pruritus and scaling
  ➢ SCLE-like rashes, annular erythema, including Sweet's-like lesions and papular erythema.
  ➢ Raynaud's syndrome
  ➢ Hyperglobulinemic purpura and inflammatory vasculitis, including PAN-like lesions.
  ➢ Vitiligo
  ➢ Abnormalities of sweating
  ➢ Amyloid
  ➢ Alopecia—diffuse and generalized.

## Revised Classification Criteria for Sjögren's Syndrome (SS)

1. **Ocular symptoms—at least one of**
   - Dry eyes for more than 3 months
   - Sensation of sand or gravel in the eyes
   - Need for tear substitutes more than 3 times a day
2. **Oral symptoms—at least one of**
   - Dry mouth for more than 3 months
   - Recurrently or persistently swollen salivary glands as an adult
   - Need liquids to swallow dry food
3. **Ocular signs—at least one of the following two tests positive:**
   - Schirmer's test, performed without anesthesia (≤5 mm in 5 mins)
   - Rose Bengal score or other ocular dye score
4. **Histopathology in minor salivary glands, focal lymphocytic sialoadenitis (focus score ≥1).**
5. **Salivary gland involvement: A positive result for at least one of the following diagnostic tests**
   - Unstimulated whole salivary flow (≤1.5 ml in 15 mins)
   - Parotid sialography showing the presence of diffuse sialectasias (punctate, cavitary, or destructive pattern), without evidence of obstruction in the major ducts.
   - Salivary scintigraphy showing delayed uptake, reduced concentration and/or delayed excretion of tracer.
6. **Autoantibodies: Presence in the serum of antibodies to Ro (SSA) or La (SSB) antigens, or both.**

### For Primary SS

In patients without any potentially associated disease, primary SS may be defined as follows:

(a) The presence of any four of the six items is indicative of primary SS, as long as either item 4 (histopathology) or 6 (serology) is positive.

(b) The presence of any three of the four objective criteria items (that is, items 3, 4, 5, 6).

### For Secondary SS

In patients with a potentially associated disease, the presence of item 1 or item 2 plus any two from among items 3, 4, and 5 may be considered as indicative of secondary SS.

- **Laboratory abnormalities**
  - ➤ Hypergammaglobulinemia and rheumatoid factor are frequently demonstrated in the serum.

- ➢ Antinuclear antibodies are present in more than 50% of patients (homogeneous factor is more frequent than speckled, and nucleolar factor is only occasionally found).
- ➢ Anti-Ro (also called SS-A) and anti-La (SS-B) are frequently found, and are an important part of the diagnostic profile of the disease.
- **Complications:** Increased risk of developing lymphoreticular malignancies.
- **Treatment**
  - ➢ Symptomatic management of dry eyes and dry mouth.
  - ➢ Corticosteroids
  - ➢ Chloroquine and hydroxychloroquine
  - ➢ Cyclophosphamide

## QUESTIONS FROM PREVIOUS EXAMINATIONS

1. SLE
2. Rheumatoid arthritis
3. Capillary microscopy; number of capillaries and dimensions; arteries and veins
4. DLE vs SLE
5. Antiphospholipid syndrome
6. Raynaud's disease
7. Calcinosis cutis
8. Le cell test
9. Gottron's sign
10. Occupational scleroderma
11. Smith's antigen
12. Lupus hair
13. Progressive systemic sclerosis
14. Clinical features, diagnosis and treatment of dermatomyositis
15. Scleromyxedema
16. ANA +ve and its significance
17. Carpet tack sign
18. HPE of morphea
19. Hailey-Hailey syndromes

## MULTIPLE CHOICE QUESTIONS

1. Gottron's papules are:                                      *(MH 2006)*
   (a) Lichenoid            (b) Psoriatic
   (c) Vesicular            (d) Pustular

2. A 42-year-old female has palpable purpura with rash over buttocks and thighs, pain in abdomen, and arthropathy. Likely diagnosis is:                           *(AI 08)*
   (a) Sweet syndrome       (b) HSP
   (c) Purpura fulminans    (d) Meningococcemia

3. Which of the following is not a feature of dermatomyositis?
                                              *(AIIMS Nov 09)*
   (a) Gottron's papules    (b) Periungual telangiectasia
   (c) Salmon rash          (d) Mechanic's hand

4. A 20-year-old woman presents with bilateral conductive deafness, palpable purpura on the legs and hemoptysis. Radiograph of the chest shows a thin-walled cavity in left upper zone. Investigations reveal total leukocyte count 12,000/mm³, red cell casts in the urine 12,000/mm³, and serum creatinine 3 mg/dl. What is the most probable diagnosis?    *(AI 2004)*
   (a) Henoch-Schönlein purpura
   (b) Polyarteritis nodosa
   (c) Wegener's granulomatosis
   (d) Disseminated tuberculosis

5. A 40-year-old woman presented with an 8-month history of erythema and swelling of the periorbital region and papules and plaques on the dorsolateral aspect of forearms and knuckles with ragged cuticles. There was no muscle weakness. The most likely diagnosis is:                    *(AIIMS Nov 2004)*
   (a) SLE
   (b) Dermatomyositis
   (c) Systemic sclerosis
   (d) Mixed connective tissue disorder

6. Palpable purpura is seen in the following *except:*    *(AI 2000)*
   (a) Cryoglobulinemia     (b) HSP
   (c) Giant cell arteritis (d) Drug-induced vasculitis

7. A 23-year-old female developed brown macular lesions over bridge of nose and cheek following exposure to light. The likely diagnosis is:                            *(AIIMS 99)*
   (a) SLE                  (b) Acne rosacea
   (c) Chloasma             (d) Photodermatitis

8. **"Pinch purpura" is diagnostic of:**                    *(AIIMS May 05)*
   (a) Primary systemic amyloidosis
   (b) Secondary systemic amyloidosis
   (c) ITP
   (d) Drug-induced purpura

9. **A 40-year-old farmer with the history of recurrent attacks of abdominal pain complains of itching when exposed to sunlight and maculopapular rash on sun-exposed areas. His symptoms are more during summer. What is the diagnosis?** *(AIIMS 01)*
   (a) Seborrheic keratosis        (b) Contact dermatitis
   (c) Psoriasis                   (d) Porphyria cutanea tarda

10. **A 45-year-old farmer has itchy erythematous papular lesions on face, neck, "V" area of chest, dorsum of hands and forearms for 3 years. The lesions are more severe in summers and improve by 75% in winters. The most appropriate test to diagnose the condition would be:** *(AI 06)*
    (a) Skin biopsy                (b) Estimation of IgE levels in blood
    (c) Patch test                 (d) Intradermal prick test

11. **'Carpet tack sign' is seen in:**                     *(DNB 12)*
    (a) Psoriasis                  (b) Discoid lupus erythematosus
    (c) Pemphigus vulgaris         (d) Erythema multiforme

## Answers

1. **Ans. (a)** Lichenoid *(Ref. Harrison's Internal Medicine, 17th edn, Table 383–2)*
2. **Ans. (b)** HSP *(Ref. Harrison's Principles of Internal Medicine, 17th edn, 2128)*
3. **Ans. (c)** Salmon rash *(Ref. Harrison's Internal Medicine, 17th edn, Table 383–2)*
4. **Ans. (c)** Wegener's granulomatosis
5. **Ans. (b)** Dermatomyositis *(Ref. Roxburgh's Skin Diseases, 7th edn, 83)*
6. **Ans. (c)** Giant cell arteritis *(Ref. Harrison's Internal Medicine, 17th edn/ Table 54–16)*
7. **Ans. (c)** Chloasma *(Ref. Roxburgh's Skin Diseases, 7th edn/239)*
8. **Ans. (a)** Primary systemic amyloidosis *(Ref. Harrison, 17th edn, Chapter 54)*
9. **Ans. (d)** Porphyria cutanea tarda *(Ref, Rook's Dermatology, 7th/ 57.13)*
10. **Ans. (a)** Skin biopsy
11. **Ans. (b)** Discoid lupus erythematosus

# 22 Skin Diseases in Pregnancy

## COMMON SKIN CHANGES IN PREGNANCY

- **Vascular changes and lesions**
  - ➤ There is increased skin blood flow during pregnancy and this makes the skin more prone to itch and to edema, manifest as tightening of rings and shoes.
  - ➤ Spider nevi and palmar erythema are common, as are hemangiomas.
  - ➤ Pyogenic granuloma may develop: This is a benign tumor with a tendency ulcerate and to bleed, and is sometimes clinically confused with melanoma. It often recurs after local destruction.
- **Pigmentary changes and pigmented lesions**
  - ➤ There is darkening of the nipples, genitalia, and linea alba.
  - ➤ The unsightly and sometimes psychologically distressing facial pigmentation of melasma (chloasma) affects many women, is worse with sunlight, and can be reduced by the use of high protection factor (SPF 25) UV B and UVA sunscreens.
  - ➤ Pigmented nevi can increase in number, size, and pigmentation.
  - ➤ Melanoma may occur and is associated with a poor prognosis in pregnant women.
  - ➤ Any rapidly changing, irregularly shaped, or irregularly pigmented mole should be biopsied to exclude a dysplastic nevus or melanoma.
- **Hair changes**
  - ➤ There is diminished shedding of hair, due to prolongation of anagen. This is perceived as thickening of the hair.
  - ➤ Increased sebum secretion makes hair appear more lustrous.
  - ➤ The synchronized shedding after parturition gives rise to the distressing postpartum telogen effluvium.
  - ➤ Hirsutism may begin or worsen in pregnancy as there is an associated increase in androgens.

- **Pilosebaceous changes**
  - ➢ The increased oestrogens of pregnancy usually improve acne, but there may be worsening of acne in some unfortunate patients, and the entire skin is usually greasier.
- **Striae**
  - ➢ Striae on the breasts and abdomen are very common in pregnancy, but do not necessarily relate to either the total weight gain or the rate of weight gain.
- **Cutaneous infections**
  - ➢ Candida of the vulva as well as the vagina may occur.
  - ➢ Cutaneous and genital warts thrive in pregnancy. Treatment of genital warts is by physical destruction as podophyllin must not be used in pregnancy.
  - ➢ Genital herpes simplex infections can pose problems as regards delivery during active infections.
- **The pregnancy dermatoses**
  - ➢ There are five major dermatoses which occur in pregnancy, and some that can be precipitated by pregnancy.
- **Pruritus of pregnancy**
  - ➢ Itching occurs in about 20% of pregnancies.

## CAUSES OF PRURITUS IN PREGNANCY

- General causes of pruritus
- Pruritic urticarial papules and plaques of pregnancy
  - ➢ Common, intense pruritus involving abdomen
  - ➢ May spread to thighs, buttocks, breasts and arms
- Prurigo of pregnancy (common)
  - ➢ Onset in second-half of pregnancy
- Herpes gestationis or pemphigoid gestationis (uncommon)
  - ➢ Autoimmune disorder with Graves' disease association
- Intrahepatic cholestasis of pregnancy (common)
  - ➢ No jaundice in mild form (prurigo gravidarum)
  - ➢ Trunk and extremity itching without rash
  - ➢ Occurs in second or third trimester and resolves with delivery
  - ➢ May recur in subsequent pregnancies or with OC pills.
  - ➢ **Treatment:** Ursodeoxycholic acid
- Pruritic folliculitis of pregnancy (uncommon)
- Non-primary pruritic conditions
  - ➢ Atopic dermatitis
  - ➢ Contact dermatitis

## SPECIFIC DERMATOSES OF PREGNANCY

- Pemphigoid (herpes) gestationis
- Polymorphic eruption of pregnancy
- Prurigo of pregnancy
- Pruritic folliculitis of pregnancy

### Herpes Gestationis

- **Pemphigoid gestationis** (PG), also known as **herpes gestationis,** is a rare, nonviral, subepidermal blistering disease of pregnancy and the puerperium.
- PG may begin during any trimester of pregnancy or present shortly after delivery.
- Lesions are usually distributed over the abdomen, trunk, and extremities; mucous membrane lesions are rare.
- Skin lesions in these patients may be quite polymorphic and consist of erythematous urticarial papules and plaques, vesiculopapules, and/or frank bullae. Lesions are almost always very pruritic.
- Severe exacerbations of PG frequently occur after delivery, typically within 24–48 hours.
- PG tends to recur in subsequent pregnancies, often beginning earlier during such gestations. Brief flare-ups of disease may occur with resumption of menses and may develop in patients later exposed to oral contraceptives.
- Occasionally, infants of affected mothers demonstrate transient skin lesions.
- Biopsies of early lesional skin show "teardrop-shaped" subepidermal vesicles forming in dermal papillae in association with an eosinophil-rich leukocytic infiltrate. Differentiation of PG from other subepidermal bullous diseases by light microscopy is difficult.
- Direct immunofluorescence microscopy of perilesional skin from PG patients reveals the immunopathologic hallmark of this disorder—*linear deposits of C3 in epidermal basement membrane.* These deposits develop as a consequence of complement activation produced by low titer IgG anti-basement membrane autoantibodies directed against BPAG2, the same hemidesmosome-associated protein that is targeted by autoantibodies in patients with BP—a subepidermal bullous disease that resembles PG clinically, histologically, and immunopathologically.
- **Treatment**
  - ➤ Many patients require treatment with moderate doses of daily glucocorticoids (i.e. 20–40 mg prednisone) at some point in their course.

> Mild cases (or brief flare-ups) may be controlled by vigorous use of potent topical glucocorticoids.
> Maternal prognosis is good.
> Infants born of mothers with PG appear to be at increased risk of being slightly premature or "small for dates".

### Polymorphic Eruption of Pregnancy (Pruritic Urticarial Papules and Plaques of Pregnancy)

- Eruption begins in third trimester usually in a primigravida
- Etiology is obscure. Related to abnormal weight gain in mother and twin pregnancy.
- Intense itching is present.
- Eruption consists predominantly of urticated papules and plaques.
- Lesions begin on abdomen closely following lines of striae
- Umbilicus is usually spared.
- **Treatment:** Topical emollients or steroids.
- No harm to the fetus.

### Prurigo of Pregnancy/Early Onset Prurigo of Pregnancy/Prurigo Gestationis of Besnier

- Begins between 25 and 30 weeks of pregnancy.
- Multiple excoriated papules over  the abdomen and extensor surfaces of the limbs
- Lesions may continue in the puerperium.
- Mother and fetus are unaffected.
- Disease may recur in subsequent pregnancies.

### Pruritic Folliculitis of Pregnancy

- Onset in second half of pregnancy
- Resolves within 2 weeks of delivery
- Erythematous follicular papules over trunk
- Lesions spread to extremities
- Mother and fetus are unaffected.

## LESS WELL DEFINED DERMATOSIS

### Impetigo Herpetiformis

- Generalized pustular psoriasis of pregnancy is a rare variant of pustular psoriasis, also called as impetigo herpetiformis.
- A rare eruption, occurring especially in pregnancy, with the features of generalized pustular psoriasis, but with a tendency to be symmetrical and grouped, and often starting in the flexures.

- Constitutional disturbance may be severe.
- Onset is usually in the last trimester of pregnancy.
- The eruption usually starts in the inguinogenital region and other flexures, with minute pustules arising on an acutely inflamed area of skin. These extend centrifugally, drying in the centre, or form plaques in which eroded greenish yellow pustules become fetid, crusted or vegetating.
- Reddish brown pigmentation is seen on healing.
- Buccal mucosa may be involved.
- Greater risk of stillbirth, neonatal abnormalities and death.
- Though the disease remits after parturition during the postpartum phase, recurrences are common in subsequent pregnancy.
- Systemic steroids are the drugs of choice for the treatment.

## Papular Dermatitis of Pregnancy

- The rash consists of widespread, 3–5 mm, intensely itchy papules with a small central crust.
- Higher fetal mortality with this eruption.

### QUESTIONS FROM PREVIOUS EXAMINATIONS

1. Herpes gestationis
2. Pupps
3. Pregnancy dermatosis
4. Impetigo herpetiformis

### MULTIPLE CHOICE QUESTIONS

1. **A pregnant female complains of sudden onset of multiple generalized vesiculobullous lesions almost all over the body associated with pain and mild fever. She also has associated bilateral knee joint pain without any redness or swelling of joints. On examination, the lesions are found to have pustular tips with surrounding red hue. She is diagnosed having pustular psoriasis. Which of the following is the most appropriate drug to be used in management of this patient?** *(AI 2008)*
   (a) Dapsone           (b) Isotretinoin
   (c) Prednisolone      (d) Methotrexate

2. Which is the characteristic lesion of pregnancy? *(AP 2008)*
   - (a) Vitiligo
   - (b) Pemphigus
   - (c) Tinea
   - (d) Chloasma

3. A 32-year-old pregnant female complained of pinkish depressed atrophic linear streaks over abdomen, buttocks, breasts, thighs, and arms, which have started appearing since a few weeks. The lesions are painless and non-itchy. What is the diagnosis?
   *(MP 11)*
   - (a) Linea nigra
   - (b) Striae gravidarum
   - (c) Melasma
   - (d) Pemphigoid gestationis

4. A 28-year-old pregnant female in 2nd trimester presented with complains of sudden onset of multiple slightly pruritic vesiculobullous lesions over abdomen and limbs. Which of the following is the most appropriate clinical diagnosis?
   *(AMU 2008)*
   - (a) Pustular psoriasis
   - (b) Pruritic folliculitis of pregnancy
   - (c) Prurigo of pregnancy
   - (d) Pemphigoid gestationis

## Answers

1. **Ans. (c)** Prednisolone
2. **Ans. (d)** Chloasma *(Ref. Oxford Textbook of Medicine, 4th edition, Chapter 13.13)*
3. **Ans. (b)** Striae gravidarum
4. **Ans. (d)** Pemphigoid gestationis.

# 23 Skin Manifestations of Endocrine Diseases

## HYPERPITUITARISM

- Dermatological features include a protruding, thickened lower lip, edematous thick eyelids, a large and furrowed tongue, triangular large ears, numerous skin tags ('fibroma molluscum'), widened skin pores, wet and oily skin due to hyperhidrosis and increased sebum production, acne and cutis gyrata of the scalp in more extreme cases.
- Hyperpigmentation develops in about half of the affected individuals due to increased levels of melanocyte-stimulating hormone (MSH), and acanthosis nigricans may occur.
- The scalp hair is initially coarse and there may be hirsutism, but later in the disease there is a decrease in gonadotrophin production, which causes the hair to become finer, with loss of secondary sexual hair.
- The nails are flat and wide and grow fast.

## HYPOPITUITARISM

- Pallor of the skin due to decreased MSH secretion results in generalized hypopigmentation, most apparent in the skin of the nipple, areola and genitalia; in contrast with anemia, the mucous membranes retain their normal color.
- There is an increased sunburn tendency and lack of tanning, and there may be a degree of carotenemia due to hypothyroidism.
- Loss of terminal hair due to decreased gonadotrophin secretion is observed in all patients, first in the axillae and later, but not invariably, in the pubic area.
- Fine wrinkling and dryness of the skin simulates advanced age.
- The face appears expressionless due to diminution of the facial skinfolds.
- The activity of sebaceous and sweat glands is reduced.

- Onycholysis, longitudinal ridging and brownish discoloration of the nail plate may be seen.
- Pituitary dwarfism is characterized by proportionate retardation.

## HYPERCORTICISM

- Truncal obesity (classically deposits of fat over the clavicles and back of the neck, the 'buffalo hump')
- Facial fullness and plethora ('moon facies') are most frequent
- Slender limbs
- Skin atrophy
- Fragility, bruising and poor healing
- Telangiectasia
- Striae (typically wide and red)
- Hirsutism
- Hypertrichosis (downy facial hair in iatrogenic hypercorticism) Acneiform lesions (often monomorphic and devoid of comedones and cysts)
- Male pattern baldness in women
- Dermatophyte and yeast infections

## ADDISON'S DISEASE/HYPOCORTICISM

- General symptoms include wasting, fatigue, orthostatic hypotension, dizziness, anorexia, abdominal pain and amenorrhea.
- Self-mutilation, presenting as gouges in the skin, has been reported as a result of psychiatric symptoms.
- Hyperpigmentation of the skin, due to increased secretion of pituitary MSH and ACTH as a response to low adrenal corticosteroid levels, is the cardinal dermatological feature. This develops insidiously and is often not recognized as abnormal by the patient.
- **Patterns of increased pigmentation**
  - ➢ Light-exposed areas—face, dorsa of hands
  - ➢ Areas subject to friction—elbows, knees, waistline, under bra straps
  - ➢ Accentuation of normally high pigmentation areas—genital, perineum, axillae
  - ➢ Areolae, umbilicus
  - ➢ Palmar creases
  - ➢ Tongue and mucous membranes
  - ➢ Scars
  - ➢ Hair and nails—longitudinal melanonychia

> Darkening of existing pigmented lesions (such as café au lait patches)
> Eruptive lentigines
> Mucous membrane lesions are usually spots or patches rather than diffuse pigmentation, and the oral pigmentation may persist after glucocorticoid replacement therapy.
> Scar pigmentation only occurs in scars acquired during adrenal insufficiency and is permanent—scars that precede the disorder or occur during therapy are unaffected.

- In women, in whom the adrenal gland is the main source of androgens, there may be loss of axillary and pubic hairs and improvement in acne.

## HYPERTHYROIDISM

- **Skin**
  > Soft, smooth, velvety
  > Increased skin temperature
  > Palmar erythema, facial flushing
  > Increased sweating
  > Pruritus
  > Hyperpigmentation
  > Pretibial myxedema
  > Vitiligo
  > Cutaneous signs of goiter: Pemberton sign and Maroni sign
  > Others—urticaria, palmoplantar pustulosis
- **Nails**
  > Fast nail growth
  > Soft nails, koilonychia
  > Distal onycholysis (Plummer's nails)
  > Thyroid acropachy
- **Hair**
  > Fine thin hair, diffuse alopecia
  > Alopecia areata

## HYPOTHYROIDISM

- The most prominent manifestation of hypothyroidism is related to dermal accumulation of mucopolysaccharides, in particular chondroitin sulphate and hyaluronic acid, which bind water in the tissue and lead to puffiness of the skin.

- The yellowish skin color is due to a combination of alterations in connective tissue of the dermis, carotenemia and vasoconstriction (due to the slowed metabolic rate).
- The connective tissue changes also cause loss of support of dermal vessels, and along with decreased levels of clotting factors, predispose to purpuric lesions or bruising.
  The hypometabolic state and low core temperature may cause cold extremities due to reflex vasoconstriction.
- **Skin**
  - ➤ Pale, cold, scaly and wrinkled skin
  - ➤ Xerosis, asteatotic eczema, itch
  - ➤ Palmoplantar keratoderma
  - ➤ Absence of sweating
  - ➤ Ivory-yellow skin color
  - ➤ Puffy edema of hands, face and eyelids
  - ➤ Purpura and ecchymoses
  - ➤ Punctate telangiectases on arms and fingertips
  - ➤ Delayed wound healing
  - ➤ Xanthomatosis (secondary to hyperlipidemia)
- **Nails**
  - ➤ Brittle and striated nails
  - ➤ Slow nail growth
- **Hair**
  - ➤ Coarse sparse scalp hair
  - ➤ Loss of pubic, axillary and facial hair
  - ➤ Loss of lateral eyebrows (madarosis)
- **Oral**
  - ➤ Large tongue
  - ➤ Gingival swelling (in congenital hypothyroidism)
  - ➤ Oral candidosis

## DIABETES MELLITUS AND SKIN

- Diabetes mellitus is a metabolic disorder characterized by elevated fasting and postprandial blood glucose levels and a variety of multisystem complications, mainly in the blood vessels, eye, kidney, nervous system and integument.
- Three main types can be distinguished.
  - ➤ Type 1, also known as insulin-dependent diabetes mellitus or juvenile-onset diabetes, is characterized by abrupt onset of symptoms, insulinopenia, dependence on insulin injections, proneness to ketoacidosis and lack of ability to produce C peptide.

➢ Type 2, non-insulin-dependent diabetes mellitus or adult onset diabetes, is characterized by lack of ketoacidosis except under stressful circumstances, ability to produce C peptide, a tendency to obesity and improvement following loss of weight.

➢ Type 3, secondary diabetes, is an additional type of diabetes, which occurs as a complication of pancreatic, hormonal or genetic disease or following ingestion of certain drugs or chemical compounds.

- **Skin symptoms due to diabetic vascular abnormalities**

  ➢ *Diabetic microangiopathy:* In diabetic microangiopathy, there is proliferation of endothelial cells and deposits of PAS-positive material in the basement membrane of arterioles, capillaries and venules with resulting decreased luminal area. Basement membrane thickening is a characteristic finding in diabetic and prediabetic patients. Microangiopathy is responsible for the retinopathy, nephropathy and possibly also neuropathy and dermopathy associated with diabetes.

  ➢ *Erysipelas-like erythema:* Well-demarcated, red areas occur on the legs or feet, and there may be underlying destructive bone disease caused by a small vessel insufficiency.

  ➢ *Wet gangrene of the foot:* This is a late manifestation of diabetic microangiopathy. Non-diabetic atherosclerotic subjects tend to develop a dry form as a result of large vessel insufficiency.

  ➢ *Diabetic rubeosis:* A peculiar rosy reddening of the face, and sometimes of the hands and feet, may be seen in long-standing diabetes.

  ➢ *Diabetic dermopathy (diabetic shin spots):* This is the most common dermatosis associated with diabetes mellitus. Lesions are predominantly situated on the shins, forearms, thighs and over bony prominences. Seen more frequently men than women. The initial lesion is an oval, dull-red papule 0.5–1 cm in diameter. It evolves slowly, producing a superficial scale, leaving an atrophic brownish scar. The color is due to hemosiderin in histiocytes near the vessels.

  ➢ *Large vessel disease:* Atherosclerosis is the second form of vascular disease frequently associated with diabetes mellitus. The patient shows intermittent claudication with pallid and cool skin distally on the extremities. The postural test discloses delayed filling of the veins. Common clinical sequelae are myocardial infarction, cerebral thrombosis, nephrosclerosis and ischemic gangrenous lesions of the legs and feet.

- **Diabetic neuropathy**
  - ➤ Elderly patients with an insidious onset of the disease are especially at risk.
  - ➤ Commonly, there is a distal symmetrical polyneuropathy with mixed motor and sensory nerve involvement.
  - ➤ The motor neuropathy of the foot is characterized by dorsally subluxed digits, distally displaced plantar fat pads, depressed metatarsal heads, hammer toes and pes cavus. Proper foot care is essential to prevent formation of indolent perforating ulcers ('mal perforans').
  - ➤ A painless and slowly penetrating ulcer of the sole and of other pressure sites is suggestive of diabetic neuropathy. The ulcer is circular and punched out in shape, occurring in the middle of a callosity.
  - ➤ Loss of temperature and pain sensation and absence of the ankle reflex (an early sign of diabetic neuropathy) indicate a neuropathic origin. Sensory abnormalities of the lower extremities include numbness, tingling, aching and burning.
  - ➤ Autonomic neuropathy may cause decreased or absent sweating of the lower extremities with compensatory sweating in other skin areas.
- **Cutaneous infections in diabetes mellitus**
  - ➤ Skin infections due to *Staphylococcus aureus* and group A *Streptococcus haemolyticus* are common in diabetic patients. Invasive Pseudomonas infection of the ear can progress through cellulitis and osteitis to cranial nerve damage and meningitis with a high mortality rate, so-called malignant otitis externa.
  - ➤ **Non-clostridial gas gangrene:** The commonest pathogens are *Escherichia coli,* Klebsiella, Pseudomonas and Bacteroides spp. in various combinations.
  - ➤ ***Candida albicans:*** *Candida albicans* infections of mouth, nail folds, genitals and intertriginous skin areas are frequent in diabetics.
- **Acanthosis nigricans:** Usually associated with insulin resistance.
- **Various skin disorders associated with diabetes mellitus**
  - ➤ Necrobiosis lipoidica
  - ➤ Disseminated granuloma annulare
  - ➤ Pruritus
  - ➤ Stiff joints and waxy skin
  - ➤ Scleredema diabeticorum
  - ➤ Vitiligo

- Lichen planus
- Hemochromatosis
- Eruptive xanthomas of the skin
- Finger pebbles
- Skin tags
- Reactive perforating collagenosis.

- **Local insulin reactions**
  - Insulin may cause immediate local reactions, starting as erythema, which turn urticarial within 30 min and subside within an hour; these are probably IgE mediated.
  - Serious generalized immediate reactions are rare. The most common reactions are delayed, starting about 2 weeks after onset of insulin therapy. An itchy nodule develops at the site of injection. It lasts for days and heals with hyperpigmentation and perhaps a scar. Delayed hypersensitivity is involved.
  - **Insulin lipodystrophy.** Insulin lipodystrophy is rare. Patients present with atrophic plaques at the sites of insulin injection. There is atrophy of the subcutaneous fat. The lesions seldom show complete spontaneous resolution. The mechanism is not known.

- **Diabetic bullae**
  - The location is the lower legs and feet, occasionally hands and fingers. They range in size from less than one centimeter to several centimeters. A typical blister arises on a non-inflamed base, and heals without scarring in 2–5 weeks.

## QUESTIONS FROM PREVIOUS EXAMINATIONS

1. Diabetes and skin
2. Skin changes in thyroid disorders.

## MULTIPLE CHOICE QUESTIONS

1. **Typical dermatological features of chronic cortisol excess include the following** *except:*
   - (a) Thick skin
   - (b) Easy bruisability
   - (c) Acne
   - (d) Purple striae
2. **Cutaneous calciphylaxis is associated with:**
   - (a) Cushing's syndrome
   - (b) Hypothyroidism
   - (c) Hyperparathyroidism
   - (d) All of the above

3. **Wrong about acanthosis nigrigans:**
   (a) May be present in patients with acromegaly
   (b) The skin, mostly in the axillae and nape of the neck is affected.
   (c) The biopsy reveals hyperkeratosis and papillomatosis with slight acanthosis.
   (d) The dark color of the lesion is due to melanin deposition.

4. **Mucocutaneous candidiasis is associated with the following *except*:**
   (a) Autoimmune polyglandular syndrome
   (b) Diabetes mellitus
   (c) Cushing's syndrome
   (d) Hyperparathyroidism

5. **Necrolytic migratory erythema is feature of:**
   (a) Pseudohypoparathyroidism
   (b) Glucagonoma syndrome
   (c) Autoimmunepolyglandular syndrome type 1
   (d) Autoimmune polyglandular syndrome type 2

6. **Telogen effluvium is feature of:**
   (a) Diabetes mellitus        (b) Thyroid disorders
   (c) Addison's disease        (d) Pituitary tumors

7. **The drug considered as a risk factor for calciphylaxis is**
   (a) Calcium
   (b) Diuretic
   (c) Warfarin
   (d) Heparin

8. **A skin lesion in pretibial region of a 28-year-old diabetic woman is shown. What is the probable diagnosis?**
   (a) Necrobiosis lipoidica diabeticorum
   (b) Granuloma annulare
   (c) *Tenia corporis*
   (d) Telangiectasis

## Answers

1. **Ans. (a)** Thick skin.

   Typical features of chronic cortisol excess include thin skin, central obesity, hypertension, plethoric moon facies, purple striae and easy bruisability, glucose intolerance or diabetes mellitus, gonadal dysfunction, osteoporosis, proximal muscle weakness, signs of hyperandrogenism (acne, hirsutism), and psychological disturbances (depression, mania, and psychoses).

   Both systemic and topical glucocorticoids cause a variety of atrophic skin changes, including atrophy. Glucocorticoids play no role in maintenance therapy in either UC or CD. Once clinical remission has been induced, they should be tapered according to the clinical activity, normally at a rate of no more than 5 mg/week. They can usually be tapered to 20 mg/d within 4–5 weeks but often take several months to be discontinued altogether. The side effects are numerous, including fluid retention, abdominal striae, fat redistribution, hyperglycemia, subcapsular cataracts, osteonecrosis, osteoporosis, myopathy, emotional disturbances, and withdrawal symptoms.

2. **Ans. (c)** Hyperparathyroidism.

| Skin lesions in endocrine disorders | |
|---|---|
| *Lesions* | *Associated conditions* |
| Acanthosis nigricans | Acromegaly, hyperprolactinemia, DM, Cushing's syndrome, excessive androgen production |
| Acne | Cushing's syndrome, hyperprolactinemia, excessive androgen production |
| Acquired ichthyosis | Hypothyroidism |
| Acquired perforating dermatosis | DM |
| Alopecia areata/universalis | Hypoparathyroidism, APS-1, hyperthyroidism |
| Asteatotic eczema | Hypothyroidism |
| Atopic dermatitis | Hyperthyroidism |
| Autoimmune bullous diseases | DM, hyperthyroidism, hypoparathyroidism |
| Calciphylaxis | Hyperparathyroidism, DM |
| Cherry angioma | Hyperprolactinemia |
| Chronic urticaria | Hyperthyroidism, DM |
| Cutis verticis gyrata | Acromegaly |
| Deep mycotic infections | DM, Cushing's syndrome |
| Dermatophyte infections | DM, Cushing's syndrome |
| Eruptive xanthoma | DM |
| Erythrasma | DM |
| Foot ulcers | DM |
| Generalized myxedema | Hypothyroidism |
| Granuloma annulare | DM |

3. **Ans. (d)** The dark color of the lesion is due to melanin deposition. Acanthosis nigrigans may be present in patients with acromegaly, hyperprolactinemia, diabetes mellitus (DM).

Cushing's syndrome, and excessive androgen production.

The skin, mostly in the axillae and nape of the neck becomes dark, soft, and velvet-like with delicate folds. The biopsy reveals hyperkeratosis and papillomatosis with slight acanthosis. The valleys between the papillae are filled with keratotic material. Slight hyperpigmentation of the basal cell layer can be seen, but the dark color of the lesion is due to hyperkeratosis rather than melanin.

**4. Ans. (d)** Hyperparathyroidism.

| | |
|---|---|
| Hyperpigmentation | Addison's disease, ectopic ACTH syndrome, Cushing's disease, hyperthyroidism, POEMS syndrome |
| Hypertrichosis | Cushing's syndrome |
| Langerhans' cell histiocytosis | Diabetes insipidus, hypopituitarism |
| Lipoatrophy/lipohypertrophy | DM |
| Loss of pigmentation | Hypopituitarism |
| Metastatic calcification | Hyperparathyroidism |
| Mucosal or cutaneous candidiasis | APS-1, DM, Cushing's syndrome |
| Necrobiosis lipoidica | DM |
| Necrolytic migratory erythema | Glucagonoma syndrome |
| Oral lichen planus | DM, hypothyroidism |
| Osteoma cuits | Pseudohypoparathyroidism |
| Palmar and plantar erythema | DM |
| Palmoplantar keratoderma | Hypothyroidism |
| Periungual telangiectasia | DM |
| Pretibial myxedema | Hyperthyroidism |
| Primary cutaneous amyloidosis (macular or lichenoid amyloidosis) | Hyperparathyroidism, pheochromocytoma |
| Psoriasis (generalized or pustular) | Hypoparathyroidism |
| Pseudomonas infections | DM |

**5. Ans. (b)** Glucagonoma syndrome.

**Necrolytic migratory erythema**

Necrolytic migratory erythema is a paraneoplastic cutaneous sign associated with a glucagon-secreting tumor, which is malignant in the majority of cases. The distinctive skin lesions of necrolytic migratory erythema are situated mainly on the face in perioral and perinasal distribution, the perineum, genitalia, shins, ankles, and feet. These are annular or circinate erythematous and flaccid vesiculopustular lesions, leading to crusted erosions. Various histopathological findings may be seen depending on the type of lesion that is biopsied. The most distinctive histopathologic feature is the pale, vacuolated keratinocytes in the upper layers of the epidermis, ending up with necrosis, leading to subcorneal or intraepidermal cleft formation. Subcorneal pustules may be evident adjacent to necrotic areas. There is usually a broad parakeratotic scale, in which Candida may be noted.

6. **Ans. (b)** Thyroid disorders.

| | |
|---|---|
| Scleredema | DM |
| Shin spots or pigmented pretibial papules | DM |
| Skin tags (acrochordon) | Acromegaly, DM |
| Staphylococcal pyoderma (carbuncule, furuncle | DM, Cushing's syndrome |
| Striae | Cushing's syndrome |
| Subcutaneous ossification | Albright hereditary osteodystrophy |
| Telogen effluvium | Hyperthyroidism, hypothyroidism |
| Ungual dystrophy | Hypoparathyroidism |
| Vitiligo | Hypoparathyroidism, DM, APS-1 hypothyroidism, hyperthyroidism |
| Xanthoma disseminatum | Diabetes insipidus |

APS: Autoimmune polyglandular syndrome, DM: Diabetes mellitus.

7. **Ans. (c)** Warfarin.

Administration of *warfarin* can result in painful areas of erythema that become purpuric and then necrotic with an adherent black eschar; the condition is referred to as warfarin-induced necrosis. This reaction is seen more often in women and in areas with abundant subcutaneous fat—breasts, abdomen, buttocks, thighs, and calves.

The erythema and purpura develop between the third and tenth day of therapy, most likely as a result of a transient imbalance in the levels of anticoagulant and procoagulant vitamin K-dependent factors.

Continued therapy does not exacerbate pre-existing lesions, and patients with an inherited or acquired deficiency of protein C are at increased risk for this particular.

8. **Ans. (a)** Necrobiosis lipoidica diabeticorum.

Large symmetric plaque with active tan-pink, well-demarcated, raised, firm borders and a yellow center. The central parts of the lesion are depressed with atrophic changes of epidermal thinning and telangiectasis against a yellow background. Necrobiosis lipoidica diabeticorum.

# 24 Skin Manifestations of Internal Malignancies and Skin Malignancies

## CUTANEOUS MARKERS OF INTERNAL MALIGNANCY

- **Cutaneous markers can be classified into 2 major types**
  - Genetically determined syndromes with a cutaneous component (genodermatoses) that predispose at risk individuals to develop cancer.
  - Paraneoplastic syndromes which occur as a result of circulating factor(s) or presumed factors produced by the underlying cancer.
- **Genodermatoses**
  - Skin diseases that come under the group of genodermatoses include:
    - Cowden's disease
    - Gardner's syndrome
    - Gorlin's syndrome
    - Multiple endocrine neoplasm type 2B
    - Neurofibromatosis
    - Peutz-Jeghers syndrome
    - Torre-Muir syndrome
    - Progeria (premature aging syndromes)
- **Paraneoplastic syndromes**
  - Cutaneous paraneoplastic syndromes can be categorized according to the type of lesion they produce (Table 24.1).

| Table 24.1: Types of cutaneous paraneoplastic syndromes | |
| --- | --- |
| *Papulosquamous* | *Erythematous* |
| • Acanthosis nigricans | • Dermatomyositis |
| • Acquired ichthyosis | • Erythema gyratum repens (erythema annulare centrifugum) |
| • Acrokeratosis paraneoplastica | • Hypertrophic osteoarthropathy and digital clubbing |

*Contd.*

**Table 24.1:** Types of cutaneous paraneoplastic syndromes *(Contd.)*

| *Papulosquamous* | *Erythematous* |
|---|---|
| • Extramammary Paget disease | • Multicentric reticulohistiocytosis |
| • Florid cutaneous papillomatosis | • Necrolytic migratory erythema |
| • Palmoplantar keratoderma | • Sweet disease |
| • Pityriasis rotunda | |
| • Sign of Leser-Trélat | |
| • Tripe palms | |
| *Bullous* | *Miscellaneous* |
| • Paraneoplastic pemphigus | • Generalized granuloma annulare (rarely) |
| • Bullous pemphigoid | • Carcinoid syndrome |
| | • Hypertrichosis lanuginosa acquisita |
| | • Trousseau's syndrome |

- **Dermatologic manifestations of malignancy** (Table 24.2)

**Table 24.2:** Dermatological manifestations of malignancy

| *Manifestation* | *Associated cancer* |
|---|---|
| 1. Erythema gyratum repens | Lung cancer (commonest underlying neoplasm) |
| 2. Necrolytic migratory erythema | Glucagonoma syndrome |
| 3. Erythema annulare centrifugum | Myeloproliferative disorders |
| 4. Porphyria cutanea tarda, acute intermittent and variegate porphyrias | Hepatocellular carcinoma |
| 5. Linear IgA disease | Lymphoproliferative malignancy |
| 6. Erythema multiforme-like eruptions | Carcinomas, lymphomas and leukemias, particularly myelomonocytic types |
| 7. Migratory thrombophlebitis (Trousseau's sign) | Carcinoma of the pancreas, stomach and lung |
| 8. Transient acantholytic dermatosis | Myelogenous leukemia and carcinoma of the genitourinary tract |
| 9. Pyoderma gangrenosum (in a superficial and bullous form) | Myeloproliferative diseases, including acute and chronic myeloid leukemia, acute lymphocytic leukemia, myeloid metaplasia, PRV, multiple myeloma, lymphoma and myelofibrosis. Also with UC. |
| 10. Sweet's syndrome | Hemopoietic malignancies |

*Contd.*

**Table 24.2:** Dermatological manifestations of malignancy (*Contd.*)

| *Manifestation* | *Associated cancer* |
| --- | --- |
| 11. Erythroderma | Mycosis fungoides and Sézary syndrome |
| 12. Leser-Trélat sign (sudden development of numerous seborrheic keratoses, in an eruptive fashion with or without pruritus) | Internal malignancy |
| 13. Seed-like keratoses of the palms and soles | Internal malignancy |
| 14. Clubbing and hypertrophic osteoarthropathy | Commonest being carcinoma of the bronchus |
| 15. Cutis verticis gyrate | Paraneoplastic phenomenon |
| 16. Scleroderma-like skin changes | Carcinoid syndrome |
| 17. Acquired hypertrichosis lanuginosa | Internal malignancy |
| 18. Generalized hyperhidrosis | Malignant disease |
| 19. Lichen planus | Neoplasia (oral squamous carcinoma) |

- **Chromosomal breakage syndromes**
  - These are a group of genetic disorders that typically are transmitted in an autosomal recessive mode of inheritance and are characterized by a defect in DNA repair mechanisms or genomic instability, and patients with these disorders show increased predisposition to cancer (Table 24.3).
  - All patients are sensitive to UV radiation, although the major feature of one of the disorders, ataxia-telangiectasia (Louis-Bar syndrome), is hypersensitivity to ionizing radiation.
  - These disorders are relatively rare and often lethal.
  - **These include**
    - Ataxia-telangiectasia (AT)
    - Bloom syndrome (BS)
    - Fanconi's anemia (FA)
    - Xeroderma pigmentosum (XP)
  - These syndromes are characterized by different types of cancer; including leukemia, lymphoma, and solid tumors (e.g. skin cancer).
  - In addition, the syndromes are associated with other traits, such as cerebellar ataxia, immunodeficiencies, growth retardation, microcephaly, skeletal abnormalities, hypogonadism, pancytopenia, and abnormal pigmentation.

**Table 24.3:** Chromosomal breakage syndromes with neoplasias caused by defective DNA repair

1. **Ataxia-telangiectasia**: 11q22.3 Roentgen therapy, ionizing radiation, UV: Decreased IgA, IgG2, IgG, IgE; No increased sister chromatid exchanges (SCE) but increased gaps and breaks, nonhomologous interchanges; 1 : 8 acute lymphocytic leukemia, lymphoma, epithelial cancer, gliomas, and breast cancer.

2. **Bloom syndrome**: 15q26.1 UV, cancer chemotherapeutic agents: Decreased IgA and IgM, and/or IgG, 12–15 times higher SCE, homologous interchanges, increased gaps and breaks 1 : 5–8 leukemia, lymphoma, adenocarcinoma, and others.

3. **Fanconi's anemia**: UV, chemotherapeutic agents for immunosuppression, diepoxybutane, other DNA cross-linking agents; Increased gaps and breaks, 30% between nonhomologous chromosomes, clones with translocations; Aplastic anemia: Pancytopenia, leukemia, acute myeloid leukemia, squamous cell carcinoma, and others.

4. **Xeroderma pigmentosum**: UV, increased gaps and breaks, increased SCE after UV, 1000-fold increased risk to skin lesions, malignant melanoma, keratoacanthomas, and others.

## Benign Tumors

### Nevus

- Nevus is the Latin word for 'maternal impression' or 'birthmark' and indicates a circumscribed, non-neoplastic skin or mucosal lesion, usually present at or soon afterbirth, and fixed.
- Nevi are classified as:
  - ➢ Epidermal nevi
  - ➢ Dermal nevi
  - ➢ Subcutaneous nevi
  - ➢ Vascular nevi

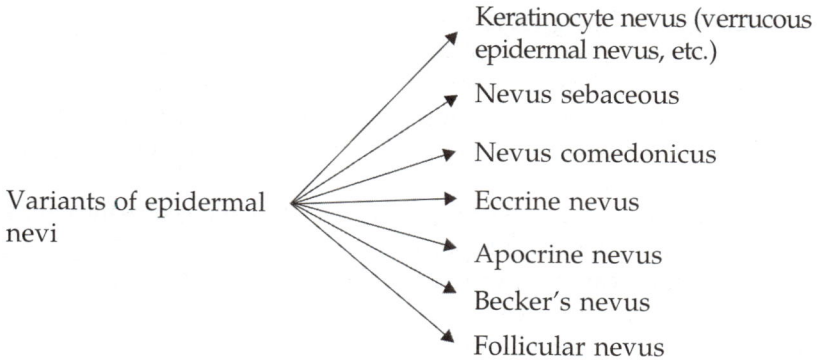

Variants of epidermal nevi:
- Keratinocyte nevus (verrucous epidermal nevus, etc.)
- Nevus sebaceous
- Nevus comedonicus
- Eccrine nevus
- Apocrine nevus
- Becker's nevus
- Follicular nevus

- Verrucous epidermal nevi are congenital, non-inflammatory cutaneous hamartomas composed of keratinocytes.
  - Their prevalence in adults is probably 0.1–0.5%.
  - Occur equally in males and females.
  - Present at birth. Develop during infancy.
  - Linear configuration common, especially along the skin tension lines.
  - Appears as typical verrucous papules that coalesce to form well-demarcated, skin-colored to brown papillomatous plaques.
  - They are divided into epidermolytic and non-epidermolytic types.
  - **Epidermolytic verrucous epidermal nevus:** Epidermolytic verrucous epidermal nevi show hyperkeratosis, acanthosis and papillomatosis with epidermolytic hyperkeratosis identical to that seen in bullous ichthyosiform erythroderma. This comprises perinuclear vacuolization of the keratinocytes, associated with premature and excessive formation of irregular keratohyalin granules, indistinct cell borders and hyperkeratosis.
  - **Non-epidermolytic verrucous epidermal nevus:** The most common histological pattern is sharply demarcated hyper-keratosis and acanthosis, often associated with papillomatosis, and occasionally by focal hypergranulosis and/or columns of parakeratosis. About 10% of lesions show a distinctive 'church-spire' pattern of acanthosis and hyperkeratosis, resembling acrokeratosis verruciformis.
- **Melanocytic nevi**
  - Melanocytic nevi are normal, benign proliferations of melanocytes. Although the risk of a nevus evolving into a melanoma is extremely small, melanocytic nevi are both risk factors for melanoma and precursors of melanoma.
  - They are classified into congenital and acquired.
  - **Congenital melanocytic nevi**
    - Nevus is present at birth.
    - Small congenital nevi are defined as under 1.5 cm in diameter, large as having a diameter between 1.5 and 20 cm and giant nevi as having a diameter of 20 cm or more (Fig. 24.1).
    - The majority are macular at birth. As the child grows the nevus usually grows in proportion.
    - A significant proportion of nevi become paler in the first 1 to 2 years of life, and at sites such as the scalp may fade to cosmetic insignificance.

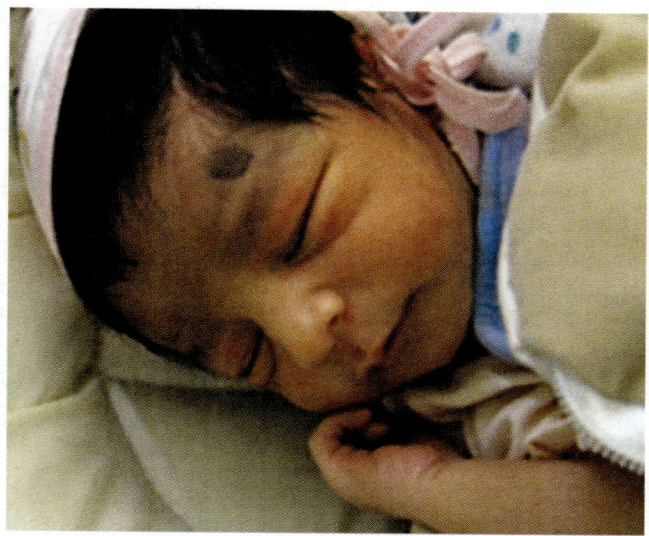

**Fig. 24.1:** Congenital melanocytic nevus on forehead

- The giant, garment or bathing-trunk nevus is very rare. The common site is the lower back and thigh area and a very large proportion of the infant's surface area may be involved. There may also be large numbers of smaller congenital nevi present elsewhere on the infant's skin; increased numbers of these will develop over time. These are called satellite nevi.

➤ *Acquired melanocytic nevus*
  - A benign cluster of melanocytic nevus cells arising as a result of proliferation of melanocytes at the dermal–epidermal junction.
  - These may all remain in contact with the basal layer of the epidermis, giving rise to the junctional nevus. In other nevi, some of the nevus cells may migrate into the dermis over time, giving rise to the compound nevus. The end stage of this process is when there are no nevus cells attached to the epidermis and all are lying free in the dermis. This pattern is that of the mature intradermal nevus.
  - *Junctional nevus* is a macular brown lesion, which may show pigment lying along the normal skin markings. It may have a slightly irregular lateral margin because of this, and may have a large diameter of up to 10 mm. The pigmentation tends to be uniform and regular.

- The *compound nevus* usually slowly becomes raised above the epidermal surface and may be round or oval. The color varies with the natural pigmentation of the patient and may be very dark, but the majority become paler with age. There is usually a little, if any pigment on the flat surrounding epidermis. It is important to recognize that slow elevation and the transformation of a macular melanocytic nevus to a palpable symmetrical, evenly pigmented symmetrical papule over time, is not a sign of malignant change but a normal maturation pattern of these nevi.
- *Intradermal nevi* are frequently raised, dome-shaped, non-pigmented nodules, most commonly seen on the face. There are often some overlying telangiectatic vessels and outgrowth of one or two coarse terminal hairs is common.

➢ *Halo nevus/Sutton's nevus*
- A melanocytic nevus surrounded by a depigmented halo of otherwise normal skin.

➢ *Meyerson's nevus*
- A melanocytic nevus that has developed an associated inflammatory reaction, which looks like eczema.

## Seborrheic Keratoses
- A benign tumor, frequently pigmented, more common in the elderly and composed of epidermal keratinocytes.
- Seborrheic keratoses are most often evident during the fifth decade, but may be present as early as the third decade.
- Equal incidence in males and females.
- Most lesions are found on the trunk with a smaller number on the limbs, head and neck.
- They are usually asymptomatic but may be itchy.
- The most common appearance is that of a very superficial verrucous plaque which appears to be stuck on the epidermis, varying from dirty yellow to black in color and having loosely adherent, greasy keratin on the surface.
- The shape is round or oval and multiple lesions may be seen.
- Size varies from 1 mm to several cm.
- On the eyelids and major flexures, seborrheic keratoses may be pedunculated and less keratotic.
- Irritation or infection causes swelling, sometimes bleeding, oozing and crusting, and a deepening of the color because of inflammation.

- **Indications for excision**
  - ➢ Cosmesis
  - ➢ Local irritation due to recurrent trauma
  - ➢ Malignancy suspected (excisional biopsy needed).
- **Treatment:** Chemical or electrocautery

## Leser-Trélat Sign

- The sudden onset of multiple rapidly growing seborrheic keratoses (SKs) associated with pruritus is known as the sign of Leser-Trélat, and may indicate an underlying visceral malignancy, a leukemia, or lymphoma.
- Associated with underlying adenocarcinoma
  - ➢ Stomach cancer
  - ➢ Colon cancer
  - ➢ Breast cancer

## Dermatosis Papulosa Nigra

- A pigmented papular eruption of the face and neck caused by a nevoid developmental defect of the pilosebaceous follicles, with histology resembling seborrheic keratoses.
- The condition is most common in black races.
- Etiology: This lesion is probably genetically determined.
- Incidence is higher in females than males.
- The individual lesions are black or dark brown, flattened or cupuliform papules 1–5 mm in diameter.
- They are most numerous in the malar regions and on the forehead. They are rare on the lower parts of the face and the chin, but in a few individuals may be found on the neck, chest and back.
- Treatment is seldom requested. Removal with the diathermy or cautery is effective.

## Skin Tags/Soft Warts/Achrochordon

- A common, benign lesion composed of loose fibrous tissue and occurring mainly on the neck and major flexures as a small, soft, pedunculated protrusion.
- These lesions are very common, particularly in women at the menopause or later.
- The lesions are pedunculated and may have a long stalk. They vary in size and are about 2 mm in diameter on average.
- They are round, soft and inelastic. The color may be unchanged, but they are frequently hyperpigmented.

- The most common site is on the sides of the neck, where they may be mixed with typical small, sessile, seborrheic keratoses. When more profuse, they can extend onto the face or down to the back and chest. Similar lesions may be found in and around the axillae and groins.
- **Treatment:** Both cautery and cryotherapy with liquid nitrogen are effective.

### Milium

- A small subepidermal keratin cyst.
- Milia are quite common at all ages from infancy onwards.
- They may arise spontaneously or follow some dermatological disorder particularly in second-degree burns, epidermolysis bullosa, porphyria cutanea tarda and bullous lichen planus.
- They may also follow dermabrasion and occur in areas of chronic topical corticosteroid-induced atrophy.
- The lesions are firm, white or yellowish, rarely more than 1 or 2 mm in diameter and appear to be immediately beneath the epidermis. They are usually noticed only on the face, and occur in the areas of vellus hair follicles, on the cheeks and eyelids particularly.
- **Treatment:** Incision of the epidermis over the milium with a cutting edge needle or sharp-pointed scalpel and squeezing out the contents is usually effective. Recurrence is uncommon. Spontaneous disappearance occurs in many milia in infants.

### Pyogenic Granuloma

- A vascular nodule that develops rapidly, often at the site of a recent injury, and which is composed of a lobular proliferation of capillaries in a loose stroma.
- Common lesion affecting both sexes with a predilection for males except for lesions that occur in the oral cavity which are more common in females.
- It may occur at any age with a peak in the second decade of life.
  Granuloma gravidarum is a variant of pyogenic granuloma that presents in the oral cavity during pregnancy.
- The tumor is vascular, bright red to brownish red or blue–black in color.
- It is partially compressible, but cannot be completely blanched and does not show pulsation. Older and darker lesions are frequently eroded and crusted, and may bleed very easily. Occasionally, the surface is raspberry-like or even verrucous.

- The base is often pedunculated and surrounded by a collar of acanthotic epidermis; the lesion may be sessile.

  The common sites are the hands, especially the fingers, the feet, lips, head and upper trunk, and the mucosal surfaces of the mouth and perianal area.
- **Treatment.** The pedunculated lesions are easy to treat by curettage with cauterization or diathermy coagulation of the base. Recurrence is common.
- Other treatment modalities that have been used include Nd:YAG laser, cryosurgery, intralesional steroids, flash lamp pulsed dye (FLPD) laser and even injection of absolute ethanol.

## Hypertrophic Scars and Keloids

- Both conditions represent an excessive connective tissue response to injury, which may be trivial.
- A keloid (cheloid, meaning 'crabclaw') is a benign, well-demarcated area of fibrous tissue overgrowth that extends beyond the original defect.
- A hypertrophic scar is similar, but remains confined to the initial defect and tends to resolve with time (Table 24.4).
- The cause is unknown, although both local and constitutional factors are involved. A scar at any site has the potential to become hypertrophic or keloidal, although the earlobes, chin, neck, shoulders, upper trunk and lower legs are especially vulnerable.
- Ear piercing is an important cause of earlobe keloids.
- Burns or scalds and infected lesions predispose to hypertrophy.
- Another risk factor is the presence of foreign material, either exogenous (e.g. suture material) or endogenous (e.g. embedded hair).
- Some races, notably Afro-Caribbeans, are more prone to develop keloids than others.
- A positive family history is obtained in 5–10%.
- Keloids are rare in infancy and old age, occurring chiefly between puberty and the age of 30 years.
- Women have a greater predisposition, and keloids may occur or enlarge during pregnancy.
- Both hypertrophic scars and keloids become raised and thickened within 3–4 weeks of the provocative stimulus.
- The lesion becomes a firm, pink or red plaque, which may grow for months or years. Lesions often assume a 'dumb-bell' configuration, but sometimes become bizarre and irregular.

- Usually, a hypertrophic scar shows signs of regression after a few months. The surface of a keloid becomes smoother and rounder, extending beyond the area of the original lesion.
- Spontaneous keloids usually develop on the presternal region or upper chest.
- **Prophylaxis and treatment:** Non-essential surgery should be avoided in the sites of predilection. If surgery is necessary, simple excision, ideally intralesional (core) excision, aiming to minimize skin tension and secondary infection, is preferable to electro-coagulation or caustic chemicals. In an individual at risk, preoperative radiotherapy to the excision site may be useful.
- Some lesions respond to pressure alone, or to occlusion with a hydrocolloid dressing.
- Small keloids can respond to self-adherent silicone sheeting/silicone gel.
- Intralesional triamcinolone (10 mg/ml) is useful, especially in early lesions. Several injections may be necessary at intervals of 3–6 weeks. Cryotherapy is also effective.
- Radiotherapy, topical retinoic acid, intralesional 5-fluorouracil and 585 nm flashlamp-pumped pulsed dye laser have been used in Table 24.5.

**Table 24.4:** Differences between keloid and hypertrophic scar

| Property | Keloid | Hypertrophic scars |
|---|---|---|
| Stays in confines of injury | No | Yes |
| Precipitated by trauma | Not always | Yes |
| Area of occurrence | Area of a little motion | Area of motion |
| Growth | For extended period | Regress in time |
| Symptomatic | Usually | Usually |
| Response to treatment | Poor | Good |
| Sodium (osmotic pressure) | Normal | Decreased |
| Magnesium (metabolic activity) | Increased | Decreased |
| Calcium (reflects collagen metabolism) | Increased | Decreased |
| Mucinous ground substance | Abundant | Scanty |
| Fibroblasts | Few | Numerous |
| Foreign body reactions | None | Frequent |
| Luxol fast blue collagen stain | Reddish | Blue |
| Mast cells | Increased | Increased |
| Pathogenesis | Unknown | Unknown |
| Contains myofibroblasts | No | Yes |
| Alanine transaminase | Increased | Normal |

**Table 24.5:** Proposed mechanisms of various pharmacologic treatments for keloids

| Pharmacologic treatment | Mechanism of action |
|---|---|
| Triamcinolone acetonide | Inhibits alpha-2 macroglobulins (inhibits collagenase breakdown of collagen): Decreases production of TGF-beta 1 |
| Interferon | Inhibits types I, III, and possibly IV collagen synthesis via reduction in cellular messenger RNA |
| 5-fluorouracil | Inhibits fibroblast proliferation by blocking DNA synthesis and transcription through competitive inhibition of thymidylate synthesis |
| Imiquimod | Stimulates immune pathways enhancing healing ability; induces local synthesis of cytokines causing down-regulation of collagen synthesis |
| Bleomycin sulfate | Inhibits TFG-beta stimulated collagen synthesis in skin fibroblasts |
| Retinoic acid | Inhibits DNA synthesis in lymphocytes and fibroblasts *in vitro* |
| Tacrolimus | Inhibits TNF-alpha and decreases expression of gli-1 oncogene, which has increased expression in keloids |
| Calcium channel blockers | Induces changes in fibroblast gene expression, resulting in decreased collagen synthesis and increased collagenase production |
| Pentoxifylline | Modulates dermal fibroblast deposition of extracellular matrix components *in vitro* |
| Colchicine | Inhibits collagen synthesis, microtubular and collagenase stimulation |

## Premalignant Skin Conditions

### *Actinic Keratosis*

- Hyperkeratotic lesions occurring on chronically light-exposed adult skin, which are focal areas of abnormal proliferation and differentiation that carry a low risk of progression to invasive SCC. Majority of actinic keratoses (AKs) occur on sun-exposed sites in fair-skinned people.
- **Etiology:** Excessive sun exposure, ionizing radiation or radiant heat and in workers exposed to pitch and other products of coal distillation.

- These lesions occur usually in middle aged or elderly subjects on habitually sun-exposed areas such as the face, scalp and dorsa of the hands. The vermilion of the lower lip but not often of the upper lip may also show keratosis.
- Knobloch syndrome (lesions are usually multiple and comprised of either macules or papules with a rough scaly surface resulting from disorganized keratinization and a variable degree of inflammation.
- Lesions vary in size from less than 1 mm to over 2 cm and are usually asymptomatic.
- Later lesions are covered with dry, rough, adherent and often yellow- or brown-colored scale. The adherent scale can only be picked off with difficulty, revealing a hyperemic base with punctate bleeding points.
- **Treatment:** Topical 5-fluorouracil, topical tretinoin, cryotherapy, curettage.

### Bowen's Disease

- A form of intraepidermal SCC characterized by a persistent, non-elevated, red, scaly or crusted plaque with a small potential for invasive malignancy.
- Common in fair skinned individuals.
- Most cases of typical Bowen's disease are found on the lower legs of elderly women.
- **Etiology:** Chronic sun exposure and exposure to arsenic.

  The initial change is a small, red and slightly scaly area, which is symptomless and gradually enlarges in a somewhat irregular fashion. The white or yellowish scale is detached without much difficulty to give a moist, reddened and at times granular surface, but without producing bleeding.
- The margin is well-demarcated and the lesion slightly raised; the surface is usually flat, but may become hyperkeratotic or crusted.
- **Treatment:** Cryotherapy; curettage and cautery; PDT (photo-dynamic therapy); laser destruction; excision; 5-fluorouracil cream; imiquimod cream; and radiotherapy.
- Surgical excision is a useful approach, particularly for small lesions in poor healing sites, perineal lesions and digital lesions.

### Erythroplasia of Queyrat

Bowen's disease of the mucosa of the penis.

## Bowenoid Papulosis of the Genitalia

- Bowenoid papulosis (BP) is characterized clinically by lesions with a benign appearance which show histological features suggestive of squamous cell neoplasia.
- Most of the lesions either regress spontaneously over time or undergo resolution after local treatment.
- BP is now generally viewed as a localized form of *in situ* SCC which develops as a consequence of infection by high-risk human papillomavirus, especially HPV 16 and HPV 18.
- Treatment of BP includes locally destructive therapies such as excisional surgery, electrocoagulation, cryotherapy, 5-fluorouracil and 5% imiquimod cream.

# Malignancies

## Mycosis Fungoides (MF) and CTCL

- It the most common type of cutaneous lymphoma.
- **Pathophysiology**
  - ➢ MF is a malignant lymphoma characterized by the expansion of a clone of CD4+ (or helper) memory T cells (CD45RO+) that normally patrol and home to the skin.
  - ➢ The malignant clone frequently lacks normal T cell antigens such as CD2, CD5, or CD7.
  - ➢ Extravasating into the dermis, the cells show an affinity for the epidermis, clustering around Langerhans' cells as seen microscopically as **pautrier microabscesses**.
  - ➢ The disease fundamentally is a systemic disease, even when the disease appears to be in an early stage and clinically limited to the skin.
- **Clinical features**
  - ➢ Pruritus is seen
  - ➢ Patch phase MF is characterized by flat, usually erythematous, macules that may have a fine scale, may be single or multiple, and may be pruritic.
  - ➢ Plaques tend to be raised, demonstrating fine-scale, well-demarcated, erythematous shapes with irregular borders. Annular or serpiginous patterns with central clearing and pruritus are common.
  - ➢ Patches and plaques may affect any area of the skin, but they often are distributed asymmetrically in the areas that a bathing suit would cover (i.e. hips, buttocks, groin, lower trunk, axillae, breasts).
  - ➢ When the disease affects the scalp, it often is accompanied by alopecia.

- ➢ Tumors are red-violet nodules that may be dome-shaped, exophytic, or ulcerated.
- ➢ Skin erythroderma
- ➢ Generalized erythroderma often is intensely symptomatic, with pruritus and scaling that can be profound. The patients experience thickening of the skin folds in the face (leonine facies), hyperkeratosis and fissuring of the palms and soles, onychodystrophy, ectropion of the eyelids, alopecia, and edema. Sun exposure may be painful as well as pruritic.
- ➢ Stage III disease is defined by the presence of generalized erythroderma.
- ➢ Extracutaneous involvement is more clinically evident as the stage and extent of MF increases.
- ➢ Peripheral lymphadenopathy is the most frequent site of extracutaneous involvement in MF.
- ➢ Liver, lung: Stage IVB disease is defined by the presence of visceral involvement (e.g. liver, lung, bone marrow).

- **Lab studies**
  - ➢ Consider HIV and human T cell lymphotrophic virus type I (HTLV-I) testing.
  - ➢ LDH is a marker of bulky or biologically aggressive disease.
  - ➢ Abnormal transaminase values may indicate hepatic involvement.
  - ➢ Flow cytometric study of the blood (include available T cell-related antibodies): Conduct this test to detect a circulating malignant clone and to assess immunocompetence by quantifying the level of CD8-expressing lymphocytes.
  - ➢ *Uric acid:* Perform this study in cases involving a bulky disease and/or biologically aggressive disease.

- **Histological findings**
  - ➢ The criteria for diagnosis include the following:
    - A band-like upper dermal infiltrate of lymphocytes and other inflammatory cells, with no grenz zone, is present.
    - Epidermotropism of mononuclear cells occurs.
    - When a clear halo surrounds an intraepidermal mononuclear cell singly or in clumps, this is called a Pautrier microabscess. Its presence is suggestive of MF, but it is not necessary for diagnosis.
    - Little spongiosis of the epidermis is found.
    - Lymphocytes have nuclei that are hyperchromatic and convoluted or cerebriform.

- **Treatment**
  - ➤ *Topical treatments*
    - In the patch or plaque phase: Topical steroids, topical retinoids, topical chemotherapy (e.g. nitrogen mustard or bischloroethylnitrosourea (BCNU), UV B or UV A treatment enhanced with psoralen (PUVA), or **total body electron beam radiation**.
    - In the tumor phase: Topical combined with systemic modalities (e.g. PUVA plus interferon).
  - ➤ *Systemic treatments*
    - Extracorporeal photopheresis (leukapheresis with PUVA treatment for the collected white blood cells with reinfusion of treated cells)
    - Recombinant alpha interferon
    - Oral retinoids
    - Fusion toxin treatment
    - Monoclonal antibody treatment
    - Systemic chemotherapy with a variety of single agents
    - Bone marrow transplantation: Allogenic transplants are reported.

## Pautrier Microabscesses

- These small, intraepidermal collections of lymphoid cells in the absence of marked spongiosis are characteristic of mycosis fungoides.
- The cells within the epidermis may show some degree of nuclear hyperchromatism or atypia. Single cell colonization of the epidermis is more commonly seen than true Pautrier microabscess formation in many cases of early mycosis fungoides.

### *Sézary Syndrome*

- Sézary syndrome (SS) is a variant of MF, occurring in about 5% of all cases of MF.
- The patient with SS has generalized exfoliative erythroderma, lymphadenopathy, and more than 1000 per $mm^3$ atypical T-lymphocytes with cerebriform nuclei circulating in the peripheral blood or other evidence of a significant malignant T cell clone in the blood such as clonal T cell gene rearrangement (identical to that found in the skin).
- Occurs in elderly usually over 60 yrs of age.
- More common in males.
- **Treatment**: Chemotherapy combined with electron beam therapy or photochemotherapy.

## Kaposi's Sarcoma

- Human herpesvirus type 8 is believed to be the cause of most cases of Kaposi's sarcoma.
- There are at least four distinct epidemiologic forms of KS:
  - The classic form that occurs in older men of predominantly Mediterranean or Eastern European Jewish backgrounds with no recognized contributing factors
  - The equatorial African form that occurs in all ages, also without any recognized precipitating factors
  - The form associated with organ transplantation and its attendent iatrogenic immunosuppressed state
  - The form associated with HIV-1 infection.
- In the latter two forms, KS is an opportunistic disease; in HIV-infected individuals, unlike typical opportunistic infections, its occurrence is not strictly related to the level of depression of CD4+ T cell counts.
- The Köebner's phenomenon has been reported to develop in classic or acquired immune deficiency syndrome-related Kaposi's sarcoma.

## Basal Cell Carcinoma

- A malignant tumor that rarely metastasizes, composed of cells similar to those in the basal area of the epidermis and its appendages.
- BCC is the most common malignant tumor of the skin and the most common cancer in some countries, including the USA and Australia.
- BCC is more common in males than females.
- More than three quarters of patients are over 40 years old.
- BCC may arise in skin damaged by sunlight and ionizing radiation. It may occur in burn scars or vaccination scars. Acute episodes of intense burning sun exposure are a greater risk factor than cumulative lifetime sun exposure.
- Mutations in the PTCH1 gene and a key role of the Hedgehog (Hh) signalling pathway in its pathogenesis.
- **Clinical features**: The most common type is the noduloulcerative variant. The early tumors are commonly small, translucent or pearly, raised and rounded areas covered by thin epidermis through which a few dilated, superficial vessels show. Tiny flecks

of pigment may be seen with a hand lens. The nodule slowly increases in size and undergoes central ulceration. The typical lesion then consists of a slowly enlarging ulcer surrounded by a pearly rolled border. This represents the so-called rodent ulcer. It is locally invasive without any metastasis to the lymph nodes.

- Other variants include pigmented BCC, superficial spreading BCC, morphea like BCC and fibroepithelioma.

  The typical BCC runs a slow progressive course.

  Invasive rodent ulcers, if neglected, may cause death. This is preceded by prolonged mutilation of the face or scalp, with destruction of the nose or eye and exposure of the paranasal sinuses or the skull, dura or brain.

- **Treatment**
  - ➢ Curettage and cautery
  - ➢ Cryotherapy
  - ➢ Conventional surgical excision
  - ➢ Moh's micrographic surgery:
    - – Moh's micrographic surgery is an expedient treatment that allows for complete microscopic examination of the tumor, maximum preservation of normal tissue, and a high degree of assurance of cure.
    - – Moh's micrographic surgery is primarily used to treat basal and squamous cell carcinomas, but can be used to treat less common tumors including melanoma.
    - – Moh's surgery is appropriate when
      - o the cancer is in an area where it is important to preserve healthy tissue for maximum functional and cosmetic result, such as eyelids, nose, ears, lips, fingers, toes, genitals;
      - o the cancer was treated previously and recurred;
      - o scar tissue exists in the area of the cancer;
      - o the cancer is large;
      - o the edges of the cancer cannot be clearly defined; and
      - o the cancer is growing rapidly or uncontrollably.

## Squamous Cell Carcinoma

- A malignant tumor arising from the keratinocytes of the epidermis.
- Cutaneous SCC is predominately a disease of white populations.
- Sun exposure is the major etiological factor.

- Additional etiological factors implicated in development of cutaneous SCC are trauma, albinism, burn scars, ionizing radiation, chronic inflammation, chronic DLE, chronic exposure to thermal radiation and scarring. Radiant heat from coal and peat fires may cause SCC in women who habitually sit with their legs close to the fire. The preceding lesion is called erythema ab igne.

- SCC is also an occasional complication of long-standing chronic granulomas such as venereal granulomas, syphilis, lupus vulgaris, leprosy and lupus erythematosus, chronic ulcers, osteomyelitis sinuses, old burn scars and hidradenitis suppurativa.

- It may complicate scarring dermatoses such as poikiloderma congenitale, dystrophic epidermolysis bullosa and porokeratosis of Mibelli.

- **Clinical features:** SCC does not often arise from healthy-looking skin. Commonly, there are signs of photodamage: Solar elastosis of the dermis, hyperkeratosis, irregular pigmentation and telangiectasia, or leukokeratosis and fissuring of the lip.

- The first clinical evidence of malignancy is induration. The area may be plaque-like, verrucous, tumid or ulcerated, but in all cases the lesion feels firm when pressed between the finger and thumb.

- The better-differentiated tumors are usually papillomatous and are capped by a keratotic crust in the earlier stages. This may be shed later to reveal an ulcer or eroded tumor with an indurated margin and a purulent, exuding surface that bleeds rather easily. The outline may be rounded, but is often irregular.

- On mobile structures such as the lip or genitalia the presenting sign may be a fissure or small erosion or ulcer which fails to heal and bleeds recurrently.

- The most common sites for SCC are those most exposed to the sun. They occur on the backs of the hands and forearms, the upper part of the face, and especially in males, on the lower lip and pinna.

- Regional nodes may become enlarged, either as a result of infection of the ulcer or from metastases.

- **'Epithelioma cuniculatum':** There is a soft bulbous mass with a squashy consistency on the distal part of the sole of the foot. Multiple sinuses open on the surface, and when pressed, greasy, rancid and foul-smelling material can be expressed.

- **Verrucous SCC:** In both the oral cavity and on the genital mucosa, a strikingly verrucous lesion may develop. These lesions, because of the site involved, may become massive, moist, cauliflower-like and often malodorous because of secondary infection. The clinically apparent relentless growth contrasts with the pathologically less aggressive appearance characterized by a lack of mitotic figures and a well-demarcated lower margin with no strands of cells becoming detached from the main bulk of the lesion.

- **Treatment**
  - ➢ *Conventional surgical excision:* Well-defined, low-risk tumors less than 2 cm in diameter, surgical excision with at least a 4-mm clinical margin. Higher-risk tumors which are more than 2 cm, moderately or poorly differentiated, extending into the subcutis or on high-risk sites including the scalp, ears, nose, lip or eyelid require wider margins of more than 6 mm.
  - ➢ *Moh's micrographic surgery:* Radiotherapy is rarely the treatment of choice but may be indicated for some very large or rapidly enlarging tumors or in patients where aggressive surgical management may not be tolerated. Also used as an adjuvant therapy.

## Malignant Melanoma

- A malignant tumor arising from the epidermal melanocyte.
- Intermittent sun exposure and use of sun beds are major etiological factors.
- The strongest phenotypic risk factor for melanoma is the presence of increased numbers of melanocytic nevi. Weaker phenotypic risk factors relate to the presence of skin that burns easily in the sun such as skin type I, high density of freckles, fair skin, blue eyes and red hair.
- Family history of melanoma is also a risk factor.
- Malignant melanoma has following variants:
  - ➢ Superficial spreading melanoma
  - ➢ Nodular melanoma
  - ➢ Lentigo maligna melanoma
  - ➢ Acral lentiginous or palmoplantar malignant melanoma
- The clinical diagnosis of melanoma is based upon recognition of a progressively changing melanocytic lesion, which is growing and becoming irregular in shape and color.
- This is based on American ABCD categories and the Glasgow seven-point checklist.
- American **ABCD** mnemonic is **A:** asymmetry, **B:** irregular border, **C:** irregular color and **D:** diameter over 1 cm.
- The Glasgow seven-point checklist is divided into three major and four minor features. These are:

*Major features*
- Change in size
- Change in shape
- Change in color

*Minor features*
- Diameter more than 5 mm
- Inflammation
- Oozing or bleeding
- Mild itch or altered sensation
- It is suggested that any lesion with one major feature in an adult be considered for removal, and that the presence of additional minor features should add to clinical suspicion.

**Malignant melanoma**
- Change in size—any adult nevus >6 mm is suspect (for reference a lead pencil diameter is 7 mm) and anything changing to >10 mm is more likely to be malignant than benign
- Caused by UV exposure
- Superficial spreading form is the most common
- Breslow thickness is the most important prognostic indicator until there is lymph node involvement
- Sentinel node biopsy is useful for staging disease

## Superficial Spreading Melanoma

- This is by far the most frequent type of melanoma.
- The commonest sites are the female leg and the male back, but any body site may be involved.
- An evolving, superficial spreading melanoma has the appearance of a flat, pigmented lesion, which becomes increasingly irregular in shape and colour over time.

## Nodular Melanoma

- This variety presents most commonly in the fifth or sixth decade and occurs more frequently in males than in females.
- The trunk is a common site.
- These lesions grow rapidly and have a poor prognosis.
- Nodular melanomas develop as an elevated, dome-shaped polypoid or even pedunculated structure. Melanin pigment may be sparse in these lesions and a raised, red central area, with only a peripheral brown ring of melanin, is a common clinical pattern; in others the more typically variable pigmentation may be seen. Ulceration and bleeding from the lesion occur frequently.

## Lentigo Maligna Melanoma

- In this histogenetic variant the preceding horizontal or *in situ* growth phase is known as a lentigo maligna (Hutchinson's melanotic freckle; melanosis circumscripta precancerosa of Dubreuilh). By comparison with the radial growth phase of the superficial spreading melanoma, lentigo maligna represents a much more prolonged period of lateral extension.
- Most occur on the face, commonly on the upper cheek, temple or forehead.
- Initially the lentigo maligna is a flat, brown or black, irregularly shaped lesion.
- These lesions will grow very slowly, over months or years, and there may be central regression while the peripheral. Margin continues to extend. In time, a raised central nodule will develop, indicating transition to the vertical growth phase.

## Acral Lentiginous Melanoma (Palmoplantar Malignant Melanoma)

- This type of melanoma comprises around 10% of all melanomas on white skin but over 50% of all melanomas on darker-skinned peoples.
- The lesions are found mainly on the sole of the foot but also on the palm of the hand, and are characterized, by a large, macular, lentiginous pigmented area around an invasive, raised tumor.

## Subungual Melanoma

- Subungual melanomas are rare.
- They are most common on the thumb or the great toe. Because they arise from the nail matrix, subungual melanomas usually produce an abnormal nail and a variable degree of pigmentation of the nail itself.
- The classical presentation is of a new, linear, pigmented band along the length of the nail, which starts to widen progressively, especially at the base, so that the pigmented band tends to be funnel shaped.
- Over time, proliferation of the melanoma cells within the nail matrix then additionally interferes with nail formation and a progressively dystrophic nail results. Eventually, pigment may spread to the surrounding normal skin as 'Hutchinson's sign' (Table 24.6).

**Treatment**

- The extent of excision will relate to the tumour thickness. At present, if the diagnosis is of a level 1 or *in situ* melanoma, a margin of only 2–5 mm of surrounding normal skin is considered adequate.
- Invasive melanomas up to 2 mm thick may be safely treated with a minimal excision margin of 1 cm. Patients with thicker tumours are more likely to develop lymph node recurrence if a 1 cm margin is used and therefore the recommended excision margin is 2 to 3 cm where anatomically possible.

| **Table 24.6:** Collagen and related disease | | |
|---|---|---|
| *Collagen type* | *Distribution tissue* | *Genetic disorders* |
| **Fibrillar collagens** | | |
| I | Ubiquitous in hard and soft tissues | Osteogenesis imperfecta Ehlers-Danlos syndrome—arthrochalasias type |
| II | Cartilage, intervertebral disk, vitreous | Achondrogenesis type II, spondyloepiphyseal dysplasia syndrome |
| III | Hollow organs, soft tissues | Vascular Ehlers-Danlos syndrome |
| V | Soft tissues, blood vessels | Classical Ehlers-Danlos syndrome |
| IX | Cartilage, vitreous | Stickler syndrome |
| **Basement membrane collagens** | | |
| IV | Basement membranes | Alport syndrome, Goodpasture's syndrome |
| **Other collagens** | | |
| VI | Ubiquitous in microfibrils | Bethlem myopathy |
| VII | Anchoring fibrils at dermal–epidermal junctions | Dystrophic epidermolysis bullosa |
| IX | Cartilage, intervertebral discs | Multiple epiphyseal dysplasias |
| XVII | Transmembrane collagen in epidermal cells | Benign atrophic generalized epidermolysis bullosa |
| XV and XVIII | Endostatin-forming collagens, endothelial cells | Knobloch syndrome (type XVIII collagen) |

## QUESTIONS FROM PREVIOUS EXAMINATIONS

1. Sézary syndrome
2. Pautrier's microabscess
3. Kaposi's sarcoma
4. Keratoacanthoma
5. Verrucous carcinoma
6. Mycosis fungoides
7. Malakoplakia
8. Leiomyoma
9. Malignant melanoma
10. Basal cell carcinoma
11. Lymphocytic infiltrate
12. Precancerous dermatosis
13. Dermatosis of senile skin
14. Astiocytosis
15. Pseudo-Kaposi's sarcoma
16. Parapsoriasis
17. Painful tumors of skin
18. Lymphomatoid papulosis
19. Leser-Trélat sign
20. Bowen's disease
21. Sjögren's syndrome
22. Acrosclerosis
23. Relapsing polychondritis
24. Scleredema of Buschke
25. Bowenoid papulosis
26. Syringoma
27. HPE of BCC
28. Moh's microsurgery technique
29. Drug-induced pseudolymphoma
30. Sézary cells
31. Juvenile xanthogranuloma
32. Steatocystoma multiplex
33. Sebaceous horn
34. Immunological typing of T cell lymphoma
35. Classify pigmented nevi
36. Vascular nevi
37. Giant cell nevus

38. Blaschko's lines
39. Pigmented nevi
40. Buschke-Ollendorff syndrome
41. Port-wine stain
42. Verrucous angiokeratoma
43. Blue nevus
44. Spider nevus
45. Halo nevus
46. Nevus flammeus
47. Nevus of Ota
48. Colloid milium
49. Pyogenic granuloma

## MULTIPLE CHOICE QUESTIONS

1. **All the following skin conditions are considered as skin markers for internal malignancy** *except:*           *(Kar 07)*
   - (a) Acanthosis nigricans
   - (b) Dermatomyositis
   - (c) Bullous pemphigoid
   - (d) Pemphigus vulgaris

2. **Best range of UV light used for treatment of skin diseases:**           *(MH 2001)*
   - (a) 100 to 200 nm
   - (b) 200 to 400 nm
   - (c) 400 to 700 nm
   - (d) More than 700

3. **Skin cancers develop due to sunlight exposure induced by:**           *(Kar 07)*
   - (a) UVA rays
   - (b) UV B rays
   - (c) UVC rays
   - (d) All of the above

4. **Which of the following is not true about mycosis fungoides?**           *(AI 07)*
   - (a) It is the most common cutaneous lymphoma
   - (b) Pautrier abscess can occur
   - (c) Diffuse erythroderma is common
   - (d) It often curable by therapy and has indolent course

5. **Which of the following is associated with maximum risk of skin malignancy?**           *(JIPMER 09)*
   - (a) Down's syndrome
   - (b) Fanconi's syndrome
   - (c) Bloom's syndrome
   - (d) Xeroderma pigmentosum

6. **Which of the following is not a premalignant condition?**
   *(Punjab 08)*
   (a) Bowen's disease        (b) Steatocytoma multiplex
   (c) Solar dystrophic keratosis (d) Lincus complex

7. **Acanthosis nigricans is associated with the following** *except:*
   *(MP 08)*
   (a) Adenocarcinoma of colon
   (b) Adenocarcinoma of breast
   (c) Adenocarcinoma of lung
   (d) Adenocarcinoma of uterus

8. **Moh's micrographic surgery is used for Rx of:**    *(Delhi 04)*
   (a) Squamous cell carcinoma of skin
   (b) Lichen planus
   (c) Pustular dermatosis
   (d) Vitiligo

9. **A 70-year-old man comes for multiple raised pigmented lesions over his back and chest. These have developed gradually over several years. There are two lesions on the mid-lower back that intermittently itch intensely and are somewhat larger and much darker than the other lesions, which number is 50 or more. What is the probable diagnosis?**    *(CMC 07)*
   (a) Solar lentigo           (b) Actinic keratosis
   (c) Seborrheic keratosis    (d) Leser-Trélat sign

10. **Which of the following is not true about mycosis fungoides?**
    *(AIIMS Nov 06)*
    (a) Most common form of cutaneous lymphoma
    (b) Pautrier's microabscesses occur
    (c) Diffuse erythroderma common
    (d) Often curable by therapy and has indolent course

11. **Pautrier's microabscesses are histological features of:**
    *(AIIMS Nov 05)*
    (a) Sarcoidosis             (b) TB
    (c) Mycosis fungoides       (d) Epithelial cell carcinoma

12. **Underlying internal malignancy is associated with the following** *except:*    *(AI 96)*
    (a) Acanthosis nigricans    (b) Bullous pyoderma
    (c) Granuloma annulare      (d) Erythema gyratum repens

13. **Actinic keratosis predisposes to:**        *(AIIMS May 02)*
    (a) Basal cell carcinoma    (b) Squamous cell carcinoma
    (c) Malignant melanoma      (d) Epithelial cell carcinoma

14. **Genodermal diseases that can cause skin malignancy:**
    *(PGI 03)*
    (a) Xeroderma pigmentosum  (b) Neurofibromatosis
    (c) Actinic keratosis         (d) PCT
    (e) Steatosis

15. **True about acanthosis nigricans:**            *(PGI 03, 08)*
    (a) Most commonly seen in obesity
    (b) Seen in axilla
    (c) Signifies internal malignancy
    (d) Associated with insulin resistance
    (e) Seen in old age

16. **A 35-year-old premenopausal patient has recently developed a 1.5 cm sized pigmented lesion on her back. Which of the following forms of tissue diagnosis will you recommend for her?**            *(AIIMS May 06)*
    (a) Needle biopsy           (b) Trucut biopsy
    (c) Excision biopsy         (d) Incisional biopsy

17. **A 48-year-old sports photographer has noticed a small nodule over the upper lip from four months. The nodule is pearly white with central necrosis, telangiectasia. The most likely diagnosis would be:**            *(AIIMS May 06)*
    (a) Basal cell carcinoma    (b) Squamous cell carcinoma
    (c) Atypical melanoma       (d) Kaposi's sarcoma

18. **Dystrophic epidermolysis bullosa is caused by a mutation of:**
    *(AIIMS Nov 2008)*
    (a) Alpha 6 integrin         (b) Collagen type 7
    (c) Laminin 4                (d) Keratin 14

19. **Which of the following is a precancerous condition of the skin?**
    *(MH 14)*
    (a) Bowen's disease          (b) Seborrheic keratosis
    (c) Leprosy                  (d) Psoriasis

## Answers

1. **Ans. (d)** Pemphigus vulgaris *(Ref. Rook's Textbook of Dermatology, 7th edn/35.3)*

2. **Ans. (b)** 200 to 400 nm *(Ref. Robbin's Pathologic Basis of Disease, 7th edn, 321, Table 9–19)*

3. **Ans. (b)** UV B rays. *(Ref. Harrison's Internal Medicine, 17th edn, Chapter 57)*

4. **Ans. (d)** It often curable by therapy and has indolent course

5. **Ans. (d)** Xeroderma pigmentosum

6. **Ans. (d)** Lincus complex
7. **Ans. (b)** Adenocarcinoma of breast *(Ref. Robbin's Pathologic Basis of Disease, 7th edn/ Table 7–12; page 335)*
8. **Ans. (a)** Squamous cell carcinoma of skin
9. **Ans. (d)** Leser-Trélat sign
10. **Ans. (d)** Often curable by therapy and has indolent course *(Ref. Rook, 7th edn/54.7)*
11. **Ans. (c)** Mycosis fungoides *(Ref. Rook, 7th edn/ 7.42)*
12. **Ans. (c)** Granuloma annulare *(Ref. Harrison's Internal Medicine, 17th edn/ Chapter 338)*
13. **Ans. (b)** Squamous cell carcinoma *(Ref. Harrison's Internal Medicine, 17th edn/Chapter 83)*
14. **Ans. (a)** Xeroderma pigmentosum *(Ref. Roxburgh, 17th edn/218)*
15. **Ans. (a, b, c, d)** *(Ref. Rook, 7th edn/34.108)*
16. **Ans. (c)** Excisional biopsy
17. **Ans. (a)** Basal cell carcinoma
18. **Ans. (b)** Collagen type 7
19. **Ans. (a)** Bowen's disease

# Sexually Transmitted Diseases

## REITER'S DISEASE

- Characterized by presence of non-suppurative polyarthritis exceeding a duration of one month associated or preceded closely by a lower urogenital or enteric infection
- Observed in young men with HLA-B27 antigen
- Most common example of reactive arthritis
- Triad of arthritis, conjunctivitis and urethritis
- *Infectious agents*
  - ➢ Chlamydia
  - ➢ Salmonella
  - ➢ Shigella
  - ➢ Yersinia
  - ➢ Campylobacter
- Constitutional symptoms are common, including fatigue, malaise, fever, and weight loss.
- *The musculoskeletal symptoms* are usually acute in onset. Arthritis is usually asymmetric and additive, with involvement of new joints occurring over a period of a few days to 1–2 weeks. The joints of the lower extremities, especially the knee, ankle, and subtalar, metatarsophalangeal, and toe interphalangeal joints, are the most common sites of involvement, but the wrist and fingers can be involved as well. The arthritis is usually quite painful, and tense joint effusions are not uncommon, especially in the knee. Patients often cannot walk without support. Dactylitis, or "sausage digit," a diffuse swelling of a solitary finger or toe, is a distinctive feature of ReA and other peripheral spondyloarthritides but can be seen in polyarticular gout and sarcoidosis. Tendinitis and fasciitis are particularly characteristic lesions, producing pain at multiple insertion sites (entheses), especially the Achilles insertion, the

plantar fascia, and sites along the axial skeleton. Spinal and low-back pain are quite common and may be caused by insertional inflammation, muscle spasm, acute sacroiliitis, or presumably, arthritis in intervertebral articulations.

- *Urogenital lesions* may occur throughout the course of the disease. In males, urethritis may be marked or relatively asymptomatic and may be either an accompaniment of the triggering infection or a result of the reactive phase of the disease. Prostatitis is also common. Similarly, in females, cervicitis or salpingitis may be caused either by the infectious trigger or by the sterile reactive process.
- *Ocular disease* is common, ranging from transient, asymptomatic conjunctivitis to an aggressive anterior uveitis that occasionally proves refractory to treatment and may result in blindness.
- *Mucocutaneous lesions* are frequent. Oral ulcers tend to be superficial, transient, and often asymptomatic. The characteristic skin lesions, **keratoderma blenorrhagica**, consist of vesicles that become hyperkeratotic, ultimately forming a crust before disappearing. They are most common on the palms and soles but may occur elsewhere as well. In patients with HIV infection, these lesions are often extremely severe and extensive, sometimes dominating the clinical picture.
- *Lesions on the glans penis,* termed **circinate balanitis**, are common; these consist of vesicles that quickly rupture to form painless superficial erosions, which in circumcised individuals can form crusts similar to those of keratoderma blenorrhagica.
- *Nail changes* are common and consist of onycholysis, distal yellowish discoloration, and/or heaped-up hyperkeratosis.
- *Less-frequent or rare manifestations of ReA include* cardiac conduction defects, aortic insufficiency, central or peripheral nervous system lesions, and pleuropulmonary infiltrates.
- *Differential diagnosis*
  - ➢ Seronegative rheumatoid arthritis
  - ➢ Septic arthritis
  - ➢ Gonococcal arthritis
  - ➢ Psoriatic arthritis
- *Management*
  - ➢ NSAID—mainstay of treatment
  - ➢ Steroids
  - ➢ Methotrexate
  - ➢ Azathioprine
  - ➢ Sulfasalazine

## CHANCROID

- *Haemophilus ducreyi,* a gram-negative bacillus, is the etiologic agent of chancroid.
- Characterized by genital ulceration and inguinal adenitis.
- After an incubation period of 4 to 7 days, the initial lesion—a papule with surrounding erythema appears.
- In 2 to 3 days, the papule evolves into a pustule, which spontaneously ruptures and forms a sharply circumscribed ulcer.
- Ulcer is painful, deep with undermined irregular edges, necrotic yellowish slough at the floor and a nonindurated base, called soft chancre.
- These ulcers are highly infectious and multiple lesions appear on the genitalia from autoinoculation.
- The ulcers are very tender and bleed easily.
- In females they appear on the labia majora, perineum and perianal area, and may also affect the vagina and cervix. Lesions are more common in uncircumcised men and are usually located in the coronal sulcus or on the inner aspect of the prepuce. Perianal lesions occur in MSM (Table 25.1).
- **Within a week approximately half of patients develop**
  - ➤ Enlarged
  - ➤ Tender inguinal lymph nodes (usually unilateral) which frequently become
    - – fluctuant (bubo)
    - – spontaneously rupture leaving extensive ulceration
- The presentation of chancroid does not usually include all of the typical clinical features and is sometimes atypical.

**Table 25.1:** Differences between syphilitic and chancroid ulcer

| Syphilis | Chancroid |
| --- | --- |
| 1. Papule | Pustule |
| 2. Usually single | Usually multiple, coalesce |
| 3. 5–15 mm diameter | Diameter variable |
| 4. Sharp edges, elevated and round | Undermined ragged irregular edges |
| 5. Superficial/deep | Excavated |
| 6. Base smooth and nonpurulent | Base purulent, bleeds easily |
| 7. Firm consistency (indurated) | Soft consistency, non-indurated |
| 8. Not painful or tender lesions with firm non-tender bilateral adenopathy | Very tender lesions with tender, suppurated unilateral adenopathy |

- Multiple ulcers can coalesce to form giant ulcers.
- Ulcers can appear and then resolve, with inguinal adenitis and suppuration following 1 to 3 weeks later; this clinical picture can be confused with that of lymphogranuloma venereum.
- Multiple small ulcers can resemble folliculitis.
- **Diagnosis may be confirmed by**
  - ➤ *Gram staining:* Gram-negative bacilli in school of fish or rail-road track appearance.
  - ➤ *Culture: H. ducreyi* is a highly fastidious coccobacillary gram-negative bacterium whose growth requires X factor (hemin).
  - ➤ *Multiplex PCR:* Highly sensitive and specific way to detect HSV, *Treponema pallidum* and *H. ducreyi.*
  - ➤ *Histological examination*
    - – The histology of the genital ulcer of chancroid is characterized by 3 layers of necrotic inflammatory tissue reaction, vascular proliferation and thrombosis and deepest layer of a dense infiltrate of plasma cells and lymphoid cells.
    - – Other differential diagnostic considerations include the various infections causing genital ulceration, such as primary syphilis, condyloma latum of secondary syphilis, genital herpes, and donovanosis.
- **Treatment**
  - ➤ A single dose of either azithromycin, 1 g orally, or ceftriaxone, 250 mg intramuscularly, is effective treatment.
  - ➤ Effective multiple-dose regimens are amoxicillin-potassium clavulanate (500/125 mg) three times a day orally for 7 days; erythromycin or tetracycline 500 mg orally four times a day for 7 days; or ciprofloxacin, 500 mg orally twice a day for 3 days.
  - ➤ Bubo should be aspirated, if fluctuant.

## LYMPHOGRANULOMA VENEREUM

- Lymphogranuloma venereum (LGV) is a sexually transmitted disease caused by *Chlamydia trachomatis* serotypes L1, L2 and L3.
- The organism enters through skin breaks and abrasions or crosses the epithelial cells of mucous membranes, and travels via the lymphatics to multiply within mononuclear phagocytes in regional lymph nodes.
- Starting as an acute genital infection, it may develop into a chronic disabling illness such as genital elephantiasis or anorectal stricture.

- **Clinical features**
  - ➤ The transient primary lesion may easily missed which could be a painless papule, vesicle, a shallow ulcer or erosion, a small herpetiform lesion (commonest), or non-specific urethritis.
  - ➤ The incubation period averages 1 to 3 weeks.
  - ➤ In male, it is usually found in the coronal sulcus, prepuce or glans. In women, it is usually found in the posterior wall of the vagina, vulva or cervix.
  - ➤ The secondary stage appears in 2–6 weeks after exposure.
  - ➤ The two characteristic features of secondary stage are constitutional symptoms and regional lymphadenopathy.
  - ➤ Constitutional symptoms include fever, chills, anorexia, headache, meningism, myalgias and arthralgias.
  - ➤ Swelling of the inguinal lymph nodes is the presentation in the inguinal syndrome which is more common in men. The nodes are firm, slightly painful and enlarge over 1 to 2 weeks and are unilateral in two-thirds of the cases. Later nodes develop multiple areas of suppuration (multilocular abscess) referred to as buboes. However, spontaneous recovery occurs in a great majority of the cases. In few they may rupture through overlying bluish hued skin forming multiple discharging sinuses.
  - ➤ If the femoral nodes are involved, it produces the **classical "Groove sign of Greenblat"** with inguinal nodes above the Poupart's ligament and femoral nodes below the ligament. This sign is pathognomonic for LGV.
  - ➤ In women, inguinal lymphadenitis is unusual, however, the iliac lymph nodes may be involved and lead to pelvic adhesions. The anorectal syndrome is a more common presentation in women.
  - ➤ In MSM engaging in receptive anal intercourse, the secondary stage presents as an anorectal syndrome. Patients complain of mucopurulent anal discharge, rectal pain and bleeding, tenesmus and constipation. Ulcerative proctocolitis similar to that in inflammatory bowel disease is seen.
  - ➤ Antibiotic treatment in the secondary stages will prevent progression of the disease to the tertiary stage. The manifestations in this stage result from fibrosis and lymphatic obstruction, which may include genital elephantiasis, genital ulcers and fistulas, urethral and rectal stricture, perineal sinuses, rectovaginal fistulae and **"frozen pelvis"**.
- **Other manifestations**
  - ➤ *Esthiomene* (Greek, "eating away") is a primary infection of the lymphatics of the external genitalia and may cause chronic

progressive lymphangitis, chronic edema, and sclerosing fibrosis of the subcutaneous tissue of these structures.

➢ Follicular conjunctivitis due to autoinoculation of infectious discharge.

➢ Primary LGV lesions of the mouth and pharynx as the result of fellatio or cunnilingus.

➢ Erythema nodosum may occur during the early stages of infection.

- **Diagnosis**
  - ➢ The diagnostic method of choice is by nucleic acid amplification tests and confirmation by real-time PCR assays for LGV-specific DNA.
  - ➢ Serological testing may be undertaken using microimmuno-fluorescent (MIF) antibody testing to the L-serovar in specialized laboratories. An MIF titre >1 : 128 is strongly suggestive of LGV, but serological testing lacks sensitivity in early infections.
  - ➢ The Frei's intradermal test, which was based on a positive hypersensitivity reaction to a purified chlamydial antigen, is now only of historical interest.
  - ➢ Chlamydia can be isolated in tissue culture using HeLa-229 or McCoy cell lines.

- **Treatment**
  - ➢ The recommended treatment is with doxycycline 100 mg twice daily or erythromycin 500 mg four times daily for 3 weeks.
  - ➢ Bubos may require repeated aspiration.
  - ➢ Long-term complications such as fistulae and strictures may require surgery to alleviate symptoms.

        **Differential diagaosis of elephantiasis of the genitalia**
          1. Filariasis
          2. Tuberculosis
          3. Fungal infections
          4. Parasites
          5. Granuloma inguinale (pseudoelephantiasis)

## DONOVANOSIS (GRANULOMA INGUINALE AND GRANULOMA VENEREUM)

- Donovanosis is a chronic, progressively destructive bacterial infection of the genital region caused by caused by *Klebsiella granulomatis* (formerly known as *Calymmatobacterium granulomatis*).

- It is an intracellular, gram-negative, pleomorphic, encapsulated (when mature) bacterium measuring 1.5 × 0.7 microns.
- **Clinical manifestations**
  - ➤ The incubation period is usually 1–4 weeks but may extend to 1 year.
  - ➤ Skin lesions have been detected in infants 6 weeks to 6 months after birth.
  - ➤ The disease begins as one or more subcutaneous nodules that erode through the skin to produce clean, friable, granulomatous, nonindurated, beefy red, sharply defined, usually painless ulcers.
  - ➤ These lesions, which bleed readily on contact, slowly enlarge by peripheral extension and may attain a large size.
  - ➤ Not associated with inguinal lymphadenopathy. But subcutaneous granulomas in the inguinal area may present as pseudobuboes.
  - ➤ The genitalia are involved in 90% of cases, the inguinal region in 10%, and the anal region in 5–10%.
  - ➤ Genital swelling, particularly of the labia, is a common feature and occasionally progresses to pseudoelephantiasis.
  - ➤ Phimosis and paraphimosis are common local complications, and progressive erosion of affected tissues may completely destroy the penis or other organs.
  - ➤ Tissue destruction may be greater in patients co-infected with HIV than in those without HIV infection.
- **Less common clinical variants include**
  - ➤ Hypertrophic form (cauliflower- or wartlike lesions)
  - ➤ Necrotic form (destructive lesions with foul-smelling exudate, often resembling amebiasis)
  - ➤ Sclerotic or cicatricial form, which has a dry base with extensive scar tissue.
- **Diagnosis**
  - ➤ The diagnosis is generally made by microscopic identification of Donovan bodies from lesions. These are found in large mononuclear cells of the monocyte/macrophage lineage whose cytoplasm contains numerous organisms, 0.5–0.7 by 1–1.5 μm in size, that show bipolar staining (380 safety-pin appearance). Giemsa, Wright's or Leishman's stains are usually used.
  - ➤ *Histology:* Histological examination shows epithelial proliferation with a heavy infiltrate of plasma cells and neutrophils, with a few lymphocytes.

- ➤ *Culture:* This is rarely undertaken or successful because the organism is extremely fastidious.
- ➤ PCR
- ➤ There is no serological test of proven reliability
- **Treatment**
  - ➤ The treatment of choice is azithromycin. There are various regimens.
  - ➤ The WHO recommend 1 g orally immediately, followed by 500 mg daily for 3 weeks or until complete lesion healing. Alternatively, azithromycin may be administered as 1 g orally at weekly intervals, for a minimum of 3 weeks.
  - ➤ Alternative antibiotics include cotrimoxazole 960 mg twice daily, ciprofloxacin 750 mg twice daily, or doxycycline 100 mg twice daily for 3 weeks.

## GENITAL HERPES

- Most common cause of genital ulceration.
- Herpes simplex type II is the most common cause of genital ulcer in developing countries.

| Disease | % |
|---|---|
| Herpes | 62% |
| Chanchroid | 12 to 20% |
| Syphilis | 13% |
| LGV and granuloma inguinale | 5% |

- Infection is predominantly subclinical
- Genital herpes is caused by HSV 2 and less commonly by HSV 1
- Incubation period is 2–5 days
- **Clinical manifestations**
  - ➤ First episode infection
  - ➤ Recurrent infections
- **First episode infection**
  - ➤ It can be either true primary infection or nonprimary first episode.
  - ➤ Patients with true primary infection have never been infected with any type of herpesvirus while patients with nonprimary first episode have been infected with either HSV 1 or 2.
  - ➤ First episode primary genital herpes is characterized by fever, headache, malaise, and myalgias.

- ➢ The cervix and urethra are involved in 80% of women with first episode infections.
- ➢ Pain, itching, dysuria, vaginal and urethral discharge, and tender bilateral inguinal lymphadenopathy are the predominant local symptoms.
- ➢ Lesions start as multiple discrete grouped vesicles on an erythematous base in genital area. The vesicles rupture rapidly to form superficial shallow erosions that are often painful. Lesions may coalesce to form erosions with polycyclic margin (Fig. 25.1).
- ➢ Lesions heal in 3–4 weeks even without treatment.
- ➢ A clear mucoid discharge and dysuria are characteristics of symptomatic HSV urethritis.
- ➢ Occasionally, HSV genital tract disease is manifested by endometritis and salpingitis in women and by prostatitis in men.
- ➢ HSV 1 and HSV 2 can cause symptomatic or asymptomatic rectal and perianal infections.
- ➢ First episodes of genital herpes in patients who have had prior HSV 1 infection are associated with less frequent systemic symptoms and faster healing than primary genital herpes.

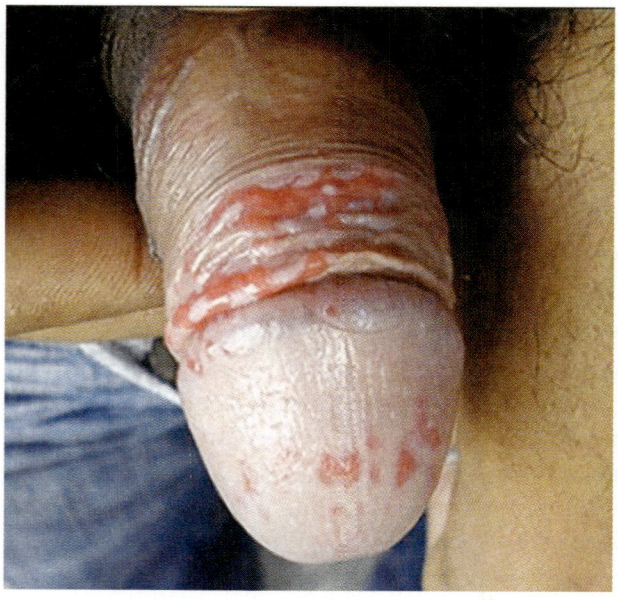

**Fig. 25.1:** Multiple shallow erythematous erosions over glans penis

- **Recurrent infection**
  - Recurrent attacks occur due to reactivation of latent virus by triggering factors like fever, emotional stress, etc.
  - These episodes are often mild with grouped vesicular lesions which rupture to form superficial erosions. Healing takes place in 7–10 days. Systemic symptoms and inguinal lymphadenopathy are usually absent.
  - The recurrence rates of genital disease differ with the viral subtype: the 12-month **recurrence rates** among patients with first-episode HSV 2 and HSV 1 infections are 90% and 55%, respectively (median number of recurrences, 4 and 1, respectively).
- **HPE**
  - In the cutaneous lesions, the cytoplasm of the infected epithelial cells becomes edematous and the cells swell, producing the so-called 'ballooning degeneration'.
  - Thick-walled vesicles are formed by the combination of intra- and intercellular edema.
  - Giant cells containing 2 to 15 or more nuclei are almost invariably present.
  - Intranuclear inclusions are seen.
- **Diagnosis**
  - **Tzanck smear:** Shows multinucleated giant cells
  - Culture: Takes 1–5 days
  - **Serological diagnosis:** Seroconversion or rising antibody titres. Type specific serological tests are better than nonspecific antibodies based ones and they are based on either Western blot or glycoprotein G (gG) assays.
  - Detection of antigen by immunofluorescence
  - Electron microscopy
  - PCR
- **Treatment**
  - *First episode:* Acyclovir 400 mg orally three times a day for 7 to 10 days or acyclovir 200 mg orally five times a day for 7–10 days or famciclovir 250 mg orally three times a day for 7–10 days or valacyclovir 1 gm orally twice a day for 7–10 days.
  - *Recurrent episode:* Acyclovir 400 mg orally three times a day for 5 days or acyclovir 200 mg orally five times a day for 5 days or acyclovir 800 mg twice a day for 5 days, or famciclovir 125 mg orally two times a day for 5 days or valacyclovir 500 mg orally twice a day for 3–5 days or valacyclovir 1 gm orally once a day for 5 days.

> *Suppressive therapy*: Indicated for frequent recurrences. Acyclovir 400 mg orally twice a day, or famciclovir 250 mg orally twice a day, or valacyclovir 500 mg orally once a day, or valacyclovir 1 gm orally once a day.

## BACTERIAL VAGINOSIS (BV)

- Characterized by an overgrowth of vaginal anaerobes and variable degrees of depletion of the normal Lactobacillus species population.
- Most common organisms associated with BV are *Gardnerella vaginalis*, Prevotella sp, Mobiluncus sp and *Mycoplasma hominis*.
- Most common cause of vaginal discharge in India.
- Complaint of offensive, fishy smelling discharge which is more marked after unprotected intercourse or at the time of menstruation. Approximately 50% of women appear to be asymptomatic.
- **Diagnosis**
  > Amsel criteria: Three of the following four criteria should be present for the diagnosis of BV
    1. Excessive homogeneous uniformly adherent vaginal discharge.
    2. Elevated vaginal pH > 4.5
    3. Positive amine test (Whiff test)
    4. Clue cells (20%)—vaginal epithelial cells covered with bacteria.
- **Treatment**
  > Metronidazole 400 mg twice a day for 5 days
  > Intravaginal clindamycin 2% cream
  > Metronidazole 0.75% gel

## WARTS

- Warts are cutaneous neoplasms that are caused by human papilloma-viruses.
- Genital warts (condylomata acuminata) are caused by HPV types 6, 11, 16, 18, 45 and 46.
- They may involve either the labia, perineum, or perianal skin. Additionally, the mucosa of the vagina, urethra, and anus can be involved, as well as the cervical epithelium. In men, the lesions often occur initially in the coronal sulcus, but may be seen on the shaft of the penis, the scrotum, perianal skin, or in the urethra.
- These appear as soft, fleshy, vascular outgrowths. Lesions are frequently pedunculated.

- More than 95% of cervical cancers contain HPV DNA of oncogenic (high-risk) types, such as 16, 18, 31, 33, and 45. HPV DNA is also present in the precursor lesions of cervical cancer (cervical intraepithelial neoplasias). Such lesions containing DNA of oncogenic types are more likely to progress than those associated with low-risk HPV types, such as 6 and 11.

DNA sequences of HPV 16 and 18, and less commonly, HPV 31, 33, 35, and 51 are found in approximately 85% of invasive squamous cell cancers and their presumed precursors (severe dysplasias and carcinoma *in situ*).

In contrast to cervical cancers, **genital warts with low malignant potential** are associated with distinct HPV types, predominantly HPV 6 and HPV 11 ("low-risk" types).

- **Pathogenesis**
  - ➤ The incubation period of HPV disease is usually 3 to 4 months (range, 1 month to 2 years).
  - ➤ The replication of HPV begins with the infection of basal cells.
  - ➤ Virions are assembled in the nucleus and released when keratinocytes are shed. This process is associated with proliferation of all epidermal layers except the basal layer and produces acanthosis, parakeratosis, and hyperkeratosis.
  - ➤ **Koilocytes**—large round cells with pyknotic nuclei—appear in the granular layer (vacuolated keratinocytes due to intranuclear inclusion bodies).
  - ➤ Episomal HPV DNA is present in the nuclei of infected cells in benign lesions caused by HPV. However, in severe dysplasias and cancers, HPV DNA is generally integrated, with disruption of the E1/E2 open reading frames. This disruption leads to upregulation of E6 and E7 and subsequent interference with cellular tumor-suppressor proteins.
  - ➤ Antibodies to E-region proteins, most notably E7, have been detected among patients with cervical carcinoma.
- **Diagnosis**
  - ➤ Mostly clinical
  - ➤ Biopsy shows koilocytes which are characteristic.
  - ➤ Speculum examination should be done to rule out vaginal and cervical warts.
  - ➤ Anoscopy to rule out anal warts and urethroscopy to rule out urethral warts.
  - ➤ *PCR:* Most sensitive method to detect HPV DNA.

> *Acetowhite test:* To identify suclinical warts. Application of 5% acetic acid to the doubtful areas for a few minutes. HPV lesions turn grayish white.

- **Treatment**
  > There are many modalities available to treat warts, but no single therapy is universally effective.
  > *Administered by provider*
    - Cryotherapy with liquid nitrogen or cryoprobe weekly for treatment of choice in pregnancy.
    - Podophyllin resin, 10–25% twice weekly for up to 4 weeks
    - Trichloroacetic acid or bichloroacetic acid, 80–90% weekly
    - Surgical excision
    - Other regimens
      o Intralesionally administered interferon
      o $CO_2$ Laser surgery
  > *Administered by patient*
    - *Podofilox,* 0.5% solution or gel twice daily for 3 days, followed by 4 days without therapy. This cycle may be repeated four times.
    - *Imiquimod* (topical interferon inducer), 5% cream 3 times/ week × 16 weeks. Applied at bedtime and the area is washed with mild soap and water the next morning.
  > Perhaps the most useful and convenient method for treating warts in almost any location is cryotherapy with liquid nitrogen.

## HPV Vaccine

- Recently developed HPV VLP vaccines dramatically reduce rates of infection and disease produced by the HPV types in the vaccines.
- These products are directed against virus types that cause anogenital tract disease and are derived from expression of the major capsid protein (L1) gene in tissue culture.
- When expressed using appropriate vectors and tissue culture systems, L1 self-assembles into a VLP that cannot be distinguished morphologically or antigenically from its wild-type counterpart but that contains no viral nucleic acid.
- Currently, **one quadrivalent product (gardasil)** containing HPV types 6, 11, 16, and 18 has been licensed and recommended for administration to girls and young women 9–26 years of age.
- Another product is **divalent (cervarix)** contains HPV types 16 and 18 and is likely to be available in the near future (Table 25.2).

| Table 25.2: Vaccines for HPV | | |
|---|---|---|
| | *Gardasil* | *Cervarix* |
| | Quadrivalent HPV vaccine | Divalent HPV vaccine |
| **Contains** | HPV types 6, 11, 16, and 18 | HPV types 16 and 18 |
| **Recommended for** | Girls and young women 9–26 years of age | Likely to be available in the near future |
| **Clinical protection** | HPV types 6 and 11 cause 90% of anogenital warts | Types 16 and 18 are responsible for 70% of cervical cancers |

- Because 30% of cervical cancers are caused by HPV types not contained in the vaccines, no changes in cervical cancer screening programs are currently recommended.
- Barrier methods of contraception may also be helpful in preventing transmission of **condyloma acuminatum** and other anogenital HPV-associated diseases.
- **Human papillomavirus (HPV) vaccination:** HPV vaccination is recommended for all women aged  9–26 years who have not completed the vaccine series.
- Ideally, vaccine should be administered before potential exposure to HPV through sexual activity; however, women who are sexually active should still be vaccinated. Sexually active women who have not been infected with any of the HPV vaccine types receive the full benefit of the vaccination.
- Vaccination is less beneficial for women who have already been infected with one or more of the four HPV vaccine types.
- A complete series consists of 3 doses.
  - ➢ The second dose should be administered 2 months after the first dose.
  - ➢ The third dose should be administered 6 months after the first dose.
- **Vaccination is not recommended during pregnancy.**
- If a woman is found to be pregnant after initiating the vaccination series, the remainder of the 3-dose regimen should be delayed until after completion of the pregnancy.

## TRICHOMONIASIS

- *Trichomonas vaginalis,* a unicellular protozoan flagellate invades the vagina, urethra and prostate and is pathogenic, causing trichomoniasis.

- Transmission is usually by sexual intercourse, with an incubation period of 4–21 days.
- Trichomoniasis characteristically causes a copious greenish yellow frothy discharge with vaginal soreness or irritation and urinary frequency. The odor of the discharge is often unpleasant, although this feature is not specific.
- The vaginal mucosal and cervical surfaces are infected and sometimes covered with punctate hemorrhages (Strawberry cervix).
- The pH of the discharge is usually higher than the normal 4.5. Many adults are asymptomatic carriers, particularly males.
- In males, it causes urethritis and rarely balanitis.
- **Diagnosis**
  - ➢ Wet mount preparation: Motile Trichomonads will be seen.
  - ➢ Culture, usually in Feinberg–Whittington medium, gives the most reliable results.
- **Treatment**
  - ➢ Metronidazole 2 gm orally as a single dose or 500 mg twice daily for 7 days. Tinidazole can be used as an alternative.
  - ➢ Sexual partners should be treated.

## GONORRHEA

- This disease is caused by *Neisseria gonorrhoeae*
- *N. gonorrhoeae* is a gram-negative, aerobic diplococcus that principally infects host columnar epithelium.
- Gonococci attach to host mucosal cells with the aid of pili and outer membrane proteins, and then penetrate between cells to the subepithelial space.
- The incubation period is short and symptoms typically have their onset 1–5 days after sexual contact with an infective person.
- In males, the usual presentation is with acute urethritis. There is rapid onset of severe burning dysuria accompanied by a purulent discharge, which is often profuse. In MSM, there may also be rectal and pharyngeal infections. Gonococcal proctitis may be asymptomatic but may also present with rectal pain, tenesmus and discharge. Infection of the oropharynx may present with exudative pharyngitis and cervical lymphadenopathy, but is also commonly asymptomatic.
- In females, the primary site of infection is the cervix, but the urethra, rectum and pharynx are other sites of infection that should be tested. Symptomatic infections manifest as excessive vaginal discharge, dysuria, deep dyspareunia and intermenstrual bleeding. However, a majority of women are asymptomatic.

- Autoinoculation of the organism from infected anogenital sites leads to acute conjunctivitis. This presents as an acutely painful red eye with purulent discharge that may progress to panophthalmitis and loss of vision.
- Gonococcal conjunctivitis is more often associated with newborn babies as ophthalmia neonatorum, which usually occurs in the first week after birth.
- Complications
- Periurethral abscess may occur in either sex and lead to fistula formation and subsequent urethral stricture.
- In females, gonorrhea should also be considered as a possible cause for a Bartholin's abscess.
- Ascending infection in men causes acute prostatitis, with symptoms of urinary frequency, stranguria and back or perineal pain.
- It may also present as unilateral or bilateral painful testicular swelling resulting from acute epididymo-orchitis.
- In women, ascending infections cause pelvic inflamatory disease. This is usually acute in onset, with lower abdominal and pelvic pain, fever, and marked adnexal and cervical motion tenderness on bimanual pelvic examination. Tubo-ovarian abscess and scarring of the fallopian tubes resulting in tubal-factor infertility may ensue.
- Acute perihepatitis (Fitz-Hugh–Curtis syndrome) may also occur with either gonorrhea, Chlamydia or mixed infections.
- Disseminated gonococcal infection (DGI): This occurs in 0.5–3% of patients from hematogenous spread. Typically, genital symptoms are absent. The classic presentation is with a dermatitis–arthritis syndrome in a patient with mild fever.
- **Diagnosis**
  - *Microscopy:* A rapid presumptive diagnosis can be made by the identification of gram-negative intracellular diplococci within phagocytes in stained smears from anogenital sites.
  - *Culture:* The gonococcus is a fastidious organism and requires appropriate methods of specimen collection and transportation to the laboratory. Specimens are plated onto nutritive, selective media and incubated in a humid atmosphere containing 5% $CO_2$. Culture remains the gold standard for diagnosing gonorrhea, and also allows the testing of isolates for antimicrobial sensitivities.
  - *Nucleic acid amplification tests (NAATs)* have been introduced as new tools to diagnose and treat *C. trachomatis* and *N. gonorrhoeae* infections.

- **Treatment**
  - ➤ Uncomplicated anogenital infection in adults
    - – Ceftriaxone 250 mg IM as a single dose
    - – Cefixime 400 mg orally as a single dose
    - – Spectinomycin 2 g IM as a single dose
    - – Ciprofloxacin 500 mg orally in a single dose
    - – Ofloxacin 400 mg orally in a single dose
    - – Levofloxacin 250 mg orally in a single dose
  - ➤ Pregnancy and breastfeeding
    - – Fluoroquinolones should be avoided
  - ➤ In addition, where regional prevalence of penicillin-resistant *N. gonorrhoeae* is ≤5%
    - – Amoxycillin 3 g plus probenecid 1 g orally as a single dose
    - – Ampicillin 2 g plus probenecid 1 g orally as a single dose

## NONGONOCOCCAL URETHRITIS

- **Etiology**
  - ➤ *C. trachomatis* 30–50%
  - ➤ *Ureaplasma urealyticum* 10–40%
  - ➤ *T. vaginalis*
  - ➤ HSV
  - ➤ Adenovirus
  - ➤ Yeasts
  - ➤ Haemophilus sp
  - ➤ Bacteroides
- Incubation period is 1–5 weeks
- In males urethritis begins with dysuria and mucoid urethral discharge. In contrast to gonococcal urethritis symptoms are usually mild.
- Most cases in females are asymptomatic
- **Diagnosis**
  - ➤ Gram's stain of urethral discharge: It shows more than 5 pus cells per oil immersion field but no gram-negative intracellular diplococci are seen.
  - ➤ Culture
- **Treatment**
  - ➤ Azithromycin 1 g oral once or doxycycline 100 mg BD for 7 days.

## TREPONEMAL INFECTIONS

- The genus Treponema includes *T. pallidum* subspecies *pallidum*, which causes venereal syphilis; *T. pallidum* subspecies *pertenue*, which causes yaws; *T. pallidum* subspecies *endemicum*, which causes endemic syphilis or bejel; and *T. carateum*, which causes pinta.
- The etiologic agents of the **endemic treponematoses** are *T. pallidum* subspecies pertenue (yaws), *T. pallidum* subspecies *endemicum* (endemic syphilis), and *T. carateum* (pinta).
- There are two types of serologic test for syphilis: Nontreponemal and treponemal. Both types of test are reactive in persons with any treponemal infection, including yaws, pinta, and endemic syphilis.

## Syphilis

- The causative organism is *Treponema pallidum*.
- The disease is classified into acquired and congenital syphilis. Both are further divided into early and late syphilis.

### Acquired Syphilis

- It has an early infectious stage and late non-infectious stage.
- The dividing line is usually taken as 2 years.
- The early infectious stage is further subdivided into primary, secondary and early latent stages.
- The late non-infectious stage is divided into late latent syphilis and tertiary syphilis (benign tertiary syphilis, cardiovascular syphilis and neurosyphilis)

### Primary Syphilis

- Incubation period is 9–90 days.
- **Typical primary chancre** usually begins as a single painless papule that rapidly becomes eroded and usually becomes indurated, with a characteristic cartilaginous consistency on palpation of the edge and base of the ulcer. It is painless, nontender, indurated ulcer with a clean looking floor and raised sharply defined border (Fig. 25.2).
- In heterosexual men, the chancre is usually located on the penis, whereas in homosexual men, it is often found in the anal canal or rectum, in the mouth, or on the external genitalia.
- In women, common primary sites are the cervix and labia. Consequently, primary syphilis goes unrecognized in women and homosexual men more often than in heterosexual men.

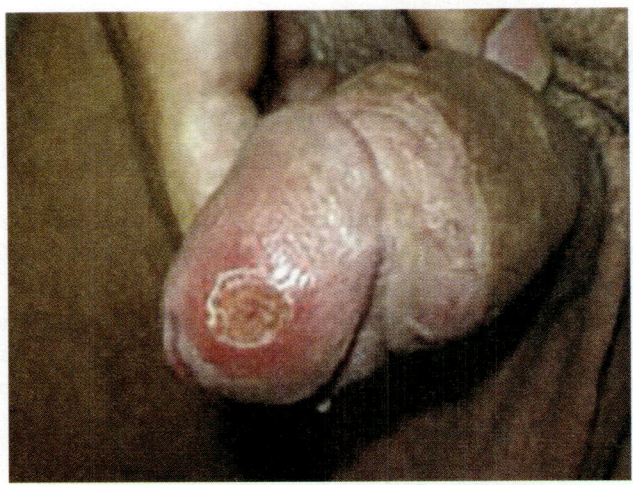

**Fig. 25.2:** Indurated ulcer with clean looking floor and raised sharply defined border (primary chancre)

- Within 1–2 weeks majority of patients develop bilateral inguinal lymphadenopathy characterized by nontender, hard, discrete, multiple nodes. Without treatment chancre heals with scarring in 3–6 weeks.
- **Chancre redux** is a recurrence of the primary sore at its original site.
- **Pseudochancre redux** describes gummatous (tertiary stage) recurrence at the site of the primary chancre.

### Secondary Syphilis

- 3–6 weeks after the appearance of primary chancre.
- Characterized by mucocutaneous lesions, constitutional symptoms and generalized lymphadenopathy.
- The skin lesions are asymptomatic, bilateral and symmetrical.
- The cutaneous lesions may be macular, papular, papulosquamous to pustular and nodular (Fig. 25.3).
- In secondary syphilis, condylomata lata, flat-topped greyish white papules, affect the vulva and anal areas as may also mucous patches, which are greyish white moist-looking lesions in the mucous membrane of the oral cavity. These lesions are highly infectious (Fig. 25.4).
- Generalized lymphadenopathy which affects frequently inguinal, posterior cervical and epitrochlear lymph nodes.
- Rarely CNS, eyes and other visceral organs are affected.

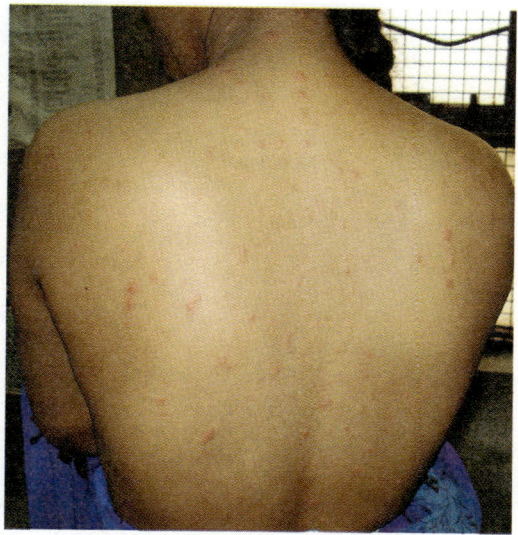

**Fig. 25.3:** Multiple papular lesions in secondary syphilis

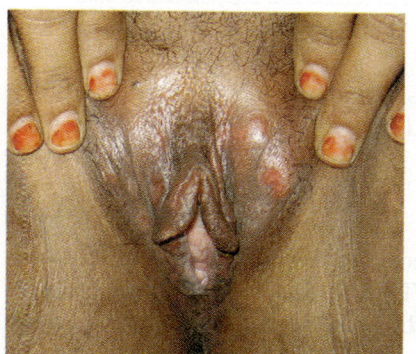 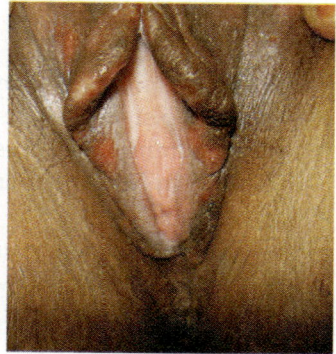

**Fig. 25.4:** Mucosal lesions of secondary syphilis

## Latent Syphilis

- Patient only has serological evidence but no clinical evidence.
- Depending on number of years that have elapsed, it is further divided into early latent syphilis (<2 yrs) and late latent syphilis (>2 yrs).

## Tertiary Syphilis

- It manifests 3–10 years after the primary stage as benign gummata of mucocutaneous and bony structures, cardiovascular syphilis or neurosyphilis (tabes dorsalis and general paresis).

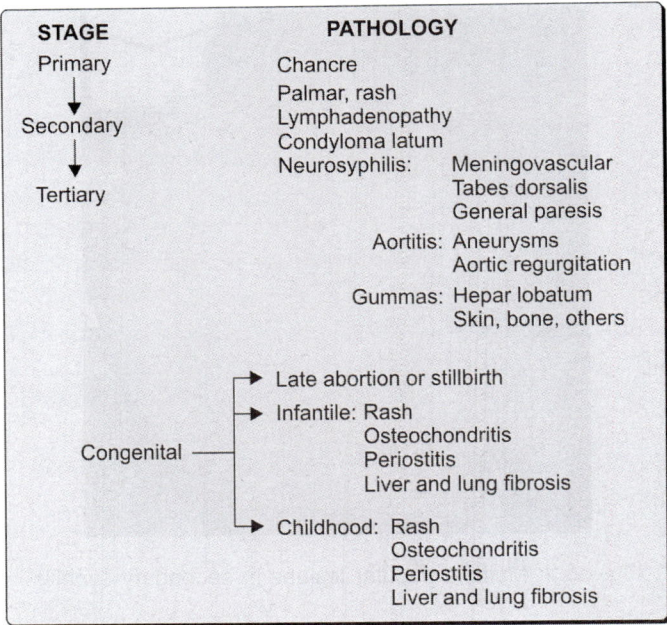

| STAGE | PATHOLOGY |
|---|---|
| Primary | Chancre |
| ↓ | Palmar, rash |
| Secondary | Lymphadenopathy |
| | Condyloma latum |
| ↓ | Neurosyphilis: Meningovascular |
| Tertiary | Tabes dorsalis |
| | General paresis |
| | Aortitis: Aneurysms |
| | Aortic regurgitation |
| | Gummas: Hepar lobatum |
| | Skin, bone, others |

Late abortion or stillbirth

Infantile: Rash
Osteochondritis
Periostitis
Liver and lung fibrosis

Congenital

Childhood: Rash
Osteochondritis
Periostitis
Liver and lung fibrosis

- **Diagnosis**
  - ➤ Dark ground microscopy of a smear of chancre of primary syphilis or the moist lesions of secondary syphilis reveal the organisms. Direct immunofluorescent staining of the smear may also demonstrate the organisms.
  - ➤ *Serological testing*
    - – The most widely used nontreponemal antibody tests for syphilis are the RPR and VDRL tests, which measure IgG and IgM directed against a cardiolipin-lecithin-cholesterol antigen complex.
    - – The RPR test is easier to perform and uses unheated serum; it is the test of choice for rapid serologic diagnosis in a clinical setting and can be automated.
    - – The VDRL test remains the standard for examining CSF.
    - – The RPR and VDRL tests are used for screening or for quantitation of serum antibody. A titre of 1 : 8 or more is said to be significant. The titer reflects disease activity, rising during the evolution of early syphilis and often exceeding 1 : 32 in secondary syphilis.
    - – A persistent fall by two dilutions (fourfold) or more after treatment of early syphilis is considered an adequate response to therapy.

- Specific treponemal tests like *Treponema pallidum* hemagglutination assay (TPHA) test, *Treponema pallidum* immobilization (TPI) test, fluorescent treponemal antibody absorption (FTA-ABS) test may be done to confirm the diagnosis.
- ➢ CSF examination and chest radiography should be done in tertiary syphilis.
- ➢ *HPE:* Endarteritis obliterans and perivascular infiltrate of lymphoid cells and plasma cells.

## Congenital Syphilis

- *Early congenital syphilis:* Features that appear within the first 2 years of life.
- *Late congenital syphilis:* Features that occur later than two years of life
- *T. pallidum* can be transmitted by an infected mother to the fetus *in utero.*
- Fetus is at greatest risk when maternal syphilis is of less than 2 years duration.
- Prenatal infection can also result in miscarriage or stillbirths.

### Early congenital syphilis

- Clinical features are similar to acquired secondary syphilis but visceral and bone involvement are more frequent.
- Signs begin to appear within 3–8 weeks of life and in all cases by third month.
- Snuffles, a form of rhinitis is most frequent and often the first finding.
- Baby appears marasmic like a wrinkled pot bellied old man.
- Bullous eruptions are seen in congenital syphilis.
- Hepatomegaly, splenomegaly, bone and joint involvement are common.
- Osteochondritis with the sawtoothed metaphysis seen on radiographs and periostitis appear with tender limbs (pseudoparalysis).

### Late congenital syphilis

- Hutchinson's triad is considered pathognomonic of congenital syphilis.
- It consists of Hutchinson's teeth, interstitial keratitis and VIII nerve deafness.
- Saddle nose, frontal bossing, saber tibia and Clutton's joints are seen (Tables 25.3 to 25.5).
- **Diagnosis**
  - ➢ *Dark ground microscopy*
  - ➢ *Serological tests*
    - The diagnosis of congenital syphilis is complicated by the transplacental transfer of maternal nontreponemal and treponemal immunoglobulin G (IgG) antibodies to the fetus.

- – This transfer of antibodies makes the interpretation of reactive serologic tests for syphilis in infants difficult.
- – Treatment decisions often must be made on the basis of identification of syphilis in the mother.
  - o Adequacy of maternal treatment.
  - o Presence of clinical, laboratory, or radiographic evidence of syphilis in the infant.
  - o Comparison of maternal (at delivery) and infant non-treponemal serologic titres utilizing the same test and preferably the same laboratory.

**Table 25.3:** Recommendations for the treatment of syphilis

| Stage of syphilis | Patients without penicillin allergy | Patients with confirmed penicillin allergy |
|---|---|---|
| Primary, secondary, or early latent | Penicillin G benzathine (single dose of 2.4 mU IM) | Tetracycline hydrochloride (500 mg PO qid) or doxycycline (100 mg PO bid) for 2 weeks |
| Late latent (or latent of uncertain duration), cardiovascular, or benign tertiary | Lumbar puncture CSF normal: Penicillin G benzathine (2.4 mU IM weekly for 3 weeks) CSF abnormal: Treat as neurosyphilis | Lumbar puncture CSF normal and patient not infected with HIV: Tetracycline hydrochloride (500 mg PO qid) or doxycycline (100 mg PO bid) for 4 weeks CSF normal and patient infected with HIV: Desensitization and treatment with penicillin if compliance cannot be ensured CSF abnormal: Treat as neurosyphilis |
| Neurosyphilis (asymptomatic or symptomatic) | Aqueous penicillin G (18–24 mU/d IV, given as 3–4 mU q4h or continuous infusion) for 10–14 days or aqueous penicillin G procaine (2.4 mU/d IM) plus oral probenecid (500 mg qid), both for 10–14 days | Desensitization and treatment penicillin |
| Syphilis in pregnancy | According to stage | Desensitization and treatment with penicillin |

**Table 25.4:** Congenital syphilis—clinical features and treatment

| Stage | Manifestations | | Treatment | |
|---|---|---|---|---|
| | Placental | Fetus | Primary | Alternative |
| Congenital (Prenatal) | Langhans' cell layer<br>Placentitis:<br>• Acute chorioamnionitis<br>• Chronic villitis<br>• Hydrops placentalis<br>• Necrotizing funisitis | Hydrops fetalis<br>Intrauterine growth retardation<br>Premature delivery<br>Stillbirth | **Aqueous crystalline PCN G**<br>100000–150 000 µ/kg/day administered as 5000 µ/kg/dose IV q12h × first 7 days of life, then g8h × 7–21 days | **Procaine PCN G**<br>50,000 µ/kg/dose qd IM × 10 days |
| | Early | Late | | |
| Congenital (postnatal) | Chorioretinitis ('Salt and pepper' fundus)<br>Dactylitis<br>Epiphysitis<br>Hepatomegaly/hepatitis<br>Parrot's pseudoparalysis<br>Pneumonia alba<br>Snuffles<br>Syphilitic pemphigus<br>Rhagades<br>Wimberger's sign | Clutton's joints<br>Frontal bossing<br>Higoumenaki's sign<br>Hutchinson's triad<br>Interstitial keratitis<br>'Mulberry' molars<br>Neurosyphilis<br>Protruding mandible<br>Saber shins<br>Saddle nose<br>Short maxillae | | |

*Contd.*

**Table 25.4:** Congenital syphilis—clinical features and treatment (*Contd.*)

| Stage | Manifestations | Treatment | |
|-------|----------------|-----------|--|
| Primary | *Cutaneous:* Balanitis of Follman, chancre redux, dory flop' sign, primary chancre, syphilis d'emblee *Other:* Regional lymphadenopathy | *Primary, secondary or early latent (<1 year):* **Benzathine PCN G** 2.4 mill U IM in a single dose | **Doxycycline** 100 mg bid PO × 14 days *or* **Tetracycline** 500 mg qid PO × 14 days *or* **Ceftriaxone** 1 g IM/IV daily × 8–10 days |
| Secondary | *Cutaneous findings:* Biette's collarette, condyloma latum, 'corona veneris' corymbiform, 'frambesiform syphilid' leukoderma colli (collar of Venus), lues maligna (ulceronodular, 'la grand verole') moth-eaten' alopecia, mucous patches (plaques fauchées en prairie), Ollendorff's sign, 'raw ham' papules, ringed (annular) plaques, rupial plaques, split papule *Other:* Acute meningitis, acute nephrotic syndrome, gastrointestinal involvement, granulomatous iritis, pharyngitis, retrobulbar optic neuritis, syphilitic hepatitis | *Late latent (>1 year) or syphilis of indeterminate duration, late benign:* **Benzathine PCN G** 2.4 mill U IM qwk × 3 qid PO × 28 days | **Doxycycline** 100 mg bid PO × 28 days *or* **Tetracycline** 500 mg |
| Latent | Asymptomatic | | |
| Tertiary (late) | *Cutaneous:* Gummas, pseudochancre redux *Neurosyphilis:* Asymptomatic, gummas, meningeal Meningovascular, parenchymatous (paresis, tabes dorsalis, Argyll-Robertson pupil) *Rheum:* Bilateral bursitis of Verneuil, Charcot joints *Vascular:* Aortitis, aortic aneurysm, coronary ostial stenosis | *Neurosyphilis, including ocular syphilis:* **Aqueous crystalline PCN G** mill U IV q4h × 10–14 days | **Procaine PCN G** 2.4 mill U qd IM *plus* **probenecid** 500 mg qid PO, both × 10–14 days |

**Table 25.5:** Features of syphilis

| | |
|---|---|
| Argyll Robertson pupil | Pupil accommodates, but does not react to light |
| Balanitis of Follman | Chancres may be atypical (multiple, painful, purulent, and destructive) |
| Biette's collarette | Thin, white ring of scales on the surface of the papules |
| Chancre redux | (Monorecidive chancre) the reappearance of a chancre after partial healing at result of insufficient treatment |
| Charcot joints | Enlarged, painless, inflamed joints, with or without deformity, in the low extremities and spine. |
| Clutton's joints | Synovitis with effusions of the knees and elbows |
| Corona veneris | Macules and/or papules along the hairline. |
| Corymbose (bomb shell) | A large central papule surrounded by satellite raised pustules. |
| Condyloma latum | Skin-colored or hypopigmented, moist, oozing papules located perianally and on genitalia. They become fattened and macerated. These are teeming with treponemes, and thus are extremely infectious. |
| Dory flop sign | When the foreskin is retracted, mucosal surface chancres flip briskly. |
| Frambesiform syphilid | Condylomata lata in intertriginous areas may proliferate forming nodular lesions that resemble raspberries. |
| Gummas | Rubbery tumors with predilection for skin or long bones, may also develop in the eyes, mucous membranes, throat, liver, or stomach lining. |
| Higoumenaki's sign | Unilateral, irregular enlargement of the clavicle at site of sternocleidomastoid attachment, secondary to periostitis. |
| Hutchinson's teeth | Centrally notched, widely spaced, peg-shaped upper incisors. |
| Hutchinson's triad | Hutchinson's teeth, CN 8 nerve deafness, and corneal opacities (secondary to interstitial keratitis). |
| Langhans' cell layer | Layer of the cytotrophoblast of the placenta: A controversial protective placental barrier until 20-wk gestation. Recently it has been demonstrated that treponemas cross the placenta in early pregnancy. |
| Leukoderma colli | (Syphilitic leukoderma/collar of pearls/collar of Venus/venereal collar), round or oval, ill-defined, depigmented macules with hyperpigmented borders occurring on the anterolateral neck and chest. |
| Lues maligna | Areas of ulcerated and necrotic tissue, occurs in secondary syphilis (more likely patients with HIV). |
| Mulberry molars | (Moon's or Fournier's molar) sixth-year molars, is seen in the first lower molar. |

*Contd.*

**Table 25.5:** Features of syphilis   *Contd.*

| | |
|---|---|
| Mucous patch | Painless, shallow, rounded gray macerated erosions, located on the oral, genital and anal mucosa. These are teeming with treponemes. |
| Ollendorff's sign | Papules tender to palpation. |
| Parrot's pseudoparalysis | Reduced movement of the extremities due to pain. |
| Pneumonia alba | Yellowish-white, heavy firm, and grossly enlarged lungs (pneumonitis). |
| Pseudochancre redux | A solitary gumma of the penis. |
| Rhagades (Parrot's lines) | Perioral fissures. |
| Rupial lesion | Ulcerative lesions with a heaped-up crust, oyster-shell-like. |
| Saber shins | Anterior tibial bowing. |
| Snuffles | Bloody or purulent mucinous nasal discharge. |
| Split papule | Lesions at the angle of the mouth or the corner of the nose which have a central linear erosion. |
| Syphilis d'emblee | Syphilis occurring without an initial sore. |
| Syphilitic pemphigus | Vesiculobullous eruption. |
| Wimberger's (cat-bite) sign | A radiographic "saw-tooth" appearance at the medial aspect of the proximal tibial metaphysis. |

- The regimen of 2.4 million units of benzathine pencillin intramuscularly weekly for three consecutive weeks results in low to undetectable cerebrospinal fluid levels of penicillin and treatment failures have been described when this regimen has been used to treat neurosyphilis.

- For these reasons, present recommendations for the therapy of neurosyphilis employ higher doses of short-acting penicillin in order to achieve better penetration and higher levels of drug in the cerebrospinal fluid. Recommended regimens include 3–4 million units of aqueous crystalline penicillin G intravenously every 4 hours for 10–14 days.

- Alternatively, 2, 4 million units of procaine penicillin can be given intramuscularly once daily along with 500 mg of probenecid orally four times daily, both 10–14 days.

- Because of concerns about slowly dividing organisms that may persist, many experts recommend subsequent administration of 2.4 million units of benzathine penicillin intramuscularly once weekly for 3 wks as additional therapy.

- Patients with a history of penicillin allergy should be skin-tested, desensitized, and treated with penicillin.

## QUESTIONS FROM PREVIOUS EXAMINATIONS

1. Giant condyloma
2. Chancroid
3. Herpes progenitalis
4. Complications of untreated gonococcus in male and female
5. Pseudobubo
6. Greenbaldt and pund cells
7. Secondary syphilis
8. Natural history of untreated syphilis
9. Clincal features of acquired syphilis
10. Neurosyphilis
11. Serological tests for syphilis
12. Genital ulcer
13. FTA ABS
14. Chracott's joints
15. Urethroscopy
16. Saddle nose
17. Interstitial keratitis
18. Prozone phenomenon
19. Sero partners
20. Darkfield microscopy
21. Chancres
22. Pseudochancre redux
23. CSF changes in syphilis
24. CSF VDRL test
25. Atonic bladder
26. Hutchinson's triad
27. Corono veneris
28. BO sign
29. Syphilis in pregnancy
30. CVS syphilis
31. Syphilis + HIV
32. Nonvenereal treponemiasis
33. Congenital syphilis
34. Heart and great vessels in syphilis
35. Darter-Korras concept
36. Aneurysms of aorta
37. AR pupil
38. Rosemenaki sign

39. Clutton's joint
40. Stigmata of congenital syphilis
41. Reagin test
42. HPE of granuloma inguinale
43. Inguinal adenitis
44. Lymphatic involvement in LGV
45. Differential diagnosis of LGV
46. Frei test
47. Esthiomine
48. Saxaphone penis
49. Fitz-Hugh–Curtis syndrome
50. *H. ducreyi*
51. LAS diagnosis of LGV
52. Condyloma acuminatum
53. Recurrent herpes genitalis
54. Vaginitis
55. Balanoposthitis
56. Zoon's balanitis
57. Balanosis xerotica obliterans
58. Trichomoniasis
59. Clue cells
60. Whiff test
61. Circinate balanitis
62. Nonspecific urethritis
63. PID
64. Chronic prostitis
65. *Ureaplasma urealyticum*
66. Keratoderma blenorrhagicum
67. Pila antigen
68. Morning drop
69. Two-glass test

## MULTIPLE CHOICE QUESTIONS

1. **Features of Reiter's disease are the following** *except:*

   *(AIIMS Nov 2008)*

   (a) Oral ulcers
   (b) Circinate balanitis
   (c) Subcutaneous nodules
   (d) Keratoderma blenorrhagicum

2. **Symptoms of urethritis, conjunctivitis and reactive arthritis in a HLA-B27 positive person are mostly associated with which of the following organisms?**    *(AIIMS Nov 2008)*
   - (a)  *Ureaplasma urealyticum*
   - (b)  *Streptococcus bovis*
   - (c)  Group B streptococci
   - (d)  *Borrelia burgdorferi*

3. **Keratoderma blenorrhagicum is seen in:**    *(AIIMS Nov 2008)*
   - (a)  Psoriasis
   - (b)  Syphilis
   - (c)  Reiter's disease
   - (d)  Disseminated gonococcal infection

4. **Molluscum contagiosum is caused by:**    *(JK 2009)*
   - (a)  Staphylococci
   - (b)  Poxvirus
   - (c)  The itch mite
   - (d)  Human papillomavirus

5. **Worldwide accepted minimum dose of mega units benzathine penicillin in tertiary syphilis:**    *(AP 07)*
   - (a)  4.8 mega units
   - (b)  6 mega units
   - (c)  7.2 mega units
   - (d)  10 mega units

6. **Chancroid is caused by:**    *(UP 09)*
   - (a)  *Haemophilus ducreyi*
   - (b)  HSV
   - (c)  *Chlamydia trachomatis*
   - (d)  *Calymmatobacterium granulomatis*

7. **Pinta is caused by:**    *(TN 06)*
   - (a)  *Treponema pertenue*
   - (b)  *Treponema carateum*
   - (c)  *Treponema pallidum*
   - (d)  *Treponema endemicum*

8. **Condyloma acuminatum caused by:**    *(MH 2001)*
   - (a)  Treponema
   - (b)  CMV
   - (c)  HPV
   - (d)  Herpes simplex

9. **Painful ulcers over genitalia are caused by:**    *(MH 03)*
   - (a)  Primary syphilis
   - (b)  Granuloma inguinale
   - (c)  Chanchroid
   - (d)  Lymphogranuloma venerum

10. **Hard chancre is seen in:**    *(DNB 09)*
    - (a)  Chancroid
    - (b)  Syphilis
    - (c)  Tularemia
    - (d)  All of the above

11. **Condyloma latum is caused by:**    *(MH 05)*
    - (a)  *Haemophilus ducreyi*
    - (b)  *Calymmatobacterium granulomatis*
    - (c)  *Treponema pallidum*
    - (d)  Herpes simplex virus

12. **Groove sign:**                                    *(JIPMER 03)*
    (a) Lymphogranuloma venereum
    (b) Lymphogranuloma inguinale
    (c) Chancroid
    (d) Gonorrhea

13. **True regarding warts include the following** *except:*    *(MH 08)*
    (a) It is a cutaneous neoplasm
    (b) It rarely regresses spontaneously
    (c) Causative agent is human papillomavirus
    (d) Urethra and vulva are affected in the females

14. **True about genital herpes includes the following** *except:*
    *(MH 08)*
    (a) Usually caused by HSV 2
    (b) Primary lesions more painful than secondary
    (c) Systemic are more commonly seen in primary than secondary
    (d) Recurrence rate is 30–40%

15. **Immunomodulator used in treatment of genital warts:**  *(AI 2008)*
    (a) ATRA                      (b) Podophylline
    (c) Imiquimod                 (d) Prednisolone

16. **Treatment of choice for genital warts in pregnancy:**  *(AIIMS Nov 09)*
    (a) Salicylic acid with lactic acid solution
    (b) Podophylin
    (c) Imiqimod
    (d) Cryotherapy

17. **HPV vaccine is:**                                 *(AIIMS Nov 09)*
    (a) Monovalent                (b) Bivalent
    (c) Quadrivalent              (d) Bivalent and quadrivalent

18. **A 30-year-old man with history of multiple exposures presents with painful indurated ulcer on the glans penis since 5 days. The undermined sloughed edges of margins were noted. The most porobable diagnosis is:**    *(AI 2008)*
    (a) Chancroid                 (b) Primary chancre
    (c) Herpes genitalis          (d) LGV

19. **Following are primary cutaneous diseases** *except:*    *(AI 09)*
    (a) Psoriasis                 (b) Reiter's disease
    (c) Lichen planus             (d) Icthiosis

20. **Ollendorff's sign is seen in:**                  *(AFMC 07)*
    (a) Primary syphilis          (b) Secondary syphilis
    (c) Latent syphilis           (d) Neurosyphilis

21. After 8 weeks of visit to female sex worker male patient develops painless ulcer over penis that bleeds on touch without any lymphadenopathy, diagnosis is: *(AMU 08)*
    - (a) Primary syphilis
    - (b) Chanchroid
    - (c) Herpes simplex virus
    - (d) Donovanosis

22. The syndromic management of urethral discharge includes the treatment of: *(AI 03)*
    - (a) *Neisseria gonorrhoeae* and herpes genitalis
    - (b) *Chlamydia trachomatis* and herpes genitalis
    - (c) *Neisseria gonorrhoeae* and *Chlamydia trachomatis*
    - (d) Syphilis and chancroid

23. The most frequent cause of recurrent genital ulceration in a sexually active male is: *(AI 03)*
    - (a) Herpes genitalis
    - (b) Aphthous ulcer
    - (c) Syphilis
    - (d) Chancroid

24. A VDRL reactive mother gave birth to an infant. All of the following would be helpful in determining the risk of transmission to the infant, *except:*
    - (a) TPHA test on the serum sample of the mother
    - (b) TPHA test on the serum sample of the infant
    - (c) VDRL on the paired serum sample of the infant and mother
    - (d) Time interval between the treatment of the mother and her delivery

25. All except one are true regarding yaws: *(AI 2008)*
    - (a) Caused by Treponema subspecies *T. pertenue*
    - (b) It cross reacts with antibody titer of syphilis
    - (c) It is transmitted sexually
    - (d) The recommended treatment is benzathine penicillin

26. Treatment of choice for neurosyphilis: *(AI 2008)*
    - (a) Procaine penicillin
    - (b) Benzathine penicillin
    - (c) Oral penicillin G
    - (d) Ampicillin

27. True regarding tertiary syphilis: *(AI 2008)*
    - (a) It is the most infectious stage of syphilis
    - (b) All patients with primary syphilis progress to tertiary stage if untreated
    - (c) Gumma are seen
    - (d) It contains high number of spirochete in the lesions

28. **A 23-year-old college student has asymptomatic and hyperpig-mented macules on both palms for 3 weeks. The most appropriate diagnostic test is:** *(AIIMS 2004)*
    (a) Venereal disease research laboratory (VDRL) test
    (b) Skin biopsy
    (c) Serum cortisol levels
    (d) Assay for arsenic in skin, hair and nails

29. **A 42-year-old engineer developed redness of the glans and radial fissuring of the prepuce 2 weeks ago. A potassium hydroxide preparation of scrapings from the glans showed pseudohyphae and buds. Which one of the following systemic illnesses should be screened for?** *(AIIMS May 2004)*
    (a) Pulmonary tuberculosis    (b) Diabetes mellitus
    (c) Systemic candidiasis    (d) Chronic renal failure

30. **A 23-year-old male has unprotected sexual intercourse with a commercial sex worker. 2 weeks later, he developed a painless, indurated ulcer on the glans, which exuded clear serum on pressure. Inguinal lymph nodes in both groins were enlarged and not tender. The most appropriate diagnostic test is:** *(AIIMS May 2004)*
    (a) Gram's stain of ulcer discharge
    (b) Darkfield microscopy of ulcer discharge
    (c) Giemsa stain of lymph node aspirate
    (d) ELISA for HIV infection

31. **'Chancre redux' is a clinical feature of:** *(AIIMS May 06)*
    (a) Early relapsing syphilis
    (b) Late syphilis
    (c) Chancroid
    (d) Recurrent herpes simplex infection

32. **Which of the following genital ulcers is painless?** *(AIIMS May 2013)*
    (a) Syphilis    (b) Herpes
    (c) Chancroid    (d) Fungal

## Answers

1. **Ans. (c)** Subcutaneous nodules *(Ref. Harrison's Medicine, 17th edn, 321; 1702)*
2. **Ans. (a)** *Ureaplasma urealyticum (Ref. Harrison's Medicine, 17th edn, 321; 1702)*
3. **Ans. (c)** Reiter's disease *(Ref. Harrison's Medicine, 17th edn, 321; 1702)*

4. **Ans. (b)** Poxvirus *(Ref. Kumar and Clarke Medicine, 6th edn, 1322)*
5. **Ans. (c)** 7.2 mega units *(Ref. Harison's Medicine, 17th edn, Table 162–2)*
6. **Ans. (c)** *Haemophilus ducreyi (Ref. Harison's Medicine, 17th edn, Chapter 139)*
7. **Ans. (b)** *Treponema carateum (Ref. Harison's Internal Medicine, 17th edn, Chapter 63)*
8. **Ans. (c)** Human papilomavirus (HPV)
9. **Ans. (c)** Chanchroid
10. **Ans. (b)** Syphilis
11. **Ans. (c)** *Treponema pallidum*
12. **Ans. (a)** Lymphogranuloma venereum
13. **Ans. (b)** It rarely regresses spontaneously
14. **Ans. (d)** Recurrence rate is 30–40% *(Ref. Harrison's Principles of Internal Medicine, page 772, Table 115–7)*
15. **Ans. (c)** Imiquimod
16. **Ans. (d)** Cryotherapy *(Ref. IADVL Textbook of Dermatology, 3rd edn, 1923; Fitzpatrick-Dermatology, 7th edn, 2129)*
17. **Ans. (d)** Bivalent and quadrivalent *(Ref. Harrisons Medicine, 17th edn, 1119)*
18. **Ans. (a)** Chancroid
19. **Ans. (d)** Reiter's disease *(Ref. IADVL Textbook of Dermatology, 2nd edn, 1441)*
20. **Ans. (b)** Secondary syphilis
21. **Ans. (d)** Donovanosis *(Ref. Harrison Medicine, 17th edn, 154)*
22. **Ans. (c)** *Neisseria gonorrhoeae* and *Chlamydia trachomatis*
23. **Ans. (a)** Herpes genitalis.
24. **Ans. (d)** Time interval between the treatment of the mother and her delivery
25. **Ans. (c)** It is transmitted sexually
26. **Ans. (a)** Procaine penicillin *(Ref. KDT, 6th edn, 698, 715, 729, 737)*
27. **Ans. (c)** Gumma are seen
28. **Ans. (a)** Venereal disease research laboratory (VDRL) test *(Ref. Harrison's Internal Medicine, 17th edn, Chapter 162)*
29. **Ans. (b)** Diabetes mellitus *(Ref. Harrison's Internal Medicine, 17th edn, Chapter 196)*
30. **Ans. (b)** Darkfield microscopy of ulcer discharge *(Ref: Jawetz Microbiology, 22nd edn, 642; Rook's Dermatology, 7th edn 68.70)*
31. **Ans. (a)** Early relapsing syphilis *(Ref. Rook, 7th edn, 30.7; 68.32)*
32. **Ans. (a)** Syphilis.

# 26 Human Immunodeficiency Virus and Skin

## HIV STRUCTURE

- **Classification**
  - ➢ Retroviridae (family)
  - ➢ Lentivirus (genus)
- **Characteristics**
  - ➢ 100 nm in diameter
  - ➢ Genome of 2 single strands of RNA
  - ➢ Nine genes
  - ➢ Reverse transcriptase
    - – RNA-dependent DNA polymerase
    - – Transcribes RNA into DNA
- **Genome of HIV**
  - ➢ Contains 6 regulatory genes
  - ➢ Contains 3 structural genes
  - ➢ Env (envelope glycoproteins)
  - ➢ gp120 and gp41
  - ➢ Gag (core and matrix proteins)
  - ➢ p55, p40 and p24
  - ➢ Pol (enzymes)
  - ➢ Reverse transcriptase (p66, p51)
  - ➢ Protease (p11)
  - ➢ Integrase (p32)
- **Types**
  - ➢ Human immunodeficiency virus, type 1 (HIV 1)
  - ➢ Human immunodeficiency virus, type 2 (HIV 2)
- **HIV 1 is divided into the following groups**
  - ➢ M (Major)
  - ➢ N (New)
  - ➢ O (Outlier)

## TRANSMISSION OF INFECTION

- Sexual intercourse with infected person
- Homosexual (MSM)
- Heterosexual
- Bisexual
- Children born to infected mothers
- Perinatal
- IV drug addicts sharing contaminated syringes/needles
- Transfusion of blood and blood products
  - Transfusion recipients
  - Hemophiliacs
  - Occupational exposure in health care setting

## MECHANISM OF PATHOGENICITY

- Envelope protein (gp120) of HIV binds with CD4 receptor on surface of:
  - T-lymphocytes
  - Macrophages
  - Dendritic cells
  - Microglial cells
- Coreceptors for attachment of HIV
  - CCR5 (T cells, macrophages, dendritic cells, microglial cells)
  - CXCR4 (T cells)
- Following attachment, virus enters cells and removes protein coat. Viral RNA is transcribed into DNA by:
  - Reverse transcriptase
- Viral DNA then integrated into host cell DNA
  - Integrase
- Integrated viral DNA
  - Referred to as "provirus"
  - Production of active infection

## CDC Classification (Table 26.1)

- Latest revision in 1993
- Clinical categories
  - A
  - B
  - C

**Table 26.1:** CDC classification system for HIV-infected adults and adolescents

| CD4 cell categories | Clinical categories | | |
| --- | --- | --- | --- |
| | A<br>Asymptomatic, acute HIV, or PGL | B<br>Symptomatic conditions, not A or C | C<br>AIDS-indicator conditions |
| 1. ≥500 cells/µl | A1 | B1 | C1 |
| 2. 200–499 cells/µl | A2 | B2 | C2 |
| 3. <200 cells/µl | A3 | B3 | C3 |

PGL: Persistent generalized lymphadenopathy

## Category B Symptomatic Conditions

- Category B symptomatic conditions are defined as symptomatic conditions occurring in an HIV-infected adolescent or adult that meet at least one of the following criteria:
  - ➤ They are attributed to HIV infection or indicate adefectin cell-mediated immunity.
  - ➤ They are considered to have a clinical course or management that is complicated by HIV infection.

  Examples include, but are not limited to the following:
  - ➤ Bacillary angiomatosis
  - ➤ Oropharyngeal candidiasis (thrush)
  - ➤ Vulvovaginal candidiasis, persistent or resistant
  - ➤ Pelvic inflammatory disease (PID)
  - ➤ Cervical dysplasia (moderate or severe)/cervical carcinoma *in situ*
  - ➤ Hairy leukoplakia, oral
  - ➤ Herpes zoster (shingles), involving two or more episodes or at least one dermatome
  - ➤ Idiopathic thrombocytopenic purpura
  - ➤ Constitutional symptoms, such as fever (>38.5°C) or diarrhea lasting >1 month
  - ➤ Peripheral neuropathy
- **Category C AIDS-indicator conditions**
  - ➤ Bacterial
  - ➤ Pneumonia, recurrent (two or more episodes in 12 months)
  - ➤ Candidiasis of the bronchi, trachea, or lungs
  - ➤ Candidiasis, esophageal
  - ➤ Cervical carcinoma, invasive, confirmed by biopsy

- ➤ Coccidioidomycosis, disseminated or extrapulmonary
- ➤ Cryptococcosis, extrapulmonary
- ➤ Cryptosporidiosis, chronic intestinal (>1 month induration)
- ➤ Cytomegalovirus disease (other than liver, spleen, or nodes)
- Encephalopathy, HIV-related
  - ➤ Herpes simplex: Chronic ulcers (>1 month in duration), or bronchitis, pneumonitis, or esophagitis
  - ➤ Histoplasmosis, disseminated or extrapulmonary
  - ➤ Isosporiasis, chronic intestinal (>1 month duration)
  - ➤ Kaposi sarcoma
  - ➤ Lymphoma, Burkitt, immunoblastic, or primary central nervous system
  - ➤ *Mycobacterium avium* complex (MAC) or *Mycobacterium kansasii,* disseminated or extrapulmonary
  - ➤ *Mycobacterium tuberculosis,* pulmonary or extrapulmonary
  - ➤ Mycobacterium, other species or unidentified species, disseminated or extrapulmonary
  - ➤ *Pneumocystis jiroveci* (formerly *carinii*) pneumonia (PCP) Progressive multifocal leukoencephalopathy (PML)
  - ➤ Salmonella septicemia, recurrent (nontyphoid)
  - ➤ Toxoplasmosis of brain
  - ➤ Wasting syndrome caused by HIV (involuntary weight loss >10% of baseline body weight) associated with either chronic diarrhea (two or more loose stools per day for ≥1 month) or chronic weakness and documented fever for ≥1 month.

## WHO Clinical Staging of HIV/AIDS and Case Definition

- The clinical staging and case definition of HIV for resource-constrained settings were developed. By the WHO in 1990 and revised in 2007.
- Staging is based on clinical findings that guide the diagnosis, evaluation, and management of HIV/AIDS, and it does not require a CD4 cell count. This staging system is used in many countries to determine eligibility for antiretroviral therapy, particularly in settings in which CD4 testing is not available.
- Clinical stages are categorized as 1 through 4, progressing from primary HIV infection to advanced HIV/AIDS (Table 26.2).
- These stages are defined by specific clinical conditions or symptoms. For the purpose of the WHO staging system, adolescents and adults are defined as individuals aged ≥15 years.

**Table 26.2:** WHO clinical staging of HIV/AIDS for adults and adolescents

**Primary HIV infection**
- Asymptomatic
- Acute retroviral syndrome

**Clinical stage 1**
- Asymptomatic
- Persistent generalized lymphadenopathy

**Clinical stage 2**
- Moderate unexplained weight loss (<10% of presumed or measured body weight)
- Recurrent respiratory infections (sinusitis, tonsillitis, otitis media, and pharyngitis) herpes zoster
- Angular cheilitis—recurrent, oral
- Ulceration
- Papular pruritic eruptions
- Seborrheic dermatitis
- Fungal nail infections

**Clinical stage 3**
- Unexplained severe weight loss (>10% of presumed or measured body weight)
- Unexplained chronic diarrhea for >1 month
- Unexplained persistent fever for >1 month (>37.6°C, intermittent or constant)
- Persistent oral candidiasis (thrush)
- Oral hairy leukoplakia
- Pulmonary tuberculosis (current)
- Severe presumed bacterial infections (e.g. pneumonia, empyema, pyomyositis, bone or joint infection, meningitis, bacteremia)
- Acute necrotizing ulcerative stomatitis, gingivitis, or periodontitis
- Unexplained anemia (hemoglobin <8 g/dl)
- Neutropenia (neutrophils <500 cells/µl)
- Chronic thrombocytopenia (platelets <50,000 cells/µl)

**Clinical stage 4**
- HIV wasting syndrome, as defined by the CDC (Table 26.1)
- *Pneumocystis pneumonia*
- Chronic herpes simplex infection (orolabial, genital, or anorectal site for >1 month or visceral herpes at any site)
- Esophageal candidiasis (or candidiasis of trachea, bronchi, or lungs)
- Extrapulmonary tuberculosis
- Kaposi sarcoma

*Contd.*

**Table 26.2:** WHO clinical staging of HIV/AIDS for adults and adolescents *(Contd.)*

- Cytomegalovirus infection (retinitis or infection of other organs): Central nervous system toxoplasmosis
- HIV encephalopathy
- Cryptococcosis, extrapulmonary (including meningitis), disseminated nontuberculosis mycobacterial infection
- Progressive multifocal leukoencephalopathy
- Candida of the trachea, bronchi, or lungs, chronic cryptosporidiosis (with diarrhea), chronic isosporiasis
- Disseminated mycosis (e.g. histoplasmosis, coccidioidomycosis, penicilliosis), recurrent nontyphoidal Salmonella bacteremia
- Lymphoma (cerebral or B cell non-Hodgkin), invasive cervical carcinoma
- Atypical disseminated leishmaniasis, symptomatic HIV-associated nephropathy, symptomatic HIV-associated cardiomyopathy
- Reactivation of American trypanosomiasis (meningoencephalitis or myocarditis).

## NACO GUIDELINES

### Case Definition for AIDS in India

Case definition for AIDS in India was revised in October, 1999. The new case definition is as follows:

### *Case Definition of AIDS in Children (Up to 12 Years of Age)*

1. The positive tests for HIV infection by ERS (ELISA/Rapid/Simple) in children above 18 months or confirmed maternal HIV infection for children less than 18 months.
2. Presence of at least two major and two minor signs in the absence of known causes of immunosuppression.

### Major signs

(a) Loss of weight or failure to thrive which is not known to be due to medical causes other than HIV infection.
(b) Chronic diarrhea (intermittent or continuous) >1 month duration.
(c) Prolonged fever (intermittent or continuous) >1 month duration.

### Minor signs

(a) Repeat common infections (e.g. pneumonitis, otitis, pharyngitis, etc.)
(b) Generalized lymphadenopathy
(c) Oropharyngeal candidiasis
(d) Persistent cough for more than 1 month
(e) Disseminated maculopapular dermatosis

## Case Definition of AIDS in Adults (for Persons Above 12 Years of Age)

1. Two positive tests for HIV infection by ERS test (ELISA/Rapid/Simple)
2. Any one of the following criteria:
   (a) Significant weight loss (>10% of body weight) within last one month/cachexia (not known to be due to a condition other than HIV infection), and chronic diarrhea (intermittent or continuous) >1 month duration or prolonged fever (intermittent or continuous) >1 month duration
   (b) Tuberculosis: Extensive pulmonary, disseminated, miliary, extrapulmonary tuberculosis.
   (c) Neurological impairment preventing independent daily activities, not known to be due to the conditions unrelated to HIV infection (e.g. trauma)
   (d) Candidiasis of the esophagus (diagnosable by oral candidiasis with odynophagia)
   (e) Clinically diagnosed life-threatening or recurrent episodes of pneumonia, with or without etiological confirmation
   (f) Kaposi sarcoma
   (g) Other conditions:
       - Cryptococcal meningitis
       - Neurotoxoplasmosis
       - CMV retinitis
       - *Penicillium marneffei*
       - Recurrent herpes zoster or multi-dermatomal herpes infection
       - Disseminated molluscum

## DIAGNOSIS OF HIV INFECTION

- HIV infection is diagnosed on the basis of blood tests using three different ELISA/Rapid/Simple tests using different antigen preparation.
- AIDS cases are diagnosed on the basis of two different ELISA/Rapid tests on different antigens and presence of AIDS-related opportunistic infections.
- Western blot test is used for confirmation of diagnosis of indeterminate ELISA tests.
- In developed countries following tests are also used:

- CD4 Lymphocyte counts
- Detection of viral specific RNA
- Viral culture

## HIV Testing in Infants

- CDC recommends that all pregnant women get tested for HIV before and/or during delivery. Knowing the HIV status of the mother allows physicians to prevent mother-to-child HIV transmission by providing antiretroviral treatment to both mothers infected with HIV and their newborn infants.
- However, it is difficult to determine if a baby born to a mother infected with HIV is actually infected because babies carry their mothers' HIV antibodies for several months. Today, health care providers can conduct an HIV test for infants between ages 3 months and 15 months.

## MUCOCUTANEOUS DISORDERS IN HIV INFECTION

1. **Infections**
   - *Fungal*
     - ➤ Candidiasis
     - ➤ Dermatophytosis
     - ➤ *Tinea versicolor*
     - ➤ Histoplasmosis
     - ➤ Cryptococcosis
   - *Viral*
     - ➤ HSV
     - ➤ HPV
     - ➤ Herpes zoster
     - ➤ Oral hairy leukoplakia
     - ➤ CMV infections
     - ➤ Molluscum contagiosum
   - *Bacterial*
     - ➤ Syphilis
     - ➤ Staphylococcal infections
     - ➤ *M. tuberculosis*
     - ➤ Atypical mycobacterial infections
     - ➤ Bacillary angiomatosis
2. **Infestations**
   - Scabies
   - Protozoan infections
   - Cryptosporidiosis

- Microsporidiosis
- Isospora
- *Pneumocystis carinii*
3. Pruritic papular eruption
4. Eosinophilic folliculitis
5. Aphthous ulceration
6. Xerosis/pruritus/ichthyosis
7. Seborrheic dermatitis
8. Psoriasis
9. Kaposi's sarcoma
10. Melanoma and non-melanoma skin cancer
11. Lymphomas
12. Drug eruptions
13. **Hair**
    - Patchy and diffuse alopecia/telogen effluvium
    - Fine hair
    - Eyelash trichomegaly
    - Alopecia (non-specific)
    - Alopecia areata and universalis
14. **Nails**
    - Clubbing
    - Half and half nails
    - Transverse (Beau's lines) and longitudinal ridging
    - Loss of the lunula
    - Leukonychia
    - Blue nails
    - Longitudinal melanonychia
    - Yellow nail syndrome
    - Periungual erythema
    - Onycholysis and onychoschizia
    - Onychomycosis

## TREATMENT

Four classes of drugs are used.
1. Nucleoside reverse transcriptase inhibitors (NRTIs)
2. Non-nucleoside reverse transcriptase inhibitors (NNRTIs)
3. Protease inhibitors (PIs)
4. Fusion inhibitors (FIs)—newer class

Recommended schedule:

Two NRTIs with a NNRTI or PI

## Viral Infections

- **Herpes simplex and herpes zoster viruses**
  - ➤ Recurrent oral and anogenital HSV infection is common in patients infected with HIV, and it may lead to chronic ulcerations (Fig. 26.1). In pediatric patients, HSV stomatitis is more common than varicella-zoster virus (VZV) and may become chronic and ulcerative. Patients with VZV may develop chronic ecthymatous VZV.
  - ➤ Acute disseminated HZV infection and the following atypical manifestations have also been described:
    - – Hyperkeratotic papules
    - – Folliculitis
    - – Verrucous lesions
    - – Chronic ulcerations
    - – Disseminated ecthymatous lesion
- **Epstein-Barr virus**
  - ➤ Epstein-Barr virus (EBV) has been implicated in the pathogenesis of oral hairy leukoplakia, which may develop in patients infected with HIV, particularly men.
  - ➤ Oral hairy leukoplakia is characterized by filiform white papules localized on the sides of the tongue.
  - ➤ This condition has no malignant potential, but it may be the initial sign of progressive immunosuppression. White plaques may be confused with oral candidiasis, lichen planus, and geographic tongue.
- **Cytomegalovirus**
  - ➤ CMV is a DNA virus in the Herpesviridae family.

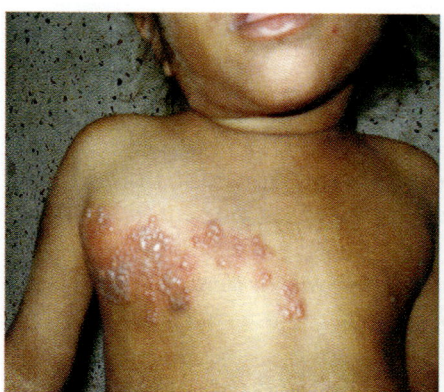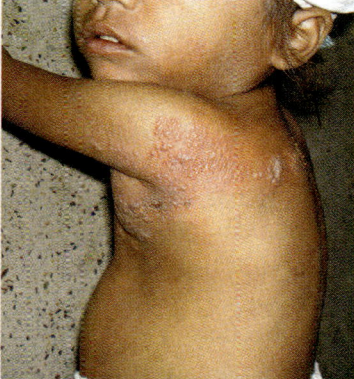

**Fig. 26.1:** Herpes zoster in HIV positive child

> Ulcers in the perineal region are the most common presentation of CMV infection in patients infected with HIV 1. The concurrent involvement of other infectious agents, such as HSV, in the same lesions confounds the role of CMV in cutaneous lesions. HSV is proposed to be the initiating infection leading to ulcer formation, with CMV secondarily localizing in the granulation tissue.

> Nonspecific maculopapular eruptions similar to those affecting patients with EBV or papulovesicular, nodular, purpuric, and ulcerative lesions of CMV infection are observed in patients who are immunocompromised. However, cutaneous lesions are rarely observed in patients infected with HIV.

> The presence of CMV infection is considered a poor prognostic sign in HIV disease.

- **Warts**
  > Widespread or recalcitrant warts may be observed on the oral mucosa, the face, the perianal region, and the female genital tract in patients infected with HIV.

  > Large plantar warts caused by human papillomoavirus-66 (HPV-66) and an epidermodysplasia verruciformis like eruption, which is believed to be associated with HPV infection, have also been reported in patients infected with HIV.

- **Molluscum contagiosum**
  > The molluscum contagiosum (MC) virus is a DNA virus in the Poxviridae family. It replicates in the cytoplasm of epidermal cells. MC lesions are small papules with central umbilication.

  > In HIV infection, MC may be widespread and atypical. The lesions may be observed on unusual sites, such as the face, neck, and scalp, and the lesions may be of unusual morphology and size.

## Fungal Infections

- **Superficial fungal infections**
  > Recurrent and persistent mucocutaneous candidiasis is common in patients with HIV infection. In the United States, recurrent vaginal candidiasis is the most common presentation of HIV infection in women.

  > In adults, generalized dermatophytosis, or *tinea capitis*, which is typically caused by *Trichophyton rubrum*, may suggest HIV infection.

  > *Pityriasis versicolor* may be persistent and recurrent in patients with HIV infection.

- **Deep fungal infections**
  - ➤ Rarely, cutaneous cryptococcosis may be observed in patients with HIV infection. Clinical manifestations include the following:
    - – Cellulitis
    - – Papules
    - – Plaques
    - – Ulcers
    - – Translucent dome-shaped papules with central umbilication, resembling MC
  - ➤ Cutaneous histoplasmosis may lead to red papules, a cellulitis like eruption, ulcerations, acneiform papules, or molluscum-like lesions in patients infected with HIV.
  - ➤ North American blastomycosis may present as a disseminated maculopapular eruption in HIV disease.
  - ➤ Systemic coccidioidomycosis may disseminate to the skin, usually as hemorrhagic papules or nodules.

## Bacterial Infections

- Impetigo and folliculitis may be recurrent and persistent in HIV disease, particularly in children. Disseminated furunculosis, gingivitis, gangrenous stomatitis, and abscess formation can occur in patients with HIV infection.
- Bacillary angiomatosis, which is caused by *Bartonella henselae* and rarely by *Bartonella quintana,* usually manifests as red papules and nodules.
- **Mycobacterial infections**
  - ➤ *Mycobacterium tuberculosis; M. avium intracellulare* complex (MAC); and rarely, *M. kansasii* may present as acneiform papules and indurated crusted plaques.
  - ➤ MAC, a common opportunistic pathogen among patients with AIDS, usually causes disseminated disease involving the lungs, lymph nodes, and gastrointestinal tract. Primary cutaneous infections with MAC are extremely rare; most cutaneous lesions are caused by dissemination. Cutaneous manifestations thus far reported include the following:
    - – Scaling plaques
    - – Crusted ulcers
    - – Ecthyma-like lesions
    - – Verrucous ulcers
    - – Inflammatory nodules

- – Panniculitis
- – Pustular lesions
- – Draining sinuses
- ➢ In patients with HIV, *M. haemophilum* can also present as violaceous draining nodules and superficial ulcers on the extremities, trunk, head, and genitalia.
- **Syphilis**
  - ➢ Co-infection with syphilis (as well as other sexually transmitted diseases) may be found in HIV-infected patients, particularly those who are homosexual or bisexual or who use illicit drugs. Syphilitic ulcers are believed to increase HIV transmission.
  - ➢ Most cases of syphilis that occur in HIV disease are clinically and serologically typical. However, syphilis seroconversion may be delayed, and standard serologic tests that aid in diagnosing syphilis may be unreliable. Also, in primary syphilis, presentation with multiple ulcers is more common in HIV-infected patients. Rapid progression of secondary syphilis to tertiary syphilis and syphilis maligna has been reported in patients infected with HIV.
- *Staphylococcus aureus* **infection**
  - ➢ Patients with HIV have been found to have increased rates of cutaneous colonization by *Staphylococcus aureus,* and in patients with advanced disease, sepsis and deep tissue infection can be common. Methicillin-resistant *S. aureus* (MRSA) soft tissue infection is an increasing problem.

## Papulosquamous Dermatosis

- Generalized dry skin syndrome is frequently observed in patients with HIV infection. Xerosis may be the initial clinical manifestation of AIDS and is often a cause of pruritus.
- Seborrheic dermatitis may be the initial cutaneous manifestation of HIV disease. The eruption, which is characterized by widespread inflammatory and hyperkeratotic lesions, may progress to erythroderma in some patients. Seborrheic dermatitis may be increased in patients with AIDS-associated dementia or CNS disease.
- The immune alterations caused by HIV infection may lead to psoriasis and Reiter's syndrome. In some instances, pre-existing psoriasis may become more severe with disseminated plaques and pustules.
- The typical skin lesions of pityriasis rosea may accompany HIV disease.

- Acquired ichthyosis may begin on the lower extremities and disseminate in advanced HIV disease.
- Eosinophilic folliculitis manifests as an idiopathic, highly pruritic, papulopustular eruption of sterile pustules involving the face, neck, trunk, and extremities.
- Pruritic papular eruption (PPE) is a common cutaneous manifestation in patients infected with HIV. It manifests as small, itchy, red or skin-colored papules on the head, neck, and upper part of the trunk. The cause is not known.

## Malignancies

- Kaposi sarcoma (KS) was the first reported malignancy associated with HIV infection and was first documented in 1981 from reports in New York, Los Angeles, and San Francisco. The worldwide prevalence of KS in patients with AIDS may approach 34%; in the United States; however, the prevalence of KS in patients with HIV disease is less than 5%. Most of the patients are homosexual men, although all patients who acquire HIV infection through sexual contact are at somewhat increased risk.
- Since the advent of highly active antiretroviral therapy (HAART), the incidence of non-AIDS-defining cutaneous cancers—in particular, basal cell carcinoma—among HIV-infected persons has exceeded that of AIDS-defining cutaneous cancers such as KS. KS remains the most common HIV-associated malignancy in sub-Saharan Africa.
- Pediatric KS is distinct, and lymph node involvement is a common manifestation.
- AIDS-related B cell non-Hodgkin lymphomas may cause skin nodules.
- Anal carcinoma and cervical intraepithelial neoplasia are papillomavirus-associated tumors associated with HIV disease. These tumors tend to be more progressive and aggressive. An increase in squamous cell carcinoma of the anal mucosa has been reported, especially in young homosexual men with HIV infection. Intraoral or multiple squamous cell carcinoma, Bowen disease, and metastatic basal cell carcinoma have occasionally been reported in patients infected with HIV.
- Malignant melanoma appears to be more aggressive in patients with HIV.
- Kaposi sarcoma

## Drug Eruptions

- Drug eruptions have been reported as the most common cause of erythroderma in patients infected with HIV.

- This elevated incidence of HIV patients with an adverse cutaneous drug eruption, including toxic epidermal necrolysis, may be due to a loss of skin-protective CD4+, CD25+ regulatory T cells.

## Management of Dermatological Manifestations in HIV

### Viral Infections

- For herpes simplex virus (HSV) and herpes zoster virus (HZV) infections in HIV-infected patients, the treatment of choice is acyclovir and other members of this drug class. These agents are activated by viral thymidine kinase. In some disseminated cases, the virus may be resistant to acyclovir because of the deficiency in viral thymidine kinase activity.
- Prolonged therapy and chronic suppressive therapy with subtherapeutic doses have also been implicated in the development of acyclovir resistance.
- In the presence of acyclovir resistance, other viral therapies, including cidofovir, foscarnet, and vidarabine, may be necessary.
- Treatment is usually not necessary for patients with oral hairy leukoplakia. If the patient is experiencing significant discomfort, systemic (1200 mg/day) and topical acyclovir, ganciclovir, or foscarnet may be recommended.
- In most cases of molluscum contagiosum, imiquimod is curative. Resolution with zidovudine therapy has been reported in HIV-associated molluscum contagiosum.
- Ablation and curettage may be useful in the treatment of molluscumcontagiosum.

### Noninfectious and Nonmalignant Cutaneous Manifestations of HIV Infection

- For xerosis, emollients and dry skin care regimens are effective.
- For seborrheic dermatitis, coal tar, sulfur, and salicylic acid shampoos; topical corticosteroids; topical tacrolimus; and 2% ketoconazole cream may be effective.
- For psoriasis and Reiter's syndrome, ultraviolet B (UVB) and psoralen with UVA (PUVA) may be useful. Systemic corticosteroids, methotrexate, and cyclosporine may increase the immune suppression and must be considered only with careful monitoring. Zidovudine is also reported to be useful in the treatment of HIV-associated psoriasis.
- For pruritic papular eruption, topical steroids, UVB, PUVA, and pentoxifylline have been reported to be effective.
- Eosinophilic folliculitis may respond to UVB, isotretinoin, or zidovudine treatment.

## Kaposi Sarcoma

- For patients with limited disease, local therapy with liquid nitrogen, alitretinoin, or intralesional vincristine may be effective.
- Surgery, radiotherapy, and systemic chemotherapy—usually with a single agent (e.g. vinblastine, vincristine, bleomycin, doxorubicin, etoposide)—may be useful in the treatment of KS; however, systemic chemotherapy has not been shown to improve the long-term survival rates. Patients who recover immune response with antiretroviral therapy have had remission of KS.
- Interferon (IFN)-alpha and IFN-beta photodynamic therapy and systemic hyperthermia have also been used.
- Cryotherapy, laser irradiation, and electrodesiccation can be useful for localized solitary lesions of KS.

## Miscellaneous Conditions

- Mucocutaneous candidiasis is usually difficult to treat; oral azole treatment may be required.
- Generalized dermatophytosis may be resistant to topical antifungal creams and may require systemic antifungal therapy.
- Bacillary angiomatosis usually responds to oral erythromycin.

## MULTIPLE CHOICE QUESTIONS

1. **Dermatologic problems in HIV infection include the following except:**
   - (a) KS
   - (b) Seborrheic dermatitis
   - (c) Alopecia
   - (d) Necrotizing vasculitis
2. **In HIV-infected patients, seborrheic dermatitis may be aggravated by concomitant infection with:**
   - (a) HSV
   - (b) *Candida albicans*
   - (c) Staphylococci
   - (d) Pityrosporum
3. **Eosinophilic pustular folliculitis, a rare form of folliculitis that is seen with increased frequency in patients with?**
   - (a) ABPA
   - (b) Asthma
   - (c) Leukemia cutis
   - (d) HIV infection
4. **Which of the following is not known to occur with more severity than usual in patients with HIV infection?**
   - (a) Psoriasis
   - (b) Ichthyosis
   - (c) Norwegian scabies
   - (d) Lichen planus

5. **Which may be the first indication of clinical immunodeficiency in HIV infected patients?**
   (a) Vitiligo
   (b) Hairy leukoplakia
   (c) Lupus vulagris
   (d) Herpes zoster

6. **Erythematous cutaneous nodules may be caused by the following in HIV infected patients:**
   (a) Bartonella
   (b) Aspergillus
   (c) HSV
   (d) Molluscum contagiosum

7. **Which of the following drug therapies in HIV patients has been associated with elongation of the eyelashes and the development of a bluish discoloration to the nails?**
   (a) Sulfa drugs
   (b) Non-nucleoside reverse transcriptase inhibitors
   (c) Zidovudine
   (d) Clofazimine

8. **The following image shows a HIV-infected patient. What is the probable diagnosis?**

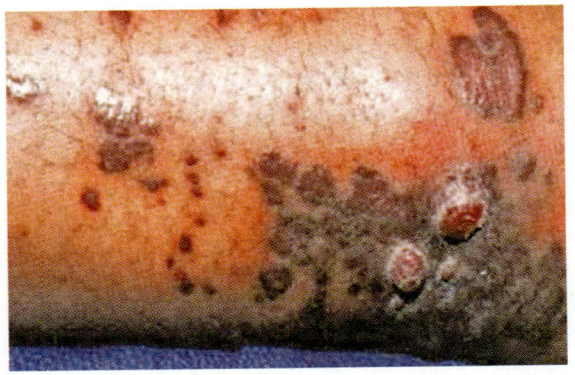

   (a) Actinic keratosis
   (b) Lupus vulgaris
   (c) Mycosis fungoides
   (d) Kaposi's sarcoma

## Answers

1. **Ans. (c)** Alopecia
   Dermatologic problems occur in >90% of patients with HIV infection. From the macular, roseola-like rash seen with the acute seroconversion syndrome to extensive end-stage KS, cutaneous manifestations of HIV disease can be seen throughout the course of HIV infection. Among the more common non-neoplastic problems are seborrheic dermatitis, folliculitis, and opportunistic infections. Extrapulmonary pneumocystosis may cause a necrotizing vasculitis. Neoplastic conditions also occur.

2. **Ans. (d)** Pityrosporum

   *Seborrheic dermatitis* occurs in 3% of the general population and in up to 50% of patients with HIV infection. Seborrheic dermatitis increases in prevalence and severity as the CD4+ T cell count declines. In HIV-infected patients, seborrheic dermatitis may be aggravated by concomitant infection with *Pityrosporum*, a yeast-like fungus; use of topical antifungal agents has been recommended in cases refractory to standard topical treatment.

3. **Ans. (d)** HIV infection

   *Folliculitis* is among the most prevalent dermatologic disorders in patients with HIV infection and is seen in ~20% of patients. It is more common in patients with CD4+ T cell counts < 200 cells/L. Pruritic papular eruption is one of the most common pruritic rashes in patients with HIV infection. It appears as multiple papules on the face, trunk, and extensor surfaces and may improve with cART. *Eosinophilic pustular folliculitis* is a rare form of folliculitis that is seen with increased frequency in patients with HIV infection. It presents as multiple, urticarial perifollicular papules that may coalesce into plaque-like lesions. Skin biopsy reveals an eosinophilic infiltrate of the hair follicle, which in certain cases has been associated with the presence of a mite. Patients typically have an elevated serum IgE level and may respond to treatment with topical anthelmintics.

4. **Ans. (d)** Lichen planus

   Pruritus is a common symptom in patients with HIV infection and can lead to prurigonodularis. Patients with HIV infection have also been reported to develop a severe form of *Norwegian scabies* with hyperkeratotic psoriasiform lesions.

   Both *psoriasis* and *ichthyosis*, although they are not reported to be increased in frequency, may be particularly severe when they occur in patients with HIV infection. Pre-existing psoriasis may become guttate in appearance and more refractory to treatment in the setting of HIV infection.

5. **Ans. (d)** Herpes zoster

   *Reactivation herpes zoster (shingles)* is seen in 10–20% of patients with HIV infection. This reactivation syndrome of varicella-zoster virus indicates a modest decline in immune function and may be the first indication of clinical immunodeficiency. In one series, patients who developed shingles did so an average of 5 years after HIV infection. In a cohort of patients with HIV infection and localized zoster, the subsequent rate of the development of AIDS was 1% per month. In that study, AIDS was more likely to develop if the outbreak of zoster was associated with severe pain, extensive skin involvement, or involvement of cranial or cervical dermatomes. The clinical manifestations of reactivation zoster in HIV-infected patients, although indicative of immunologic compromise, are not as severe as those seen in other immunodeficient conditions. Thus, while lesions may extend over several dermatomes, involve the spinal cord, and/or be associated with frank cutaneous dissemination, visceral involvement has not been reported. In contrast to patients without a known underlying immunodeficiency state, patients with HIV infection tend to have recurrences of zoster with a relapse rate of ~20%. Valacyclovir, acyclovir, or famciclovir is the treatment of choice. Foscarnet may be of value in patients with acyclovir-resistant virus.

6. **Ans. (a)** Bartonella

   Diffuse skin eruptions due to *Molluscum contagiosum* may be seen in patients with advanced HIV infection. These flesh-colored, umbilicated lesions may be treated with local therapy. They tend to regress with effective cART. Similarly, *condyloma acuminatum* lesions may be more severe and more widely distributed in patients with low CD4+ T cell counts. Imiquimod cream may be helpful in some cases. Atypical mycobacterial infections may present as erythematous cutaneous nodules, as may fungal infections, *Bartonella, Acanthamoeba*, and KS. Cutaneous infections with *Aspergillus* have been noted at the site of IV catheter placement.

7. **Ans. (c)** Zidovudine

   HIV infection and its treatment may be accompanied by cosmetic changes of the skin that are not of great clinical importance but may be troubling to patients. Yellowing of the nails and straightening of the hair, particularly in African-American patients, have been reported as a consequence of HIV infection. Zidovudine therapy has been associated with elongation of the eyelashes and the development of a bluish discoloration to the nails, again more common in African-American patients. Therapy with clofazimine may cause a yellow-orange discoloration of the skin and urine.

8. **Ans. (d)** Kaposi's sarcoma

   Image shows Kaposi's sarcoma in a patient with AIDS. Patch, plaque, and tumor stages are seen in this patient.

# Signs in Dermatology

**Albright's dimple sign**

This is seen in Albright's hereditary osteodystrophy in which there is presence of a dimple over the knuckle of the typically affected fourth metacarpal and can be enhanced by clenching of the fist.

**Antenna sign**

It is seen in keratosis pilaris in which individual follicles show a long strand of keratin glinting when examined in tangentially incident light.

**Asboe-Hansen sign (blister spread sign)**

Gustav Asboe Hansen first described it in 1960, when he demonstrated enlargement of bulla by applying finger pressure to small, intact, and tense bulla in patients with pemphigus and bullous pemphigoid. In the traditional bulla spread sign, pressure is applied to the blister from one side, whereas in eliciting Asboe-Hansen sign pressure is applied at the center of the blister and perpendicular to the surface due to smaller size of the lesion.

**Auspitz sign**

It is named after Heinrich Auspitz, described in psoriasis, where there is pinpoint bleeding on removal of scales from the lesions of psoriasis. The test by which Auspitz sign is elicited is called Grattage test. Other dermatoses where Auspitz sign can be positive is Darier's disease and actinic keratosis.

**"Breakfast, lunch, and dinner" sign**

The bites of bed bugs (Cimex lectularius) usually follow a linear pathway in a group of three to five blood meals and are often referred to as "Breakfast, lunch, and dinner" or "Breakfast, lunch, and supper" sign.

**Buschke-Ollendorff sign**

This is a sign to be elicited in case of secondary syphilis and cutaneous vasculitis, where there is deep dermal tenderness on pressing the lesion (e.g. papular lesions of syphilis) with a pinhead.

**Butterfly sign**

This refers to sparing of the mid-scapular region in patients having prurigonodularis with neurodermatitis as they are unable to reach the region for scratching.

### Buttonhole sign

In type 1 neurofibromatosis (von Recklinghausen's disease), neurofibromas can be invaginated with the tip of index finger back into the subcutis and again reappear after release of pressure. Other condition where one can find positive buttonhole sign are anetoderma and dermatofibroma.

### Carpet tack sign (tin tack sign, cat tongue sign)

When the adherent scale is removed from the lesions of discoid lupus erythematosus, the undersurface of the scale shows horny plugs that have occupied patulous hair follicles. This sign is also seen in seborrheic dermatitis.

### Chagas'-Mazza-Romaña's sign

In about eighty percent of cases of Chagas' disease (American trypanosomiasis), conjunctiva is the portal of entry for *Trypanosoma cruzi*. Unilateral swelling of eyelids and orbit after conjunctival inoculation is called eye-sign or Chagas'-Mazza-Romaña's sign or Romaña's sign.

### Coral bead sign

Papules seen around the nail fold in multicentric reticulohistiocytosis are called coral bead sign.

### Coudability sign

It was first described by Shuster in cases of alopecia areata in 1984. Coudability sign is normal-looking hairs tapered at the proximal end in the perilesional hair-bearing scalp and can easily be made to kink when bent or pushed inward.

### Coup d'ongle sign

Scraping the surface of the lesions in pityriasis versicolor will accentuate the scaling.

### Crowe's sign

Axillary freckling seen in type I neurofibromatosis is known as Crowe's sign.

### Deck-chair sign

It was classically described in papuloerythroderma of Ofuji, wherein there is flat-topped red papules that become generalized erythrodermic plaques without the involvement of abdominal skin folds.

### Darier's sign

Rubbing a lesion of mastocytoma causes urtication, flare, swelling and sometimes blister formation due to release of histamine. In contrast, pseudo-Darer's sign is seen in smooth muscle hamartoma where there is increase in induration and piloerection after firm stroking. Other conditions where one could find positive Darier's sign are leukemia cutis, juvenile xanthogranuloma, and Langerhans' cell histiocytosis.

## Dermatographism ("skin writing")

It is a form of physical urticaria that consists of local erythema due to capillary vasodilatation, followed by edema and a surrounding flare due to axon reflex induced dilation of arterioles, which is observed after the firm stroking of skin. The cause of this phenomenon is thought to be hypersensitivity of the mast cells rather than an increase in the mast cells, as observed in mastocytosis.

## Dimple sign (Fitzpatrick sign)

Squeezing the skin adjacent to a dermatofibroma causes a dimpled appearance on its surface, also termed a positive "pinch sign" or "dimple sign,".

## Dory-flop sign

It is described in relation to syphilitic chancre on the coronal border of the prepucial skin in an uncircumscribed male, whereupon on retracting the foreskin the entire ulcer flips out all at once because it is too hard to bend due to underlying button-like induration.

## Flag sign

i. The presence of sharply demarcated alternating bands of normally pigmented and hypopigmented zone of hair indicating episodes of normal nutrition and intermittent malnutrition respectively, seen in kwashiorkor- or marasmus-type malnutrition.

ii. It is a histopathological sign described in actinic keratosis, in which the basal layer is more basophilic than normal owing to crowding of atypical keratinocytes. Hyperkeratosis and parakeratosis are present, the latter overlying the abnormal cells in the epidermis. Owing to sparing of the epithelium of acrosyringia and acrotrichia, orthokeratosis appears at the ostea of these structures, giving rise to a characteristic pattern of alternating ortho- and parakeratosis, often referred to as the "flag" sign.

## Forscheimer's sign

Seen in 20% of rubella patients, where there is an enanthem of dull-red macules or petechiae confined to the soft palate during the prodromal period or on the first day of the rash. Can also be seen in infectious mononucleosis.

## Friar tuck sign

Friar tuck was a companion of Robin Hood in the legendary stories who had alopecia of the vertex with sparing of occipital region. This is described in relation to trichotillomania, where patient plucks his own hair either in a wave-like pattern across the scalp or centrifugally from a single starting point. Hairs over the occipital area are mostly spared in trichotillomania and is referred as friar tuck sign.

### Gorlin's sign

It is the ability of patients of *Ehlers-Danlos syndrome* to touch the tip of the nose with the tip of their tongue.

### Gottron's sign

It is a characteristic finding in dermatomyositis typified by scaly erythematous eruption seen on the dorsa of hands, metacarpo-phalangeal joints, and proximal interphalangeal joints.

### Groove sign

Groove sign has been described in relation to chlamydial infection, i.e. lymphogranuloma venereum (LGV) called groove sign of Greenblatt and is considered pathognomonic for LGV. Enlargement of both inguinal and femoral group of lymph nodes separated by Poupart's ligament produces a groove known as the "Groove sign of Greenblatt."

### Hamburger sign

This sign has been described in relation to trichotillomania, wherein there is vertically oriented split of hair shafts and proteinaceous material and erythrocytes are present in the split resembling a Hamburger within a bun.

### Hanging curtain sign

It is seen in patients with pityriasis rosea. When the skin is stretched across the long axis of the herald patch, the scale is noted to be finer, lighter, and attached at one end, which tends to fold across the line of stretch.

### Hertoghe's sign (Queen Anne's sign)

It is defined as loss of lateral one-third of eyebrows (superciliary madarosis). It is seen in leprosy, myxedema, follicular mucinosis, atopic dermatitis, trichotillomania, ectodermal dysplasia, discoid lupus erythematosus, alopecia areata, syphilis, ulerythema ophryogenes, systemic sclerosis, HIV infection, and hypothyroidism.

### Higoumenaki's sign

It refers enlargement of the sternal end of the (right) clavicle, frequently observed in patients with late congenital syphilis.

### Holster sign of dermatomyositis

Confluent macular violaceous erythema present on the lateral side of hip and thighs is called "Holster sign".

## Hutchinson's sign (named after Sir Jonathon Hutchinson)

- Melanonychia with pigmentation of proximal nail fold seen in subungual melanoma.
- Presence of papulovesicular lesions on the tip of nose indicates involvement of cornea as both are supplied by nasociliary nerve, a branch of trigeminal nerve.
- Micro-Hutchinson's sign: pigmentation of the periungual tissues that could not be seen with the naked eye and can be visualized by dermoscopy. Micro-Hutchinson's sign is a highly characteristic dermoscopic feature of early nail apparatus melanoma, although the sensitivity is not high.

## Hypopyon sign

Hypopyon sign describes the presence of small, discrete, vesicles either flaccid or tense that become secondarily infected and pus accumulates in the lower half of the pustule. It is a clinical sign seen in pyodermas and secondarily infected vesicobullous disorders (e.g. pemphigus, bullous pemphigoid, and linear IgA dermatosis), where there is a transverse fluid level comprising of purulent material at the bottom when the patient is in a standing position and is called hypopyon sign.

## Ingram's sign

Inability to retract the lower eyelid in patients of progressive systemic sclerosis due to underlying sclerosis is called Ingram's sign.

## Leser-Trélat sign

First described by Edmund Leser and Ulysse Trélat, characterized by sudden eruption of numerous seborrheic keratosis, usually associated with pruritus and is considered as a marker of internal malignancy.

## Love's sign

Exact localization of tenderness with the help of pinhead in glomus tumor is called Love's sign.

## Milian's ear sign

Erysipelas and cellulitis have traditionally been defined as acute inflammatory processes of infectious origin that primarily affect the dermis (in the case of erysipelas) or deeper dermis and subcutaneous tissue in cellulitis.

It is a sign used to distinguish between erysipelas and cellulitis of the facial region, where there is involvement of ear in erysipelas and sparing in cellulitis, as there is no deeper dermal tissue and subcutaneous fat.

### Mizutani's sign (round finger pad sign)

It is seen in Raynaud's phenomenon associated with systemic sclerosis. This sign refers to disappearance of the peaked contour on fingerpads and replacement with a hemisphere-like fingertip contour especially on ring fingers.

### Nikolsky's sign

This sign is named after the Russian dermatologist Piotr Vasilievich Nikolskiy who described it in 1894. It refers to easy peeling of skin on applying tangential pressure over a bony prominence and classically seen in pemphigus, toxic epidermal necrolysis, and staphylococcal scalded skin syndrome. Nikolsky's sign can also be elicited in the oral cavity with the help of cotton-tipped applicator.

### Nose sign (Pavithran's nose sign)

It is seen in exfoliative dermatitis in which there is complete absence of erythema and scaling of the nose and perinasal areas. It is hypothesized that sparing of nose in exfoliative dermatitis could be due to greater sun exposure of nose or it could be explained by the mechanism of island of normal skin.

### Osler's sign

Blue black pigmentation in the sclera near insertion of rectus muscle in patients who have alkaptonuria (endogenous ochronosis).

### Pastia's sign

Linear petechial eruption in the skin folds especially on the ante-cubital fossa and axillary fold seen in streptococcal scarlet fever is called Pastia's sign.

### Patrick Yesudian sign

Palmar melanotic macules (palmar freckling) seen in type 1 neuro-fibromatosis was first reported by Patrick Yesudian and hence the name.

### Prayer sign

It is described in relation to diabetic cheiroarthropathy, wherein the patient is requested to bring both the palmar surface of the hands together as at prayer. Prayer sign is said to be positive when patient is unable to bring both the palmar surface together completely and it indicates limited joint mobility. Limited joint mobility is secondary to nonenzymatic glycosylation of collagen and its deposition in the small joints of the hand.

### Promontory sign

It is a histopathological finding where there is appearance of a small vessel protruding into an abnormal vascular space has been termed "promontory sign." It has been described in Kaposi sarcoma, patch and plaque stage of angiosarcoma.

## Pup-tent sign

It is seen in nail lichen planus, in which the nail splits and elevates longitudinally with downward angle of lateral nail edge.

## Pseudo-Darier sign in congenital smooth muscle hematoma

- Darier's sign refers to the urtication and erythematous halo that are produced in response to rubbing or scratching of lesions of cutaneous mastocytosis.
- Pseudo-Darier's sign is a transient piloerection and elevation or increased induration of a lesion induced by rubbing and is observed in congenital smooth muscle hamartomas. A positive pseudo-Darier's sign can be helpful in clinically distinguishing congenital smooth muscle hamartoma from congenital hairy nevus.

## Raccoon sign

The most common cutaneous manifestation of neonatal lupus erythematosus is erythematous, slightly scaly eruption on the face and periorbital skin (raccoon sign/owl-eye/eye mask). Periorbital hemorrhage due to laxity of blood vessels seen after proctoscopic examination (postproctoscopic periorbital purpura) in patients having systemic amyloidosis is also called as raccoon eyes/sign/panda sign.

## Sandwich sign

In dermatophytosis, fungi are present in the horny layer between two zones of cornified cells, the upper being orthokeratotic and lower consisting partially parakeratotic cells.

## Scratch sign (coup d'ongle sign, Besnier's sign, stroke of the nail)

This sign is to be elicited in patients having pityriasis versicolor, wherein the barely perceptible scales are made to stand out by scratching the lesion with fingernail.

## Shawl sign

Confluent macular violaceous erythema on the posterior neck and shoulders in patients of dermatomyositis is called Shawl sign.

## Samitz's sign

Dystrophic and ragged cuticle seen in dermatomyositis is called Samitz sign.

## Stafne's sign

Stafne's sign is seen in progressive systemic sclerosis. Widening of the periodontal ligament space secondary to increase in the collagen synthesis and increase in the bulk of the ligament, this is accommodated at the expense of alveolar bone, thus causing an increase in the width of the periodontal ligament space.

## Thumb sign (Steinberg sign)

In patients of Marfan syndrome, the thumbs protrude from the clenched fist beyond the ulnar border of hand.

## Umbilical sign

Umbilical sign is seen in Marfan syndrome. It is the unusual ability to touch the umbilicus with the right hand, crossing the back, and approaching from the left side, indicating increased length of upper extremity.

## "V" sign

Confluent macular violaceous erythema on the anterior neck and chest in patients of dermatomyositis is called "V" sign.

## Wimberger's sign

Wimberger's sign is the presence of bilateral, symmetrical, and well-defined metaphyseal defects on the medial surface of upper tibia, can result in pseudoparalysis, and is considered pathognomonic of congenital syphilis.

## Winterbottom's sign

It is seen in early stages of African trypanosomiasis caused by *Trypanosoma brucei rhodensiense* and *Trypanosoma brucei gambiense* known as sleeping sickness. Winterbottom's sign is enlargement of lymph nodes in the posterior cervical chain.

## Wrist sign (Walker's sign)

The distal phalange of the first and fifth fingers of the hand overlaps when wrapped around the opposite wrist seen in patients having Marfan syndrome.

# Index